Flipping Health Care through Retail Clinics and Convenient Care Models

Amer Kaissi
Trinity University, USA

A volume in the Advances in Healthcare Information Systems and Administration (AHISA) Book Series

Medical Information Science
REFERENCE
An Imprint of IGI Global

Managing Director: Lindsay Johnston
Production Editor: Christina Henning
Development Editor: Austin DeMarco
Acquisitions Editor: Kayla Wolfe
Typesetter: John Crodian
Cover Design: Jason Mull

Published in the United States of America by
Medical Information Science Reference (an imprint of IGI Global)
701 E. Chocolate Avenue
Hershey PA, USA 17033
Tel: 717-533-8845
Fax: 717-533-8661
E-mail: cust@igi-global.com
Web site: http://www.igi-global.com

Library of Congress Cataloging-in-Publication Data

Kaissi, Amer, 1976- author.
Flipping health care through retail clinics and convenient care models / by Amer Kaissi.
p. ; cm.
Includes bibliographical references and index. ISBN 978-1-4666-6355-8 (h/c) -- ISBN 978-1-4666-6356-5 (eISBN) -- ISBN 978-1-4666-6358-9 (print & perpetual access) I. Title. [DNLM: 1. Ambulatory Care Facilities--trends--United States. 2. Delivery of Health Care--organization & administration--United States. 3. Physicians, Primary Care--supply & distribution--United States. W 84 AA1]
R728
362.12068--dc23

2014021284

This book is published in the IGI Global book series Advances in Healthcare Information Systems and Administration (AHISA) (ISSN: 2328-1243; eISSN: 2328-126X)

British Cataloguing in Publication Data
A Cataloguing in Publication record for this book is available from the British Library.

For electronic access to this publication, please contact: eresources@igi-global.com.

Advances in Healthcare Information Systems and Administration (AHISA) Book Series

Anastasius Moumtzoglou
Hellenic Society for Quality & Safety in Healthcare and P. & A. Kyriakou Children's Hospital, Greece
Anastasia N. Kastania
Athens University of Economics and Business, Greece

ISSN: 2328-1243
EISSN: 2328-126X

Mission

The **Advances in Healthcare Information Systems and Administration (AHISA) Book Series** aims to provide a channel for international researchers to progress the field of study on technology and its implications on healthcare and health information systems. With the growing focus on healthcare and the importance of enhancing this industry to tend to the expanding population, the book series seeks to accelerate the awareness of technological advancements of health information systems and expand awareness and implementation.

Driven by advancing technologies and their clinical applications, the emerging field of health information systems and informatics is still searching for coherent directing frameworks to advance health care and clinical practices and research. Conducting research in these areas is both promising and challenging due to a host of factors, including rapidly evolving technologies and their application complexity. At the same time, organizational issues, including technology adoption, diffusion and acceptance as well as cost benefits and cost effectiveness of advancing health information systems and informatics applications as innovative forms of investment in healthcare are gaining attention as well. **AHISA** addresses these concepts and critical issues.

Coverage

- Virtual Health Technologies
- Nursing Expert Systems
- E-Health and M-Health
- Medical Informatics
- Role of Informatics Specialists
- IS in Healthcare
- Clinical Decision Support Design, Development and Implementation
- Telemedicine
- Measurements and Impact of HISA on Public and Social Policy
- IT Applications in Health Organizations and Practices

IGI Global is currently accepting manuscripts for publication within this series. To submit a proposal for a volume in this series, please contact our Acquisition Editors at Acquisitions@igi-global.com or visit: http://www.igi-global.com/publish/.

The Advances in Healthcare Information Systems and Administration (AHISA) Book Series (ISSN 2328-1243) is published by IGI Global, 701 E. Chocolate Avenue, Hershey, PA 17033-1240, USA, www.igi-global.com. This series is composed of titles available for purchase individually; each title is edited to be contextually exclusive from any other title within the series. For pricing and ordering information please visit http://www.igi-global.com/book-series/advances-healthcare-information-systems-administration/37156. Postmaster: Send all address changes to above address.

Titles in this Series

For a list of additional titles in this series, please visit: www.igi-global.com

Flipping Health Care through Retail Clinics and Convenient Care Models
Amer Kaissi (Trinity University, USA)
Medical Information Science Reference • copyright 2015 • 300pp • H/C (ISBN: 9781466663558) • US $245.00 (our price)

Healthcare Informatics and Analytics Emerging Issues and Trends
Madjid Tavana (La Salle University, USA) Amir Hossein Ghapanchi (Griffith University, Australia) and Amir Talaei-Khoei (University of Technology, Sydney, Australia)
Medical Information Science Reference • copyright 2015 • 325pp • H/C (ISBN: 9781466663169) • US $235.00 (our price)

Laboratory Management Information Systems Current Requirements and Future Perspectives
Anastasius Moumtzoglou (Hellenic Society for Quality and Safety in Healthcare, Greece & P. & A. Kyriakou Children's Hospital, Greece) Anastasia Kastania (Athens University of Economics and Business, Greece) and Stavros Archondakis (Military Hospital of Athens, Greece)
Medical Information Science Reference • copyright 2015 • 335pp • H/C (ISBN: 9781466663206) • US $245.00 (our price)

Cloud Computing Applications for Quality Health Care Delivery
Anastasius Moumtzoglou (Hellenic Society for Quality and Safety in Healthcare, Greece & P. & A. Kyriakou Children's Hospital, Greece) and Anastasia N. Kastania (Athens University of Economics and Business, Greece)
Medical Information Science Reference • copyright 2014 • 342pp • H/C (ISBN: 9781466661189) • US $245.00 (our price)

Achieving Effective Integrated E-Care Beyond the Silos
Ingo Meyer (empirica, Germany) Sonja Müller (empirica, Germany) and Lutz Kubitschke (empirica, Germany)
Medical Information Science Reference • copyright 2014 • 366pp • H/C (ISBN: 9781466661387) • US $245.00 (our price)

Social Media and Mobile Technologies for Healthcare
Mowafa Househ (College of Public Health and Health Informatics, King Saud Bin Abdulaziz University for Health Sciences, Saudi Arabia) Elizabeth Borycki (University of Victoria, Canada) and Andre Kushniruk (University of Victoria, Canada)
Medical Information Science Reference • copyright 2014 • 372pp • H/C (ISBN: 9781466661509) • US $245.00 (our price)

IGI GLOBAL
DISSEMINATOR OF KNOWLEDGE
www.igi-global.com

701 E. Chocolate Ave., Hershey, PA 17033
Order online at www.igi-global.com or call 717-533-8845 x100
To place a standing order for titles released in this series, contact: cust@igi-global.com
Mon-Fri 8:00 am - 5:00 pm (est) or fax 24 hours a day 717-533-8661

This book is dedicated to my wife and best friend, Wafaa, whose love and support never wavered, and to my two little cheerleaders, Maria and Adam, who kept on asking "how many pages do you still have left?" and who left numerous encouraging notes on my desk and in my pancakes. They have been my inspiration. Through this book, I hope to inspire them to go on to bigger and better things in their lives and their careers.

Table of Contents

Section 2
New Trends in Healthcare Delivery

Section 3
Future Developments

Foreword

Several years back, I wrote an article for *HealthLeaders Extra* called, “Are You Ready for Big-Box Healthcare?” In that article I postulated that retail healthcare (or as some call it, retail medicine) would prove to be a significantly disruptive force in the hospital and health system sector of the industry. Specifically, I spoke to the rise of convenient care clinics in retail settings, and how that trend would augur seismic change in the field. That day has arrived, and both the history of the movement and the market implications are well-chronicled and astutely dissected in this timely book by Dr. Amer Kaissi. This is not only a thoroughly researched book about a formidable competitive movement in healthcare, it is an insightful text on the sweeping changes that have already altered the market landscape, and will continue to radically modify the nature of health care delivery in America. Consequently, this is a necessity ready for anyone who is serious about navigating/leading organizations in a consumer-driven, post-ACA world.

As noted throughout this book, we are in the throes of change that this industry has not experienced in its long and somewhat staid history. The fundamental delivery model of today – to a large extent – looks much like the delivery construct of decades ago. However, with the successful introduction of insurance exchanges – both public and private – the basic economic architecture of health care is shifting from third-party financing (either employers or government) with remotely engaged consumers/patients to direct, line-of-sight accountability and involvement by the end users, namely the consumers/patients. We are – in the language of the pundits who monitor such things – moving away from defined benefit to defined contribution. As Dr. Ezekiel Emmanuel recently predicted, “By 2025, fewer than 20% of workers in the private sector will receive traditional employer-sponsored insurance.” That is a dramatic modification of our current framework, and represents nothing short of a tectonic change for this industry, with monumental implications on how health leaders manage the operational and financial aspects of the business. Phrased another way, exchanges change everything.

Unfortunately, many people within our industry have allowed political dynamics to cloud and obscure their view of market realities. In so doing, they have missed -- or are missing -- the broader trends that have been in motion for years. In focusing narrowly on the polemics and polarization surrounding the introduction and implementation of the Affordable Care Act and its cornerstone component -- health insurance exchanges/marketplaces -- they have missed the sweeping movement toward rising consumerism and increasing retail orientation. And that represents a major managerial misstep.

Yet, as Dr. Kaissi articulately outlines in this book, the movement toward a retail orientation has been in play for many years, as evidenced by the remarkable growth and performance of convenient care clinics, urgent care centers, retail clinics, and so forth. These enterprises basically represent a move away from the traditional delivery framework toward a model which offers increased access, heightened convenience, lower prices, improved service, and generally predictable outcomes. They are –to sum it up – the embodiment of a consumer-oriented construct, and as such and are the hard-wired harbingers of a sweeping movement that will alter the entire landscape of health care as we know it today.

To that end then, those who read this book should not only appreciate the significance of this operational facet of a "new-world delivery model," but should pull up and recognize this movement for what it is, namely an element of a much larger trend. Health care – finally and fittingly – is poised to enter the market-driven realm in which virtually every other industry in America operates; a place where convenience matters, service is key, prices are transparent, value is paramount, and the consumers are in charge. As some who have awaited this moment for decades would say, "it's about time."

American health care is far from optimal. It is expensive, it is complex, it is difficult to navigate, and it produces outcomes that consistently lag behind those of most developed nations. Yet, perhaps the basis for an anecdote is on the horizon. There is an adage in marketing parlance, "the customer is always right." As we move toward a retail-oriented, consumer-driven model that adage may well be the core component of a prescription that introduces economic involvement and end-user engagement as much-needed medicine for the world's largest health care system. If that is the case, this book is a valuable and timely read in better understanding the basic ingredients of that operational prescription.

Preston Gee
Christus Health, USA

Preston Gee *is the Vice President of Strategic Marketing for Christus Health in Dallas, Texas, where he oversees the marketing function for the system. Gee is a recognized thought leader in the health industry, particularly in the areas of consumer-driven health care, service line strategy, and most recently in the realm of health insurance exchanges/marketplaces. Over the course of his career, Gee has published numerous articles on planning and strategy for virtually every major publication in the health care industry. He is a frequent speaker on current trends and emerging strategies. He is the author or co-author of several books on strategy and service line management. His latest book, The Service Line Solution: Melding Population Health with Rising Consumerism, will be published in January of 2014. His career includes SVP of Strategic Planning and Marketing at Trinity Health, Senior Director at Phase 2 Consulting in Austin, Texas, and SVP of Strategic Planning for St. David's Health System n Austin. Gee started his career with The Quaker Oats Company in marketing and new product development. He holds a BS and MBA degrees from Brigham Young University in Provo, Utah, and is a past recipient of Modern Healthcare's "Up and Comer's Award."*

Preface

The idea for writing this book came to me two years ago when my then 5-year-old son started complaining from an earache and mild fever on a Saturday morning. Since he has had a history of fighting ear infections, my wife and I knew immediately what it was and what needed to be done: a quick diagnosis and an immediate dose of antibiotics, with some fever and pain medication. The problem, though, was that our pediatrician's office was closed all weekend long. We would have to wait until Monday morning to call and schedule an appointment for Monday afternoon, at best. That meant that he would have to miss a day of school and, most importantly, one of us would have to take a day off work and stay with him at home and take him to the pediatrician. The visit would cost us about $80 out of pocket (we have a high-deductible health plan provided by my employer). It would last anywhere between one and two hours, and then we will have to drive to the nearest retail pharmacy to get the prescription filled. He would probably get his first dose of antibiotics by Monday evening, not nearly enough to fight the infection on time for Tuesday morning. Another lost day of productivity for child and parent!

Up to about eight years ago, this would have been our only option, unless we wanted to waste half a day waiting in the hospital Emergency Room and pay $500 to treat an ear infection. However, on that Saturday morning in 2012, we had at least two other options, both allowing us to get faster and more convenient care than the pediatrician's office. First off, we could take him to one of the many walk-in pediatric or adult urgent care centers that have mushroomed all over our area in the last few years. The wait time would be anywhere from 15 minutes to two hours, depending on our luck, but at least we would get to see a physician that same day and have the precious antibiotics in his system before the end of the day. The visit would cost about $110, again all out of pocket. The second option was to take him to RedicClinic, a nearby retail clinic that had opened at our local H-E-B grocery store. He would be seen by a nurse practitioner within 15 minutes, and we could fill the prescription at the store pharmacy. The visit would cost about $75.

As we discussed our options, I remembered a new service that Aetna, my employer-provided health plan, had recently made available. It was called WhiteGlove Health, a sort of house-call service. I ran the idea by my wife, but she did not warm up to it: a nurse practitioner would come to treat him *here at home*? She preferred the more traditional urgent care center, and to a lesser extent, the retail clinic that we had used once before. So I used the "I work in the healthcare field and know about this stuff" card and convinced her to give WhiteGlove a try. In truth, I was mainly adding the dollar signs in my head: the usual cost of membership for that service is $400 per year, but my employer had generously offered that service for free. The fee is $35 per visit, but WhiteGlove was offering a special discount that month for $10! I called WhiteGlove, scheduled the visit, and paid the fee by credit card over the phone. Two hours later, the nurse practitioner showed up on our doorstep with two large bags. She was professional, kind, and very efficient. She started with a series of questions about my son's medical history and symptoms, proceeded with a quick ear check, and confirmed our suspicions of ear infections in both ears. Then, to our surprise, she prepared the antibiotics solution right there in our living room and gave him his first dose. She then produced a free "well-kit" that contained chicken noodle soup, Jell-O, ginger ale, Motrin, and Mucinex. Before leaving, she asked us to take a quick 10-question patient satisfaction survey on her iPad. Not surprisingly, my wife checked "strongly satisfied" for all questions. With four more doses of antibiotics in, my son was feeling better by Sunday evening. We woke up on Monday morning to a regular beginning of another week. No school days missed, no days off from work needed. Crisis averted.

This book is not one that tackles the fundamental problems that ail our healthcare system and offers radical solutions to address them. Rather, it discusses some relatively new basic healthcare services that many American families and individuals find themselves pondering and exploring on evenings and weekends, when family physician or pediatrician offices have already called it a day. The title, *Flipping Healthcare through Retail Clinics and Convenient Care Models*, is inspired by the concept of "flipping the classroom" in academia. The flipped classroom is a pedagogical model where roles are reversed: students are expected to learn class materials on their own through pre-recorded lectures before coming to class, and to use class time to test their knowledge, inquire about in-depth issues, and interact with the professor and their classmates. In that sense, students are transformed from passive recipients to active learners. Similarly, convenient care trends have such as WhiteGlove "flipped" healthcare roles by turning passive patients into active consumers who need and demand more convenient, faster, and cheaper primary care, and who are starting to get that care with a quick trip to the strip mall or grocery store, or thorough a phone call or a mouse click.

The methodological framework of the book relies heavily on thorough and systematic reviews of the academic literature (peer-reviewed articles published in scientific journals), the grey literature (reports published by various organizations, associations, and individuals), the popular literature (articles in newspapers, magazines, online sites, blogs, etc.), and the general Internet. Moreover, I conducted in-depth interviews with 12 key informants who are well-recognized experts in the various areas of convenient care. I also used previous and current academic research on retail clinics that I am involved in, and recalled dozens of presentations attended at various conferences and numerous conversations that I have had with a large number of people over the years. The intended audience of the book includes healthcare practitioners, managers, policymakers, researchers, students in healthcare administration and policy programs, as well as members the general public who have specific interests in healthcare-related issues.

In Chapter 1, I discuss how the American healthcare system lags behind systems of other developed countries on the important measures of cost, quality, access, and convenience. These problems have resulted in an unsustainable, inefficient, oversized, fragmented, and provider-centric system that rewards treatment over prevention and quantity over quality. While cost of care per capita and as a percentage of the Gross Domestic Product is much higher than in other countries, quality of care measured in terms of life expectancy at birth, infant mortality rates, and preventable mortality rates is questionable. Moreover, the U.S. is the only developed country that does not provide coverage to 99.9% of its citizens. A large number of uninsured patients are expected to receive coverage under various provisions of the Patient Protection and Affordable Care (PPACA), but many others will remain uninsured or underinsured. The system has been built and designed around the convenience and preference of the providers of care, not the patients and consumers seeking it, as evidenced by many physician offices closing on weekday evenings and weeknights, and long waiting lines and times. Because of these various inadequacies, hospital emergency rooms have been acting as the safety net of the healthcare system, but evidence suggests that this net has been gradually breaking: overcrowding, long wait times, ambulance diversions, patient boarding, and patients leaving without being seen by a provider are common occurrences. These problems will only be exacerbated by the expected shortage of physicians and other primary care providers.

In Chapter 2, shortages of physicians in general and primary care physicians in specific are addressed. Primary care is the backbone of healthcare systems. There is strong empirical evidence linking primary care to improved quality and reduced costs. However, the primary care system in the United States is stricken with chronic systematic problems that are likely to aggravate in the near and long-term future. A large proportion of Americans have difficulty accessing a physician due to cost issues. Moreover, there is a substantial current and expected shortage of primary care physicians and other providers. The Patient Protection and Affordable Care Act (PPACA) will expand insurance coverage to an additional 32 million Americans by the year 2019, which will increase demand for primary care services and exacerbate those shortages. Recent legislation, including the PPACA, has attempted to address the shortages by increasing the supply of providers, but with limited success. Solutions to increase access have taken the form of Community Health Centers (CHCs), as well as the restructuring of care models to foster teamwork, the use of information technology, the provision of after-hours care, as well as the use of non-physician providers such as nurse practitioners and physician assistants.

In Chapter 3, I highlight the importance of the role played by non-physician providers. The imminent primary care physician shortage, as well as other cost-related and access-related hurdles, have created a pressing need to prepare and train non-physician providers who can provide adequate primary care services. Nurse Practitioners (NPs) and Physician Assistants (PAs) have delivered services in a variety of healthcare settings for a long time, but there is a recent urgency about the importance of the role that they can play in the healthcare system. While there is strong evidence that care provided by these providers is of high quality and leads to improved patient satisfaction, some questions remain about potential cost savings. Despite a boom in the numbers of providers, their supply will likely be insufficient to meet the healthcare demands. Barriers such as restrictive scope of practice and unjust payment policies have stifled progress, and physician opposition is still a major factor in some states. Opportunities exist in some federal and state legislation to expand the scope of practice and revamp payment policies, while the recently enacted Patient Protection and Affordable Care Act (PPACA) can provide some relief towards improving the pipeline of NPs and PAs. Moreover, the use of other providers such as pharmacists and grand-aides can help fill the gap.

Chapter 4 describes the convenient care trends that are the main focus of the book. With the availability of non-physician providers to treat limited-scope conditions, several alternatives to traditional care provided in the physician office during regular business hours have started to surface in the last decade. While the settings where the care is delivered are different, the common characteristics among these alternatives are to have non-physician providers deliver care that is more convenient and less costly than that delivered in regular physician offices. These convenient care alternatives include urgent care centers, retail clinics, worksite clinics, house call services, and online services, among others. These services could be described as "disruptive innovations," or powerful changes in which a larger population of less-skilled providers can provide care in more convenient, less expensive settings that historically was only provided by expensive specialists in centralized, inconvenient locations. Given the myriad of problems faced by the American healthcare systems, these innovations are well positioned to change the way healthcare is delivered for generations to come.

In Chapter 5, the first of the convenient care trends, urgent care centers, are highlighted. Urgent care centers represent a unique innovation that has been in the making for the last 30 years. As such, they are considered more "mainstream" than other recent innovations. Urgent care centers provide unscheduled or walk-in care, are open for extended hours on weeknights and weekends, and provide services that go beyond what primary care physicians provide, such as occupational medicine, laboratory tests, and fracture care such as splinting and casting, with some providing intravenous fluids, routine immunizations, and primary care services. Half of all urgent care centers are located in freestanding clinic buildings and the other half are in retail shopping centers, and all are convenient and easy to find and access. Most centers are staffed by full-time physicians with at least one physician present at the center all the time, but care is typically delivered by non-physician providers. They tend be located in high-density urban areas and states with larger populations. Consumers appreciate the convenience of walk-in, extended hours, while physicians and other providers see them as an opportunity to practice medicine in a more controlled environment. The owners of urgent care centers are large organizations, health systems, and individual physicians operating in a highly fragmented industry. Urgent care centers seem to provide care that is of higher quality and lower cost than hospital emergency rooms, although the empirical evidence is scarce. Given the expanding industry, strong growth in company numbers, greater employment opportunities, and rising per-capita usage of urgent care centers, the urgent care industry is in the growth phase of its life cycle.

Retail Clinics, a major trend in convenient care today, are addressed in great depth in Chapter 6. They are walk-in clinics located in grocery stores, drugstores, and general merchandise retailers such as Wal-Mart, Target, CVS, Walgreens, etc. They offer a limited scope of diagnostic and treatment services for common medical conditions, as well as preventative and wellness services. Most retail clinic visits are for simple conditions and services such as upper respiratory infections, urinary tract infections, immunizations, and tests. Care is delivered by a nurse practitioner or physician assistant, and many clinics have up-front menu-style pricing, a feature that is unparalleled in the American healthcare system. The clinics operate on a walk-in basis with no appointments needed and very short wait times, and are open on evenings and weekends when most physician offices are closed. They charge an average of $70 per visit and accept all types of insurance plans. Retail clinics first appeared on the healthcare scene in 2000. Since then, there have been periods of slow growth, exponential growth, relative stagnation, and more measured growth. Many quality assurance programs are in place at the clinics and are enforced internally as well as by external bodies and agencies, such as the Convenient Care Association and the Joint Commission. When retail clinics first emerged, the main operators were investor-owned and venture-backed companies that were independent from the retailers. However, in recent years, drug store-owned clinics (such as CVS-owned MinuteClinics and Walgreen-owned Take Care) and hospital-owned clinics have become more prevalent. Empirical evidence suggests that retail clinics provide higher or equal quality, lower cost, and more convenient services than alternative care sites. However, the evidence around the effect of retail clinics on coordination and continuity of care is mixed, and some experts have warned that retail clinics may lead to new utilization and higher overall costs. The future of retail clinics in terms of numbers and usage rates looks very bright, with some operators expanding the scope of services to include management and treatment of chronic conditions.

In Chapter 7, I expound on the development of worksite clinics. Prior to the 1980s, many large employers operated onsite company clinics to treat work-related injuries. However, many of these clinics closed in the 1980s and 1990s because of the decline in heavy industry and manufacturing sectors and the reduction in workplace hazards. Recently, there has been a significant resurgence of worksite clinics. The new generation of clinics is markedly different in that their main focus is on primary care, health promotion, and wellness rather than occupational injuries. Worksite clinics are typically located on employers' campuses and serve on-campus employees, employees' dependents, and retirees. Most are staffed by non-physician providers that can address occupational health and safety issues, administer travel and influenza vaccinations, conduct new employee drug screenings, provide health and wellness education, and refer employees to in-network physicians. Clinics associated with larger employers employ physicians on a full-time or part-time basis. Worksite clinics provide care at lower costs than alternative care sites, and employers enjoy the increased productivity and decreased absenteeism of employees. However, the evidence on Return on Investment (ROI) is mixed. Some worksite clinics are operated by the employers themselves while others are operated by local health systems or physicians groups, but many choose to outsource clinic operations to external vendors. Worksite clinics seem to be well positioned to thrive in a post-reform healthcare environment.

In Chapter 8, other convenient care trends such as online services, house call services, and additional emerging models are discussed. Under the umbrella of telehealth, there are three key modes of delivery: First, real time (synchronous) delivery requires a live telecommunication connection and uses phones, video conferencing, and chat sessions. Second, "store & forward" (asynchronous) delivery captures digital media and transmits to it to providers via images, video, audio, x-rays, etc. Third, remote monitoring (synchronous or not) is a combination of real-time and store and forward, and it uses connected devices. Patient demand for telehealth services seems to be on the rise, and several companies, such as Hello Health, virtuwell, Zipnosis, and American Well, among others, are meeting this demand. However, significant legal and reimbursement hurdles still need to be overcome. Despite the scarce research evidence, care delivered in online clinics and through e-visits seems to follow clinical guidelines, and costs are significantly lower than other settings of care. However, some concerns related to overprescribing of antibiotics are raised. House call services by nurse practitioners are on the rise again. One such service, WhiteGlove, offers access to nurse practitioner care at home or at the office from 8:00 am to 8:00 pm all days of the week. It is available on a membership basis for individuals and for employees of certain companies with specific health plans.

In Chapter 9, I address the role that hospital systems have played in convenient care models and discuss the implications of healthcare reform. Convenient care models have mostly originated from outside the traditional healthcare organization circles. Large hospital systems are not known for being nimble and innovative, as many are inhibited by fixed budgets and low tolerance for risk. However, recently, hospital systems have joined the trends and developed their own retail clinics, urgent care centers, and online clinics. In fact, several hospital systems now have a "convenient care strategy" to reduce demand on their overwhelmed emergency rooms and better serve their patients. These strategies also help the systems better position themselves to deal with provisions of the Patient Protection and Affordable Care Act (PPACA), such as value-based purchasing and bundled payments. More specifically, PPACA will require hospitals to take on substantial financial risks for population health management, with specific implications such as increasing access, focusing on primary care and post-acute providers along the continuum of care; dedicating resources and expertise to reduce cost and increase value; better coordinating services and reducing readmissions; investing in health information systems and robust analytics programs to track large amounts of data on care quality and costs and assess risk and price services. Convenient care models that are appropriately aligned and integrated with the new arrangements will embody excellent opportunities for hospital systems to provide easy-access entry-points for new patients to substitute expensive traditional care settings with less costly alternatives and to deliver high-quality and expedient care that will keep patients in their network.

In Chapter 10, I evaluate the convenient care models discussed in previous chapters and attempt to predict what the future will hold for them. The convenient care models receive high scores on convenience, costs, and quality when compared to hospital emergency rooms and primary care physician offices, despite issues related to possible fragmentation of care. However, improving access to care, especially among uninsured and underserved populations, is not an advantage currently offered by convenient care. Given that the majority of the uninsured population will be receiving coverage under the Patient Protection and Affordable Care Act (PPACA), this might be less of an issue in the near future. The American healthcare system appears to be at a tipping point. Consumerism is rising, demands for price and quality transparency are increasing, and regulatory forces are forcing providers to focus on value over quantity. In this new healthcare reality, traditional healthcare providers such as hospitals and physicians will have to rethink their roles and business models, and new convenient care models will continue to emerge. Healthcare consumers in the United States should feel optimistic about the prospects of healthcare delivery. Newer, more convenient, cheaper, and better performing care models will continue to emerge and spread. The race between hospitals and health systems under legislative pressures and giant retailers spotting strategic opportunities will accelerate innovations and enable convenient care models to move from the margins to become the mainstream way of providing preventative services, treating minor conditions and managing some chronic conditions.

Amer Kaissi
Trinity University, USA

Acknowledgment

I am deeply grateful for several individuals for their advice and help. Dr. James. W. Begun at the University of Minnesota, always my mentor and advisor, offered valuable advice when I first embarked on this project. Tom Charland of Merchant Medicine gave me access to the invaluable retail clinic database that he has collected and invited me on several occasions to attend the ConvUrgent Care Symposium in which I gained valuable insight on the industry. Thirteen key informants (Dr. Ateev Mehrotra, Mr. Kevin Palattao, Mrs. Lauren Cates, Dr. Lee Resnick, Mr. Mark Clayton, Mr. Steven Jones, Mr. Steven Lazzari, Mrs. Tammy Mallow, Dr. Bill Rice, Dr. Tom Pascuzzi, and Mr. Webster Golinkin) were very gracious and agreed to share their expertise and time with me. Austin De Marco, the Managing Editor at IGI, was instrumental in keeping me on track for hard and soft deadlines. My previous boss, Professor Mary Stefl, and my current boss, Professor Edward Schumacher, at the Department of Health Care Administration at Trinity University were very supportive and understanding in terms of the time demands that this project required. Graduate Research Assistants at the Department of Health Care Administration at Trinity University, Kelsey Goodell, Nousha Parkhill, and Annemarie Witecki, provided vital research support for various parts of this book.

My parents deserve much of the credit and my gratitude to them is infinite. Finally, I am always indebted to the countless blessings of the Almighty God for the accomplishment of this and any other project in my life.

Amer Kaissi
Trinity University, USA

Section 1

Current State and Challenges of the American Healthcare System

Chapter 1
The American Healthcare System

ABSTRACT

This chapter provides an overview of the American healthcare system in terms of cost, quality, access, and convenience. Problems that have resulted in an unsustainable, inefficient, oversized, fragmented, and provider-centric system are discussed. While cost of care per capita and as a percentage of the Gross Domestic Product is much higher than in other countries, quality of care measured in terms of life expectancy at birth, infant mortality rates, and preventable mortality rates is questionable. The U.S. is the only developed country that does not provide coverage to 99.9% of its citizens. A large number of uninsured patients are expected to receive coverage under various provisions of the Patient Protection and Affordable Care (PPACA), but many others will remain uninsured or underinsured. Moreover, problems in hospital emergency rooms such as overcrowding, long wait times, ambulance diversions, patient boarding, and patients leaving without being seen by a provider are addressed. The author predicts that these problems will only be exacerbated by the expected shortage of physicians and other primary care providers.

Seeing modern healthcare from the other side, I can say that it is clearly not set up for the patient. It is frequently a poor arrangement for doctors as well, but that does not mitigate how little the system accounts for the patient's best interest. Just when you are at your weakest and least able to make all the phone calls, traverse the maze of insurance, and plead for health-care referrals is that one time when you have to because your life may depend on it.— Ross I. Donaldson, 2009

INTRODUCTION

The American healthcare system lags behind systems of other developed countries on important measures of cost, quality, access and convenience. These problems have resulted in an unsustainable, inefficient, oversized, fragmented and provider-centric system that rewards treatment over prevention and quantity over quality. In this chapter, we review the evidence on the deficiencies in the healthcare

DOI: 10.4018/978-1-4666-6355-8.ch001

system, and show-case the poster-child of inefficient and inappropriate care, the hospital emergency room.

1. COSTS

The United States (U.S.) spends more per capita on healthcare services than any other country in the world. In fact, its annual spending is two and a half times the average for OECD (Organization for Economic Co-operation and Development) countries. In 2010, the U.S. spent $8,233 on healthcare per capita, whereas the second and third highest-spending countries, Norway and Switzerland, spent only $5,388 and $5,270, respectively (OECD, 2012). Healthcare expenditures constituted 17.9% of the Gross Domestic Product (GDP) in the U.S. in 2010, about one and a half times as much as any other country, and nearly twice the OECD average. From 2011 till 2021, national health spending is projected to grow at an average rate of 5.7% annually and the health share of GDP to increase to 19.6% (Keehan et al., 2012). Compared to the average spending in Switzerland, Canada, Germany, France and Japan, the U.S. spends 168% more on hospitals/nursing homes, 236% more on ambulatory healthcare, 155% more on pharmaceutical and medical goods, and 296% more on public health and administration (OECD, 2012). About 45% of healthcare expenditures in the United States are in the form of public coverage programs, mainly Medicare and Medicaid. Medicare is the federal government's health program for people over the age of 65, while Medicaid is a joint federal-state program for the poor.

2. QUALITY

The numerous deficiencies in the primary healthcare system contribute to negative outcomes in all aspects of health in the U.S. For example, the U.S. lags behind other rich countries on important general health measures. Life expectancy at birth in the U.S. is 78.6 years, compared to 80.7 years in the United Kingdom, 80.9 years in Canada, 82 years in France and 83 years in Japan (World Bank, 2013). Infant mortality rate in the U.S. is 6 per 100,000 live births, compared to 4/100,000 in the United Kingdom, 5/100,000 in Canada, 3/100,000 in France, and 2/100,000 in Japan (World Bank, 2013).

Some have suggested that this is more related to obesity rates, income inequality, and homicide and car accident rates, rather than the healthcare system itself. For example, obesity rates have increased substantially over the past 20 years and are highest in the U.S. compared to other countries. In 2010, 36% of adults and 35% of children were overweight or obese. Nonetheless, a study that compared deaths that could be prevented by the healthcare system found that the U.S. had around 84,000 preventable deaths and ranked last out of 16 countries examined (Mahon & Fox, 2011). Other studies of preventable deaths in OECD countries concluded that the U.S. has more preventable deaths than the United Kingdom, Canada, Western Europe and the

OECD average (Gay, Paris, Devaux, & de Looper, 2011).

3. ACCESS

There were about 47 million Americans without health insurance in 2012, up from 38 million in 2000. The U.S. is the only developed country that does not provide coverage to at least 99.9% of its citizens (Kaiser Family Foundation, 2013). Most of the uninsured are in working families: about 62% have at least one full-time worker in their family and 16% have only part-time workers. Uninsured workers tend to work in low-wage or blue-collar jobs and to be employed by small firms or in service industries. Most people without insurance cannot afford to purchase it because of low income. About 40% of them have family incomes below the federal poverty level and about 10% have family incomes below 400% of the federal poverty level (FPL; $22,350 a year for a family of four in 2011). More than half of uninsured adults have no regular source of healthcare to seek when they are sick. Concerns about high medical bills lead them to delay or forgo needed care. Safety nets of community clinics and public hospitals provide services to the uninsured, but they are unable to fully substitute for the access to care that insurance provides. Because of delaying or forgoing needed care, the uninsured are less likely than those with insurance to receive preventive care and services for major health conditions and chronic diseases, and as a result are more likely to suffer serious consequences and to be hospitalized for avoidable conditions. More than 50% of uninsured individuals are strained by their medical bills and are unable to pay for other basic necessities because of these bills (Kaiser Family Foundation, 2012). A large majority of uninsured patients are expected to receive coverage under various provisions of the Patient Protection and Affordable Care Act (PPACA, discussed in Chapter 9), passed into law in 2010.

In addition, there are 25 million people who were underinsured in the U.S., up from 16 million in 2003. The underinsured is a label given to people who have some form of health insurance, but who spend 10% or more of their income on medical expenses. Among people who have insurance, 20% have had problems paying their medical bills, 26% are paying off their bills over time, and 11% are unable to pay their bills at all (Pollitz, Cox, Lucia, & Keith, 2014). Moreover, the underinsured tend to delay or avoid care, which makes their health-seeking behavior very similar to that of the uninsured.

4. CONVENIENCE

The healthcare system in the U.S. has been built and designed around the convenience and preference of the providers of care, not the patients and consumers seeking it. For example, most physician offices and medical group practices are open only Monday to Friday, from 8:00 am to 5:00 pm. Access to after-hours care, i.e. care for medical problems that arise between the hours of 5:00 p.m. and 8:00 a.m. and on weekends and holidays is not considered standard practice. After-hours care can be provided in-person, by phone or by e-mail. When compared to other industrialized nations, access to after-hours primary care services is severely lacking in the United States. In a recent survey of eleven countries, only 29% of primary care practices in the U.S. had an arrangement where patients could be seen after hours without going to an emergency room (ER). The rates in other countries were 97% in the Netherlands, 89% in the United Kingdom (UK) and New Zealand, 78% in France and 43% in Canada (Schoen et al., 2009). A recent analysis of the 2010 Health Tracking Household Survey found that among people with a usual source of primary care, only 40% reported that their practice offered extended hours. Moreover, among people who attempted after-hours contact with their primary care provider, about 20% reported it was "very difficult" or "somewhat difficult" to reach a clinician (O'Malley, 2013). This is especially important as numerous studies have shown that after-hours access does not only affect convenience, but also quality and cost of care provided. Offering after-hours access to select primary care services has the potential to eliminate many costly emergency department visits and to improve continuity of care (Margolius & Bodenheimer, 2011; Niska, Bhuiya, & Xu, 2010; Carret, Fassa, & Domingues, 2009; Pitts, Carrier, Rich, & Kellermann, 2010; Rust et al., 2008). For example, Jerant, Bertakis, Fenton and Franks (2012) found that patients reporting a usual source of care offering evening and weekend office hours had lower total healthcare expenditures than those without extended-hours access, an association related to lower prescription drug use and office visit-related expenditures, with no negative effects on mortality. Similarly, patients who reported less difficulty contacting a clinician after hours had significantly fewer emergency department visits (30.4%) compared to patients who experience more difficulty (37.7%). Patients with less difficulty also reported lower rates of unmet medical need (6.1%) compared to those with more difficulty (13.7%) (O'Malley, 2013). The main barriers for providing convenient after-hours access are outdated modes of thinking about patient preferences, as well as the primary care physician shortages (discussed in Chapter 2) which have left many offices unable be open after-hours even if they wanted to (Schoen et al., 2009).

5. HOSPITAL EMERGENCY ROOMS

Hospital emergency rooms are the safety net of the American healthcare system. However, evidence suggests that the net has been gradually breaking. In 2006, a report from the Institute of Medicine (IOM) sounded the alarm bells: "a national crisis in emergency care has been brewing and is now beginning to come into full view. Emergency departments (EDs) across the country are overcrowded. Ambulances are turned away, and patients, once they are admitted, may wait in hallways for hours or even days before inpatient beds open up for them. Often the specialists that patients need to see are not available. And the system that transports patients to the hospitals is fragmented and inconsistent in the level of quality it provides."(IOM, 2006, p.1). Eight years later, there is no sign that the crisis has been averted. The demand on hospital emergency rooms has constantly increased over the last 15 years, whereas the supply of hospital emergency rooms and their associated beds has been on the decline. Between 1997 and 2007, total annual visits increased 23.1% while the number of emergency rooms decreased by 5% (Tang, Stein, Hsia, Maselli, & Gonzales, 2010).

Contrary to its original purpose of treating life-threatening and emergent conditions, the American hospital emergency room has turned into the "true provider of 'last resort' for uninsured people and other patients who are unable to afford other medical providers in the community" (Cunningham, 2011, p.2). The main reason behind that transformation is the Emergency Medical Treatment and Active Labor Act (EMTALA), which was enacted under the Consolidated Omnibus Budget Reconciliation Act of 1986. After evidence of "patient dumping" in some emergency rooms surfaced, Congress passed EMTALA to provide enforceable standards of emergency care (Consolidated Omnibus Budget Reconciliation Act, 1986). The law requires hospitals that participate in Medicare to evaluate, stabilize the condition of, and, if necessary, admit any patient who present to the emergency room with an emergency condition, regardless of the patient's ability to pay (Bitterman, 1992). At its core, EMTALA gave Americans a right to healthcare, but it limited this right to emergency rooms. Moreover, it did not provide adequate financial support to offset the cost of uncompensated care provided to uninsured patients. Therefore, while EMTALA was designed to improve access to care, it may have reduced it instead. The increased demands on emergency rooms have stretched their capacity and have resulted in a multitude of problems in the emergency room: overcrowding, long wait times, ambulance diversions, patient boarding, and patients leaving without being seen by a provider (Institute of Medicine, 2003). At the same time, the number of medical and surgical specialists willing to take emergency room calls without compensation has dramatically declined (Asplin & Knopp, 2001).

The main patient complaints about hospital emergency rooms relate to overcrowding and long wait times. In many communities, the emergency room is often the only medical facility that is open after hours and on weekends. Two thirds of all emergency room visits occur outside normal business hours (O'Malley, Gerland, Pham, Berenson, 2005). Therefore, many patients use the emergency room not just for emergency and life-threatening conditions, but also for urgent and non-urgent minor ailments conditions. Emergency room visits are classified into five categories, depending on the level of immediacy (in minutes) assigned upon arrival by the triage staff: (1) Immediate (patient needs to be seen immediately); (2) emergent (patient needs to be seen within 15 minutes upon arrival); (3) urgent (patient needs to be seen within 15-60 minutes); (4) semi-urgent (patient needs to be seen within 1-2 hours) and non-urgent (patient needs to be seen within 2-24 hours) (Niska, et al., 2010). In 2008, 4% of emergency room visits were for patients that needed to be seen immediately; 12% were emergent; 39% were urgent; 21% were semi-urgent, and 8% were non-urgent (Cunningham, 2011). These numbers indicate that about 68% of emergency room visits can, theoretically, be taken care of in other lower-acuity settings such as urgent care centers, primary care physician offices, retail clinics and others. A recent review of the literature concluded that the average fraction of all visits that were judged to be non-urgent was 37% (Uscher-Pines, Pines, Kellermann, Gillen, & Mehrotra, 2013).

The overuse or inappropriate use of the emergency room has resulted in long wait times to see a provider. Between 2003 and 2009, mean wait time to see a provider increased 25% (Hing & Bhuia, 2012). The total amount spent in the emergency room (from arrival to discharge/ hospital admission) has also increased. In 2001, 45% of visits lasted a total of 2 hours, increasing to 60% in 2008. Overcrowding and long wait times have resulted in many patients not receiving care within the medically-recommended time frames. For immediate patients (those who should be seen in less than one minute), the average wait times is 28 minutes, whereas for emergent patients (those who should be seen in 1 to 14 minutes), the average wait time to see a in the emergency was 37 minutes, more than twice as long as recommended for their level of urgency. Wait times for other conditions were 50 minutes for urgent conditions, 68 minutes for semi-urgent conditions, and 76 minutes for non-urgent conditions (Government Accountability Office, 2009). As waiting times increase, patient satisfaction decreases. For patients who wait between 30 and 60 minutes in the emergency room, 46% rate their visit as positive, whereas for patients who wait more than one hour, that proportion drops to 28% (Cunningham, 2011). Some patients who wait for a long time leave the emergency room without being seen. This is an especially serious problem because many of them may be seriously ill, require immediate evaluation, or at risk of poorer outcomes. The proportion of patients left without being seen (LWBS) according to a recent study reached 20% in some hospitals (Hsia et al., 2011).

Faced with overwhelming numbers of patients with reduced bed and provider capacity, hospitals resorted to diverting ambulances. In 2006, about 25% of hospitals reported going on diversion (Government Accountability Office, 2009). Others hospitals responded by "boarding": admitting patients in hallways and in other spaces while waiting for an inpatient bed to become available. In 2009, 78% of visits occurred in emergency rooms that reported using boarding (Hing & Bhuiya, 2012).

Total spending on emergency room visits has been rising at a very fast rate. In 2008, about $47.3 billion was spent on emergency care, accounting for 4% of all healthcare expenditures (Agency for Healthcare Quality and Research, 2008). Moreover, cost of care per episode is very high when compared to other settings. Episodes of care initiated in hospital emergency rooms are estimated to cost $570, compared to $156 at urgent care clinics and $166 in physician offices (Mehrotra, Liu, Adams, et al., 2009).

In summary, many patients arriving to the emergency room by ambulance sometimes find themselves being diverted to hospitals that may be further away. Those that arrive, by ambulance or other means, wait for a long time to see a provider, which significantly reduces their satisfaction. Some patients leave without being seen, while those that need attention might end up in a hallway bed. Given the exorbitant costs of treatment, the emergency room is an inconvenient, expensive and inefficient venue for dealing with urgent conditions and primary care needs.

6. CONCLUSION

The American healthcare system is on the brink of financial collapse. Healthcare represents a significant drain on the economy, but most patients do not receive needed basic care due to lack of insurance or inadequate insurance. At the same time, the quality of care delivered in some settings is questionable, and most delivery models are inconvenient and unsatisfactory to the patients. These problems are exacerbated by the expected shortage of physicians and primary care providers, which will be discussed in the next chapter.

REFERENCES

Agency for Healthcare Quality and Research. (2008). *Emergency room services - Median and mean expense per person with expense and distribution by source of payment*. Summary Data Table From the Medical Expenditure Panel Survey -Household Component.

Asplin, B. R., & Knopp, R. K. (2001). A room with a view: On-call specialist panels and other health policy challenges in the emergency department. *Annals of Emergency Medicine*, *37*(5), 500–503. doi:10.1067/mem.2001.115174 PMID:11326186

Bitterman, R. A. (1992). A critical analysis of the federal COBRA hospital "antidumping law": Ramifications for hospitals, physicians, and effects on access to healthcare. *University of Detroit Mercy Law Review*, *70*, 125–190.

Carret, M. L., Fassa, A. C., & Domingues, M. R. (2009). Inappropriate use of emergency services: A systematic review of prevalence and associated factors. *Cadernos de Saude Publica*, *25*(1), 7–28. doi:10.1590/S0102-311X2009000100002 PMID:19180283

Consolidated Omnibus Budget Reconciliation Act, Pub. L. No. 99-272; 1986. 100 Stat. 82, codified as amended, 42 US Code, sec. 1395d(d).

Cunningham, P. (2011). *Nonurgent Use of Hospital Emergency Departments*. Statement Before the U.S. Senate. Health, Education, Labor and Pensions Committee Subcommittee on Primary Health and Aging Hearing on — Diverting Non-urgent Emergency Room Use: Can It Provide Better Care and Lower Costs?

Donaldson, R. (2009). The Lassa ward: One man's fight against one of the world's deadliest diseases. New York: St. Martin's Press.

Gay, J. G., Paris, V., Devaux, M., & de Looper, M. (2011). *Mortality amenable to healthcare in 31 OECD countries: estimates and methodological issues*. OECD Health Working Papers, No. 55, OECD Publishing.

Government Accountability Office. (2009). *Hospital emergency departments: Crowding continues to occur, and some patients wait longer than recommended time frames*. Report to the Chairman, Committee on Finance, U.S. Senate. GAO-09-347.

Hing, E., & Bhuiya, F. (2012). *Wait time for treatment in hospital emergency departments: 2009 NCHS data brief, no 102*. Hyattsville, MD: National Center for Health Statistics.

Hsia, R. Y., Asch, S. A., Weiss, R. E., Zingmond, D., Liang, L. J., Han, W., & Sun, B. C. (2011). Hospital determinants of emergency department left without being seen rates. *Annals of Emergency Medicine*, *58*(1), 24–32, 32.e3. doi:10.1016/j.annemergmed.2011.01.009 PMID:21334761

Institute of Medicine. (2003). *A shared destiny: community effects of uninsurance*. Washington, DC: National Academies Press.

Institute of Medicine. (2006). *The future of emergency care in the United States health system*. Washington, DC: National Academies Press.

Jerant, A., Bertakis, K. D., Fenton, J. J., & Franks, P. (2012). Extended office hours and healthcare expenditures: A national study. *Annals of Family Medicine*, *10*(5), 388–395. doi:10.1370/afm.1382 PMID:22966101

Kaiser Family Foundation. (2012). *The uninsured and the difference health insurance makes*. Retrieved from http://kff.org/health-reform/fact-sheet/the-uninsured-and-the-difference-health-insurance/

Kaiser Family Foundation. (2013). *Key facts about the uninsured population*. Retrieved from http://kff.org/uninsured/fact-sheet/key-facts-about-the-uninsured-population/

Keehan, S. P., Cuckler, G. A., Sisko, A. M., Madison, A. J., Smith, S. D., & Lizonitz, J. M. et al. (2012). National health expenditure projections: Modest annual growth until coverage expands and economic growth accelerates. *Health Affairs*, *31*(7), 1600–1612. doi:10.1377/hlthaff.2012.0404 PMID:22692089

Mahon, M., & Fox, B. (2011). *New study: U.S. ranks last among high-income nations on preventable deaths, lagging behind as others improve more rapidly* [Press Release]. The Commonwealth Fund Retrieved from http://www.commonwealthfund.org/News/News-Releases/2011/Sep/US-Ranks-Last-on-Preventable-Deaths.aspx

Margolius, D., & Bodenheimer, T. (2011). Redesigning after-hours care. *Annals of Internal Medicine*, *155*(2), 131–132. doi:10.7326/0003-4819-155-2-201107190-00011 PMID:21768588

Mehrotra, A., Liu, H., Adams, J. L., Wang, M. C., Lave, J. R., & Thygeson, M. et al. (2009). Comparing costs & quality of care at retail clinics with that of other medical settings for 3 common illnesses. *Annals of Internal Medicine*, *151*(5), 321–328. doi:10.7326/0003-4819-151-5-200909010-00006 PMID:19721020

Mehrotra, A., Wang, M. C., Lave, J. R., Adams, J. L., & McGlynn, E. A. (2008). Retail clinics, primary care physicians, and emergency departments: A comparison of patients' visits. *Health Affairs*, *27*(5), 1272–1282. doi:10.1377/hlthaff.27.5.1272 PMID:18780911

Niska, R., Bhuiya, F., & Xu, J. (2010). National hospital ambulatory medical care survey: 2007 emergency department summary. National health statistics reports; no 26. Hyattsville, MD: National Center for Health Statistics.

O'Malley, A. S. (2013). After-hours access to primary care practices linked with lower emergency department use and less unmet medical need. *Health Affairs*, *32*(1), 175–183. doi:10.1377/hlthaff.2012.0494 PMID:23242631

O'Malley, A. S., Gerland, A. M., Pham, H. H., & Berenson, R. A. (2005, November). *Rising pressure: hospital emergency departments as barometers of the health-care system*, (issue brief no. 101). Center for Studying Health System Change. Retrieved from http://www.hschange.com/CONTENT/799/?words=au167

Organization for Economic Co-operation and Development. (2012). *OECD Health Data*. Retrieved from http://www.oecd.org/health/health-systems/health-at-a-glance.htm

Pitts, S. R., Carrier, E. R., Rich, E. C., & Kellermann, A. L. (2010). Where Americans get acute care: Increasingly, it's not at their doctor's office. *Health Affairs*, *29*(9), 1620–1629. doi:10.1377/hlthaff.2009.1026 PMID:20820017

Pollitz, K., Cox, C., Lucia, K., & Keith, K. (2014). *Medical debt among people with health insurance*. Kaiser Family Foundation. Retrieved from http://kff.org/private-insurance/report/medical-debt-among-people-with-health-insurance/

Rust, G., Ye, J., Baltrus, P., Daniels, E., Adesunloye, B., & Fryer, G. E. (2008). Practical barriers to timely primary care access: Impact on adult use of emergency department services. *Archives of Internal Medicine*, *168*(15), 1705–1710. doi:10.1001/archinte.168.15.1705 PMID:18695087

Schoen, C., Osborn, R., Doty, M. M., Bishop, M., Peugh, J., & Murukutla, N. (2007). Toward higher-performance health systems: Adults' healthcare experiences in seven countries, 2007. *Health Affairs*, *26*(6), 717–734. doi:10.1377/hlthaff.26.6.w717

Tang, N., Stein, J., Hsia, R. Y., Maselli, J. H., & Gonzales, R. (2010). Trends and characteristics of US emergency department visits, 1997-2007. *Journal of the American Medical Association*, *304*(6), 664–670. doi:10.1001/jama.2010.1112 PMID:20699458

Uscher-Pines, L., Pines, J., Kellermann, A., Gillen, E., & Mehrotra, A. (2013). Emergency department visits for nonurgent conditions: Systematic literature review. *The American Journal of Managed Care*, *19*(1), 47–59. PMID:23379744

World Bank. (2013). *Life expectancy at birth.* Retrieved from http://data.worldbank.org/indicator/SP.DYN.LE00.IN

KEY TERMS AND DEFINITIONS

Access to Care: The ability of patients to receive healthcare services, depending on the availability of healthcare facilities and providers and the patient's insurance status/ability to pay.

Cost of Care: The amount in dollars spent on healthcare services within a certain healthcare system.

Healthcare System: The complete network of agencies, facilities, and all providers of health care in a certain country or geographic area.

Hospital Emergency Room: A hospital unit staffed and equipped for the reception and treatment of patients with conditions requiring immediate medical care.

Quality of Care: The extent to which healthcare services provided to individuals and patient populations improve desired health outcomes.

Chapter 2
Primary Care and Physician Shortages

ABSTRACT

In this chapter, the author provides an overview of the primary care system. Primary care is the backbone of healthcare systems and is defined as "the provision of integrated, accessible healthcare services by clinicians who are accountable for addressing a large majority of personal healthcare needs, developing a sustained partnership with patients, and practicing in the context of family and community" (Donaldson, 1996, p. 1). The primary care system in the United States is stricken with chronic systematic problems related to access, cost, and provider shortages. The chapter explicates the impact of recent legislation, including the Patient Protection and Affordable Care Act (PPACA) on these issues. It also highlights some solutions to increase access such as Community Health Centers (CHCs), the restructuring of care models to foster teamwork, the use of information technology, the provision of after-hours care, as well as the use of non-physician providers such as nurse practitioners and physician assistants.

The idealized version of primary health care envisions a kindly gentleman-black tote bag in hand-visiting his patient's home, admonishing the patient for his or her naïveté, and offering a prescription with the proverbial "take two and call me in the morning." Yet this rose-colored account of access to primary care fails to reflect reality for most residents of the United States who need health care. Many residents do not have a primary care doctor, and the ones that do may experience the rushing through a primary care examination that often took weeks to schedule.— Hansen-Turton, Ware, and McClellan, 2010

DOI: 10.4018/978-1-4666-6355-8.ch002

INTRODUCTION

Primary care is the backbone of healthcare systems. In this chapter, we define primary care and discuss its functions, stress the critical role that is plays in the American healthcare system, explain some of the major cost-related and access-related problems that currently afflict primary care and their implications for the healthcare system at large, and explicate some of the current and potential solutions to these problems.

1. DEFINITION AND FUNCTIONS OF PRIMARY CARE

The term "primary care" is thought to have first appeared in a British official white paper called the Dawson Report and published around 1920 (Starfield, Shi and Macinko, 2005). The Report mentioned "primary health care centers" as the core of regional healthcare services in the United Kingdom. Subsequently, primary care started to play an increasingly important role in that country as well as many others, but not in the United States (U.S.), where specialization of the physician workforce was in full strength. Many U.S. general practitioners (generalists) took advantage of the GI Bill of Rights after returning from service in World War II and obtained additional training in other specialties. In response, family physicians reacted to this disproportionate increase in specialization by instituting credentialing standards for family practice. Therefore, in the 1960s-1970s, primary care came to include general internal medicine and general pediatrics, and required longer post-graduate training. These developments led the way to the recognition of primary care as separate "specialty" (Starfield, Shi and Macinko, 2005).

Nowadays, primary care can be defined as "the provision of integrated, accessible health care services by clinicians who are accountable for addressing a large majority of personal healthcare needs, developing a sustained partnership with patients, and practicing in the context of family and community"(Donaldson, 1996, p.1). In addition to primary care, healthcare systems are comprised of secondary care, tertiary care and emergency care. Secondary care is consultative, short-term, and mainly aims to assist primary care providers with diagnostic or therapeutic decisions, whereas tertiary care is care for patients with unusual disorders that primary care providers are not experienced enough to treat (Starfield, 1994). Emergency care is care provided to stabilize and treat patients with acute illnesses or injuries (See Chapter 1) (Marx, 2010).

Primary care can be understood in three different ways: as the specialty of individual providers, as a specified set of functions, and as a general orientation of healthcare delivery systems (Friedberg, Hussey and Schneider, 2010). First, as a specialty, primary care providers are identified based on their training as general pediatricians, general internists, family physicians, or other generalists, including non-physician providers. According to this definition, specialists cannot serve primary care functions (Friedberg, Hussey and Schneider, 2010). The Health Resources and Services Administration (HRSA, 2013) adopts a broader definition of primary care services as basic health services which consist of "health services related to family medicine, internal medicine, pediatrics, obstetrics, or gynecology, that are furnished by physicians and where appropriate, physician assistants, nurse practitioners, and nurse midwives"; diagnostic laboratory and radiologic services; preventive health services; preventive dental services; emergency medical services; and pharmaceutical services (HRSA).

Primary Care Physicians (PCPs) typically complete a four-year graduate degree in medical school, followed by a three-year program of clinical residency (American Academy of Family Physicians, 2012). To gain entrance into medical school, students must pass the Medical College Admissions Test (MCAT). While in medical school, students spend around 9,000 hours in lectures, clinical study, laboratories, and direct patient care over the course of the four years. During that period, they take two "step" examinations, called the United States Medical Licensing Examination (USMLE), in addition to core clerkships, or periods of clinical instruction. Students that pass these requirements are granted the Medical Doctor (M.D.) degree and are entitled to start clinical training in a residency program. Some students enroll in colleges of osteopathic medicine and earn a doctor of osteopathic medicine (D.O.) degree. Medical graduates planning to specialize in primary care complete residencies in internal medicine, family medicine or pediatrics, which require three years of training (American Academy of Family Physicians, 2012). Some PCPs choose to pursue additional residency training beyond those three years. For example, a pediatrician can specialize in cardiology. That physician is no longer considered a primary care physician, but rather is considered a cardiologist (Government Accountability Office, 2008).

Second, as a set of healthcare functions, patients receive primary care when they have a usual source of care that serves four specific functions: "... first-contact, continuous, comprehensive, and coordinated care provided to populations undifferentiated by gender, disease, or organ system" (Starfield, 1994, p. 1129). First contact includes the accessibility of a provider and the extent to which the population actually uses his/her services. Longitudinality is person-focused care over time, and it includes the degree to which both provider and people in the population agree on their mutual association as well as the extent to which patients relate to that provider over time for their care. Comprehensiveness necessitates that the primary care provider offer a full range of services and the extent to which he/she actually recognizes population needs as they occur. Coordination involves a comprehensive health information system, as well as the extent and speed with which the information is recognized and used in patient care (Starfield, 1994).

Third, as a general orientation of healthcare delivery systems, primary care is measured in terms of the ratios of PCPs to specialists, ratios of PCPs to patients, and percentages of patient populations that have access to usual sources of care serving primary care functions (Friedberg, Hussey and Schneider, 2010). Included in this system-level definition are financial barriers to access, communication and care transition between PCPs and other providers, as well as local cultural and behavioral norms.

2. IMPORTANCE OF PRIMARY CARE

It is well agreed on that primary care is a crucial component of any healthcare system. There is strong empirical evidence linking primary care to improved quality. In a comprehensive review of the literature, Starfield et al. (2005) concluded that "primary care improves health by showing, first, that health is better in areas with more primary care physicians; second, that people who receive care from primary care physicians are healthier; and, third, that the characteristics of primary care are associated with better health" (p. 459). More specifically, patients who have regular access to primary care have fewer preventable Emergency Room (ER) visits and hospital admissions (Bindman, et al., 1995; Hochheiser, Woodward and Charney, 1971; Hurley, Freund and Taylor, 1988; Parchman and Culler, 1994; Wasson, Sauvigne and Mogielnicki, 1984). They also have increased trust and treatment compliance with physician orders (Fiscella, et al. 2004), as well as improved outcomes, more complete immunizations, better blood pressure, reduced mortality and improved quality of life (especially for poor patients), among other outcomes (Ferrer, Hambidge and Maly, 2005; Goldberg and Newhouse, 1987; Lohr, Brook, Damberg, et al., 1986).

In addition to its effect on quality of care, primary care is strongly associated with reduced costs. Starfield et al. suggest that, based on their reviews, the supply of PCPs is associated with lower total costs of health services, "possibly partly because of better preventive care and lower hospitalization rates" (p.473). Other studies have shown that PCPs order fewer tests, spend fewer resources and are less likely to overtreat patients than subspecialists providing routine care (Cherkin, Rosenblatt, Hart, Schneeweiss and LoGerfo, 1987; Greenfield, et al., 1992).

3. PROBLEMS IN PRIMARY CARE

Primary care in the United States represents a paradox: it is more important than ever and yet it is plagued with problems that leave providers feeling overwhelmed and undervalued (Grundy, Hagan, Hansen and Grumbach, 2010).

Cost Barriers

Experts agree that the primary care system in the United States is stricken with chronic systematic problems that are likely to aggravate in the near and long-term future. As discussed in Chapter 1, a large proportion of Americans have difficulty accessing a physician due to cost issues. In a study of primary care in eleven developed countries, American physicians were by far most likely to report that their patients have difficulty paying for medications or other out-of-pocket costs, which point to huge cost barriers (Shoen, Osborn, Doty, et al., 2007). A recent survey of American consumers shed some light on this issue (Deloitte Center for Health Solutions, 2011). First off, people with no insurance were twice as likely as those with insurance to postpone seeking healthcare services when they are sick or injured (40% vs. 23%), cite cost as the reason for the delay (83% vs. 41%), report that their healthcare spending severely limits their spending on other essentials (21% vs. 8%), and experience financial difficulties due to healthcare -related costs (43% vs. 21%) (Deloitte Center for Health Solutions, 2011). It is also important to note that for many low-income patients, the cost barriers are not just related to the actual cost of the service received. For example, blue-collar workers with 8:00 to 5:00 schedules and hourly pay cannot afford the loss in income from taking time off work to go to the physician's office, even if they have health insurance or access to a primary care provider.

Cost hurdles are not limited to the uninsured: about 60% of the population report that their monthly healthcare spending limits their household's ability to spend money on other essentials, such as housing, groceries, fuel, and education; 25% report not seeing a physician when sick or injured; and 19% report delaying or skipping treatment recommended by a physician. When asked about the reason for not seeing a physician/medical professional when sick or hurt, 49% of Americans reported that the cost was too high, while 13% reported that their insurance did not cover the service/treatment that they needed (Deloitte Center for Health Solutions, 2011).

An important portion of the insured population that is facing increasingly higher out-of-pocket cost pressures are employees enrolled in consumer-driven health plans offered by their employers. A consumer-driven health plan is a combination of a pretax payment account with a high-deductible health plan. These plans are often referred to as three-tier payment systems: a health savings account (HSA), out-of-pocket payments, and an insurance plan (Yi, 2010). The first tier is an account that allows employees to pay for services using pretax dollars, and the account may be funded by the employer or the employee. The second tier is the "coverage gap," or the difference between the amount of money in the individual's pretax account and the deductible. The amount that is not covered by the pretax account must be covered by the employee. When expenses exceed the deductible amount, the high-deductible health insurance plan becomes active. These plans, as the name suggest, have higher annual deductibles and a higher annual out-of-pocket maximum than traditional plans (Yi, 2010).

Individuals enrolled in consumer-driven health plans tend to demonstrate cost-conscious behaviors more than those with traditional coverage. For example, they are more likely to say that they had checked whether their plan would cover care; they ask for a generic drug instead of a brand name; they talk to their physician about treatment options and costs; they talk to their physician about prescription drug options and costs; they develop a budget to manage health care expenses; they check the price of service before getting care; and they use online cost-tracking tools (Fronstin, 2011). Similarly, recent research suggests that those who made their own HSA contributions in addition to their employer's contribution were very likely to report that costs affected their care-seeking behavior, whereas those who contribute to their HSA or who pay out-of-pocket for care were very likely to report financial burdens in seeking care (Reed, Graetz, Fung, Newhouse and Hsu, 2012).

Access Barriers

The other major problem affecting primary care is that of timely access to needed providers and services. Given the importance of the role played by primary care services, it is imperative for any healthcare system to have a robust and evenly distributed supply of PCPs and other providers (National Association of Community Health Centers, 2008). However, the American healthcare system is currently suffering from a shortage of PCPs that is likely to worsen over the next decades.

It is important to note that physician shortages are not limited to primary care and affect virtually all specialties. And while there is agreement today that physician shortages are inevitable, healthcare planners had forecasted physician surpluses as recently as the 1990s. It wasn't until the early 2000's that studies started to warn that physician deficits could be as great as 200,000 physicians by 2020 (Cooper, 2001; Cooper 2004). The Association of American Medical Colleges (AAMC) proposed a 30% increase in medical school enrollment to address future shortages (AAMC, 2002), while the Council on Graduate Medical Education (COGME) predicted a decrease in the ratio of full time equivalent (FTE) physicians per 100,000 population (COGME, 2005). In 2008, AAMC released updated numbers projecting a shortage of 125,000 physician FTEs by 2025 (AAMC, 2008).

Several general factors related to the supply and demand of physician services have contributed to these projected shortages. On the supply side, the number of graduates from U.S. medical schools did not change between 1980 and 2005 (AAMC, 2008). In addition, due to caps on Graduate Medical Education (GME) Medicare funds put in place by the Balanced Budget Act of 1997, the numbers of physicians starting clinical residency programs have remained constant at 25,000 per year (AAMC, 2008). The total number of hours worked by U.S. physicians has been constantly declining due to an increase in female physicians, among other factors. Female physicians are expected to make up to 54% of the workforce by 2025, and it is well documented that they work fewer hours per week, are more likely to work part-time, take more extended leave, value time for family and personal life more, and retire earlier than their male counterparts (AAMC, 2002). Physicians' aging and generational issues also play an important role. More than one third of the physician workforce is over 55 years old and is expected to retire within 20 years, while the newer generations replacing them tend to work fewer hours and are more focused on quality of life issues (AAMC, 2010).

The demand for physician services is also expected to skyrocket due to several reasons. The U.S. population will grow by 50 million between 2006 and 2025, and the number of people over 65 years will reach 71 million by 2030 (AAMC, 2010), resulting in increased demand for physician care. Concurrently, the obesity epidemic has exploded in the last 20 years, with 34% of adults (33.8%) and 17% of children and adolescents reported obese (CDC, 2012). This crisis will only worsen in the future, thus creating huge pressures on healthcare providers in the form of chronic diseases such as diabetes, hypertension and heart diseases, among others.

Reasons Behind PCP Shortages

The above-discussed factors will affect most medical specialties. However, primary care will withstand the worst of all the shortages with an estimated additional 46,000 physicians needed by 2025 (Bodenheimer, 2012). PCP shortages represent 37% of all shortages, mainly because demand will outpace supply faster for primary care than for any other specialty. Not accounting for healthcare reform (which will be discussed in the next section), the number of primary care practitioners will only increase by 2-7% from 2005 to 2025, whereas their workload will increase by 29% during the same time period (Bodenheimer, 2012). One main factor behind these numbers is the decreased interest in primary care specialization among medical students and residents, a trend that has been well documented in the literature. The percentage of medical graduates entering family medicine decreased by 6% from 2000 to 2005 (Pugno, Schmittling, Fetter, et al., 2005), with 75% of internal medicine residents choosing some form of sub-specialization instead of general medicine (West, Popkave, Schultz, et al., 2006). Similarly, a mere 2% of students in a sample of 1,177 students planned to specialize in internal medicine in 2007 (Hauer, Durning, Keman, et al., 2008), whereas only 2,660 medical students matched into internal medicine residencies in 2008, compared to 3,884 in 1985 (National Residency Matching Program, 2008). This has resulted in the ratio of PCPs to specialists in the U.S. reaching 30/70, which is dramatically lower than ratios in other developed countries (Leigh, Tancredi, Jerant, Romano and Kravitz, 2012).

The widening gap in incomes between primary care and other specialties is the main reason behind these discrepancies. Medical students graduating from public medical schools have on average $120,000 in debt, whereas those graduating from private ones have about $160,000 in debt (American College of Physicians, 2006). A recent study has estimated that with an annual salary of $130,000 per year, PCPs face a net income deficit of $800 per month in the first 3-5 years of practice (Palmeri, Pipas, Wadsworth et al., 2010). From college graduation through age 65, the difference in career wealth between PCPs and cardiologists is estimated to be a whopping $2.6 million (Vaughn, DeVrieze, Reed and Schulman, 2010).

The current system of reimbursement of physicians in the U.S. has played a key role in these disparities. Under fee-for-service, physicians receive a fee for each service provided, thus creating an incentive to provide as many services as possible. The main service provided by primary care physicians is office visits, which cannot be increased without reducing time spent with patients. Specialist physicians, on the other hand, provide several procedures in addition to office visits, and are therefore able to increase the volume of the services provided, especially with recent technological innovations (GAO, 2008). Moreover, the Resource-Based-Relative-Value Scale (RBRVS) pricing method has failed to address the gap, as it has resulted in higher fees for procedure-based services than for office visits (Bodenheimer, Berenson, and Rudolf, 2007). For example, the fee for a 30-minute office visit for an established patient with a complex medical condition is $103.42 according to Medicare; whereas the fee for a procedural service of similar duration, such as a diagnostic colonoscopy, is $449.44 (GAO, 2008). Experts hint that this is related to the disproportionate representation of specialists vs. PCPs on the Relative Value Scale Update Committee (RUC), the American Medical Association (AMA) committee that makes payment recommendations to the Centers for Medicare and Medicaid Services (CMS) (Sanders, 2013).

In addition to income, other related factors have played a role in steering medical students and residents away from a career in primary care. Smith (2011) suggested that "most U.S. medical students gain a discouraging view of practice in primary care as they observe harried primary care physicians who have too much to do and too little time in which to do it. They hear disparaging remarks about primary care from residents and faculty members, who extol narrowly focused expertise. Students see the same values expressed in the wider society, which compensates subspecialists at far higher levels than primary care physicians. Students are intimidated by the breadth of knowledge required for primary care- but simultaneously concerned that primary care might be boring. And schools have difficulty finding high-quality ambulatory care teaching sites where students can learn the art and science of primary care" (p.496).

Medicare has also contributed to the problem as it promoted the growth of residencies in specialty fields by providing about $10 billion each year to teaching hospitals, without requiring any emphasis on training PCPs. Most hospitals have a strong financial incentive to train specialists, and therefore have shifted away from training PCPs overtime (Sanders, 2013).

Effects of Health Care Reform on PCP Shortages

In March of 2010, President Barrack Obama signed the Patient Protection and Affordable Care Act (PPACA) into law. One of the main provisions of the law is the expansion of insurance coverage to an additional 32 million Americans by the year 2019. This expansion will take place through several requirements (discussed in details in Chapter 9). Medicaid will be expanded in some states to cover poor citizens with incomes less than $14,400/person or $29,330/family; young adults will remain on their parent's insurance plans till age 26; insurance companies will be prohibited from excluding people with pre-existing conditions; and all individuals will be mandated to buy health insurance or pay a penalty (PPACA, 2010). In addition, health insurance exchanges will be set up in some states, individuals and families will receive tax credits to offset private insurance costs; and large companies will have to provide insurance to their employees or pay a tax of $2,000/employee.

Given the magnitude of the expected increase in coverage, analysts have warned that the forecasted PCP shortages will skyrocket in the next few years. Several estimates have been provided. Hofer, Abraham and Moscovice (2011) suggest that the number of annual primary care visits will increase between 15.07 million and 24.26 million by 2019. This will require 4,307-6,940 additional PCPs. Kirch, Henderson and Dill (2011) estimate that coverage expansions will increase the shortages from 25,000 to 45,000 PCPs by 2020. More recently, Petterson et al. (2012) estimated that the total number of office visits to PCPs will increase from 462 million in 2008 to 565 million in 2025. This increase will require an additional 52,000 PCPs by 2025: of these, 33,000 PCPs are required to meet population growth; 10,000 are required to meet population aging; and 8,000 are required to meet the legislated insurance expansion.

The effect of these shortages could be far-reaching. Ku, Jones, Shin, Bruen, and Hayes, (2011) summarized it by stating that the "[N] ewly insured population will demand more primary care services. If the new demand exceeds the supply of care, the result could be increased waiting times and access barriers. This pressure on services could affect not only Medicaid patients but also privately insured and Medicare patients, since each community is served by a limited pool of providers. Patients who cannot get timely primary care in health centers or physicians' offices may spill over into more expensive emergency rooms or experience delays that result in otherwise avoidable hospitalizations for conditions that could be treated in ambulatory care settings" (p. 495).

The Massachusetts Experience

National observers attempting to discern the potential impact of the expansion in coverage as a result of the PPACA can draw lessons from the expansion of coverage in the state of Massachusetts. In 2006, Massachusetts enacted a landmark legislation to provide universal coverage to its residents (The Commonwealth of Massachusetts, 2006). The law established new requirements to promote the expansion of health insurance coverage in the state. All adults in the state became required to purchase health insurance or face a financial penalty (equal to up to 50% of the lowest cost premium an individual would have qualified for through the Commonwealth Health Insurance Connector, the state's health insurance exchange program).

In addition, the state's Medicaid and Children's Health Insurance Program (CHIP) was expanded to cover children with family incomes up to 300% of the Federal Poverty

Level (FPL). Provisions related to the private insurance market created coverage and affordability standards specifying what is considered minimum credible coverage and the maximum amount residents are expected to pay for it. Moreover, employers that have 11 or more employees had to contribute toward health insurance coverage for their employees or pay up to $295 annually per employee (Kaiser Family Foundation, 2012).

As a result of these provisions, the rate of uninsured non-elderly residents in Massachusetts dropped from 10.9% to 5.5% in the year following reform, and currently ranks as the lowest in the country. However, access to care, especially to PCP visits, has been problematic. For example, the wait time for an appointment with an internal medicine physician increased from 17 days in 2005 to 31 days in 2008 (Massachusetts Medical Society, 2008). In 2009, 20% of adults reported problems finding a physician who would see them, because the provider was not taking new patients or did not accept the patient's insurance. To find appropriate care, patients turned to "safety net" providers. Community health centers (discussed later in this chapter) experienced a 50,000 visit increase between 2008 and 2010, while safety net hospitals reported 100,000 more visits between 2009 and 2010 (Kaiser Family Foundation, 2012). Supply of PCPs continues to be an issue, and there are widespread reports of physicians with limited capacity straining to see more patients. As a result, Dr. Mario Motta, the President of the Massachusetts Medical Society declared that universal coverage does not equal universal access (Gula, 2009). It is important to note though that recent reports have also shown greater percentages of adults receiving preventive care visits and reporting a usual source of care than before the reform, while the number of unnecessary emergency department visits and hospital inpatient stays has decreased (Kaiser Family Foundation, 2012).

Impact of PCP Shortages

The impending PCP shortages have led to some apocalyptic prognoses about the future of the healthcare system. The American College of Physicians (2006) warned: "Primary care is on the verge of collapse.... Without primary care, the healthcare system will become increasingly fragmented, over-specialized, and inefficient, leading to poorer quality and higher costs"(p. 2-3). Bodenheimer and Pham (2010) echoed by stating that "if the primary care foundation of the healthcare system is not strengthened, true access and cost containment may be impossible" (p.799). Kaissi (2012) added that "primary care in the United States is in a deepening crisis as physician shortages and reduced patient access loom" (p.576).

Some of the effects of the PCP shortage are already apparent in the healthcare system. The National Association of Community Health Centers (2009) estimated the number of Americans that are "medically disenfranchised" to be at 60 million, or 19.8% of the population. These are people that lack adequate access to primary care because of PCP shortages in their communities. While the majority of the medically disenfranchised is low-income, uninsured and minority populations, some of them are people with health insurance. The Association warned that "the number of medically disenfranchised grew three times faster than population growth [between 2007 and 2009]- a sign that access to primary care is worsening and even reaching the doorsteps of middle class America" (p.1).

Barriers to access to PCP offices are causing many Americans to use the hospital Emergency Room (ER) as their primary source of care (as discussed in Chapter 1). In 2006, the California Medical Foundation reported that lack of access to primary care is the main reason for use of emergency rooms (ERs). Two-thirds of patients that visited the ER stated they would have visited a PCP instead had they been able to obtain an appointment (California Medical Foundation, 2006). Similarly, a 2008 study concluded that, among patients that have a usual source of primary care, there are four main timely access barriers associated with ER use: inability to get through on the phone to the PCP office; inability to get an appointment soon enough at the PCP; waiting too long at the PCP's office; and the PCP's office not being open when the patient could go (Rust, Jiali, Baltrus, Adesunloye, and Fryer,. 2008). In addition, seniors on Medicare are reporting difficulty finding a new PCP (Friedberg, Hussey and Schneider, 2010).

Physician Misdistribution

The PCP shortage problem does not affect all geographic areas in the same way. There is strong evidence that some areas, such as rural and economically-disadvantaged urban areas, have significantly lower access to PCP services. About 21% of the U.S. population lives in rural areas, but only 10% of physicians practice in these areas. The ratio of PCPs to population is only 46 per 100,000 people in rural areas, compared to 100 per 100,000 people in urban ones (Council on Graduate Medical Education, 2007). Areas with ratios of population to primary care practitioners that is greater than 2000:1 are designated as "Primary Care Health Professional Shortage Areas" by the federal Health Resources and Services Administration (HRSA). About 60 million people lived in these areas in 2009, and more than 16,000 additional primary care providers are needed to meet population needs in them (Rieselbach, Crouse and Fiona, 2010).

Another aspect of physician misdistribution will relate to the implementation of the PPACA. While the increase in demand resulting from expanded coverage will be felt in all areas of the country, some states such as Texas, Mississippi, Nevada, Idaho and Oklahoma will feel greater strains than others (Hofer, Abraham and Moscovice (2011). More recent estimates concludes that under PPACA, seven million people will be living in areas where expected increase in demand for primary care providers will be greater than baseline supply by 10%, and an additional 44 million people will be living in areas where expected increase in demand for primary care providers will be greater than baseline supply by 5% (Huang and Finegold, 2013).

4. LEGISLATION

In the last few years, some legislation has passed to increase the number of PCPs or their capacity, with limited success. In an effort to train more residents in primary care and in rural areas, the Medicare Prescription Drug, Improvement and Modernization Act of 2003 sought to redistribute nearly 3,000 residency options among American hospitals. But recent analyses have revealed that the effort failed to boost primary care or rural training (Chen, Xierali, Piwnica-Worms, Phillips, 2013). Although there was a net increase in primary care training after the redistribution, non-primary care training grew twice as much and "had a net negative effect on primary care production by diverting would-be primary care physicians to subspecialty training" (Chen, et al., 2013, p.106). Similarly, only 12 rural hospitals received additional positions, representing less than 3% of all positions redistributed (Chen, et al., 2013)

More recently, the Preserving Patient Access to Primary Care Act of 2009 created new residency positions for primary care physicians and more opportunities to train in ambulatory care settings (Preserving Patient Access to Primary Care Act, 2009), while the Resident Physician Shortage Reduction Act of the same year expanded by 15% the number of Medicare-supported physician residency training positions with preference to primary care (Resident Physician Shortage Reduction Act, 2009).

The PPACA, while contributing to the increase in demand for primary care services through coverage expansions as previously discussed, includes some provisions that can strengthen the primary care pipeline. Specifically, the act will increase payments to primary care by:

- Increasing "Medicaid payments in fee-for-service and managed care for primary care services provided by primary care doctors (family medicine, general internal medicine or pediatric medicine) to 100% of the Medicare payment rates for 2013 and 2014. States will receive 100% federal financing for the increased payment rates. (Effective January 1, 2013)" (Kaiser Family Foundation, 2010, p. 10)
- Providing "a 10% bonus payment to primary care physicians in Medicare from 2011 through 2015 (Effective for five years beginning January 1, 2011)" (Kaiser Family Foundation, 2010, p. 10).

The act will also improve workforce training and development by:

- Establishing "a multi-stakeholder Workforce Advisory Committee to develop a national workforce strategy (Appointments made by September 30, 2010)" (Kaiser Family Foundation, 2010, p. 12).
- Increasing "the number of Graduate Medical Education (GME) training positions by redistributing currently unused slots, with priorities given to primary care and general surgery and to states with the lowest resident physician-to-population ratios (effective July 1, 2011); increase[ing] flexibility in laws and regulations that govern GME funding to promote training in outpatient settings (effective July 1, 2010); and ensure the availability of residency programs in rural and underserved areas; establish[ing] Teaching Health Centers, defined as community-based, ambulatory patient care centers, including federally qualified health centers and other federally-funded health centers that are eligible for payments for the expenses associated with operating primary care residency programs. (Funds appropriated for five years beginning fiscal year 2011) (Kaiser Family Foundation, 2010, p. 12).
- Increasing "workforce supply and support training of health professionals through scholarships and loans; support[ing] primary care training and capacity building; provide state grants to providers in medically underserved areas; train and recruit providers to serve in rural areas; establish[ing] a public health workforce loan repayment program; provid[ing] medical residents

with training in preventive medicine and public health; promote training of a diverse workforce; and promot[ing] cultural competence training of health care professionals (Effective dates vary) Support the development of interdisciplinary mental and behavioral health training programs (effective fiscal year 2010)" (Kaiser Family Foundation, 2010, p. 12).

In summary, the PPACA focuses on increasing the number of medical trainees who are likely to pursue primary care and encourages physicians to practice primary care, especially in rural and underserved areas. However, analysts warn that the benefit may not be immediate or significant. The National Institute on Health Care Reform (2011) offered these sobering remarks: "Even if PPACA policies are highly effective in bringing new practitioners into the workforce, they may be insufficient given the timeline to train new physicians and other primary care practitioners. Currently, about 300,000 physicians practice primary care and about 3,000 new U.S.-educated physicians enter primary care each year, adding about 1 percent to the primary care physician workforce annually. (This is not a net gain of physicians, as it does not take into account physicians exiting the workforce.) If the cumulative effect of PPACA provisions increased the annual number of new primary care physicians by 20 percent-an optimistic assumption—new U.S.-educated physicians would generate an additional 0.3 percent of the primary care physician workforce, or about 600 additional physicians, annually. Under this scenario, by 2020, a decade after the passage of health reform, an estimated 6,000 new physicians would enter the primary care workforce, still well under the American Association of Medical Colleges' (AAMC) predicted need of about 45,000 primary care physicians" (p. 2-3).

5. CURRENT AND POTENTIAL SOLUTIONS

Several potential solutions have been proposed to address the above-discussed problems in primary care services, while some measures have already been in place. One significant approach for addressing both costs and access problems are Community Health Centers (CHCs). CHCs have been delivering highly needed primary care services in the U.S. for over 45 years. These centers are local, not-for-profit, community owned centers that serve about 20.2 million patients and deliver over 80 million visits annually (National Association of Community Health Centers, 2013). The total number of health centers receiving federal grants has reached 1,128 in 2011. These centers share some main characteristics in that they:

- "Locate in or serve areas designated as medically underserved and where too few physicians locate;
- Serve all without regard to ability to pay or insurance coverage;
- Customize their services to meet the specific health care and cultural needs of their patients;
- Offer services that make accessing health care easier (such as transportation, translation, and community outreach services) and that increase the effectiveness of the health care they receive (such as case management, health and nutrition education, and home visits);

- Offer comprehensive services that often include services not normally seen in primary
- Care settings (such as dental, behavioral health, and pharmacy services);
- Offer enhanced access to care through evening and weekend hours and locations convenient to residents; and
- Operate through patient-majority governing boards, ensuring that the centers are responsive to the most pressing local health care needs and are fully community-oriented"(National Association of Community Health Centers, 2009).

CHCs focus mostly on serving the underserved uninsured and poor populations: 36% of their patients are uninsured, and 39% are on Medicaid/SCHIP. It is important to note, however, that 14% of the patients have private insurance, 8% are on Medicare, and 2% have other kind of public insurance (National Association of Community Health Centers, 2013), which suggests that CHCs play a role that goes further than just providing care to people who don't have coverage. As Adashi, Geiger and Fine (2010) suggest: "Beyond their commitment to the uninsured, the CHCs have always welcomed the insured in need of high-quality primary care" (p.2047). It is important to note that recent legislation has given a significant boost to CHCs. The American Recovery and Reinvestment Act of 2009 (ARRA) of 2009 provided $2 billion in one-time funding to CHCs, as well as additional funds to strengthen primary care providers and health information technology in these facilities (National Association of Community Health Centers, 2009). The PPACA underwrote CHCs and will enable them to serve nearly 20 million new patients while allowing them to add about 15,000 providers to their staff (Adashi, Geiger and Fine, 2010).

To address the geographic misdistribution of physicians, proposals have focused on four main approaches (Bodenheimer and Pham, 2010). First, a major increase in funding for the National Health Services Corps (which provides scholarships and debt forgiveness for medical students) can significantly increase the number of PCPs in underserved areas. Second, medical schools should make a more conscious effort to attract and admit students from rural areas, since these are more likely to practice in these kinds of areas. Third, the number of minority physicians should be increased, as these are more likely to practice in minority communities. And fourth, funding for Title VII of the Public Health Service Act should be increased, since physicians receiving grants from this training program are more likely to practice in underserved areas (Bodenheimer and Pham, 2010).

Traditional solutions to primary care have focused almost exclusively on increasing the number of medical students entering primary care specialties. However, in a critical review of the literature on cost and quality, Friedberg, Hussey and Schneider (2010) concluded that the most cost-effective solutions to primary care are those that go beyond just increasing the numbers of primary care providers. They suggest that solutions should focus on giving primary care providers new resources, as well as reorienting entire health care delivery systems towards primary care. For example, interventions based on the Chronic Care Model (CCM) can enable providers to serve the full set of primary care functions, and provide higher quality care for patients with asthma, congestive heart failure, depression and diabetes. In addition, interventions based on the Medical Home Model (discussed in Chapter 9) and emphasizing care coordination, the use of non-physician providers, and electronic health records have a great potential. System-level solutions such as reallocating capital investments away from high-technology procedures and towards community-based primary care and payment reform to address the gaps between PCP and specialists' pay "may go a long way towards achieving reorientation, even if workforce composition is slow to respond" (Friedberg, Hussey and Schneider, 2010, p. 771).

Similarly, Margolius and Bodenheimer (2010) suggest that a paradigm shift is needed in primary care. They advance that "[c]urrently the goal of many physicians, when they enter their practice in the morning, is to see scheduled patients and get home in time to have dinner with the kids. A different goal would be for a primary care physician to enter the practice and ask: 'What can the primary care team do today to make our panel of patients as healthy as possible?' This paradigm shift has two major components. First, the team, not simply the physician, assumes some responsibility for the health of patients. Second, the team not only is focused on patients who have an appointment that day, but also is concerned about all patients receiving care from the practice" (p.780). Therefore, the focus is on teams comprised of physicians, medical assistants, advanced-practice clinicians, nurses, pharmacists, etc., as well as on providing routine and follow-up care through phone calls or email messages (Margolius and Bodenheimer, 2010). Casalino (2010) echoes this approach and suggests that most PCP visits can be taken care of by phone or e-mail, which would leave PCPs with only 8-10 patient visits per day. A recent study based on simulation methods went as far as suggesting that PCP shortages could be totally eliminated through the use of primary care teams or "pods," better sharing of data and electronic communication channels, and the use of non-physician providers (Green, Savin, and Lu, 2013). More specifically, the authors propose that timely access to primary care to all patients can be ensured by implementing partial pooling of patients by 2-3 physicians, diverting one fifth of all patients to non-physician providers, and using electronic communication with patients (Green, Savin, and Lu, 2013).

Another innovative solution to improve access, especially for hourly workers who cannot afford to take time off work as well as busy professionals who work late hours, is to provide care after hours. After-hours care is care provided by the patient's PCP for medical problems that arise between the hours of 5:00 p.m. and 8:00 a.m., and on weekends and holidays. This care can be delivered in-person, by phone or by e-mail, or through some combination of these methods (O'Malley, 2013). As mentioned in Chapter 1, the availability of this type of care can reduce the fragmentation of care, improve patient outcomes and reduce the number of unnecessary Emergency Room (ER) visits (O'Malley, 2013; O'Malley, Samuel, Bond and Carrier, 2012). Moreover, patients who have a usual source of care on evenings and weekends have lower total health expenditures, due to lower prescription drug and office-related expenses, without adverse effects on mortality (Jerant, Bertakis, Fenton and Franks, 2012). However, studies have shown that only 29% of U.S. physicians have arrangements in their practice where patients can be seen after hours (Schoen et al., 2009), whereas only 40% of patients with a usual source of care reported that their practice offered such extended hours (O'Malley, 2013). PCPs can offer after-hours care in a variety of ways: by working "in small practices (solo or two-person) where a physician is available around-the-clock," by forming "partnerships with other practices, so that physicians can rotate after-hours shifts," by joining "a small, local cross-coverage network. For example, in the Adirondack Regional Medical Home Pilot, providers cover each other's patient panels," by "joining a large cross-coverage network, such as the Geisinger Health System in Pennsylvania, which has staffed after-hours clinics and urgent care centers," and by entering "a contractual relationship with an urgent care center or after-hours clinic" (O'Malley, Samuel, Bond and Carrier, 2012, p. 1-2).

6. SUMMARY

Primary care plays a crucial role as the backbone of the American healthcare system. Appropriate availability of primary care providers and services improve quality of care and health outcomes, and reduce overall healthcare costs. However, many Americans cannot find a PCP in their area or struggle to find an appointment in a timely manner, while others cannot afford to receive needed primary care services due to lack of coverage, insufficient insurance and high out-of-pocket costs. These problems have significantly worsened in the last few years while showing no signs of easing as imminent PCP shortages will further reduce access. The recently passed PPACA will moderate some of the cost barriers by providing coverage to previously uninsured population and improving the coverage of those with inadequate plans. However, it is likely to exacerbate the access problem by further increasing demand for PCP and specialist services, while not doing enough to significantly improve the supply of PCPs. Existing approaches such as Community Health Centers have an important role to play, but substantial and timely progress cannot be achieved without the use of radically new and innovative approaches such as care teams, non-physician providers, electronic communication and after-hours care (Figure 1). In the next two chapters, we focus on the current and potential role of non-physician providers, as well as new forms of healthcare delivery that extend beyond the traditional PCP office.

Figure 1. Problems and solutions in primary care delivery

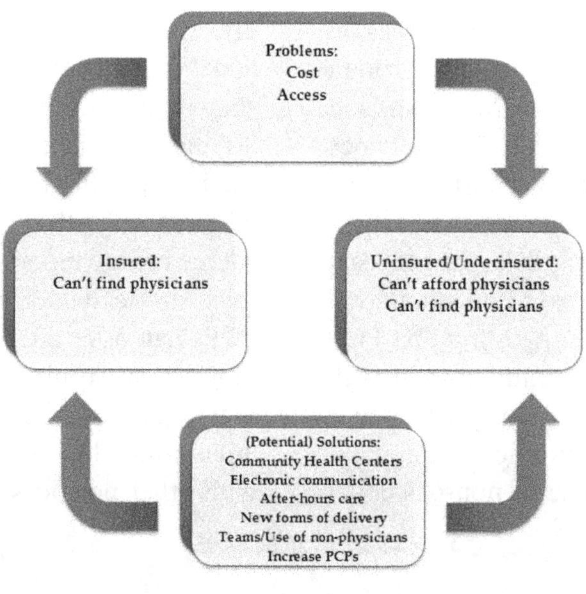

REFERENCES

Adashi, E. Y., Geiger, H. J., & Fine, M. D. (2010). Health care reform and primary care-The growing importance of the community health center. *The New England Journal of Medicine*, *362*(22), 2047–2050. doi:10.1056/NEJMp1003729 PMID:20427777

American Academy of Family Physicians. (2012). Ensuring a quality physician-led team for every patient. *Primary Care*, 21.

American College of Physicians. (2006). *The impending collapse of primary care medicine and its implications for the state of the nation's health care: A report from the American College of Physicians*. Philadelphia: American College of Physicians.

Association of American Medical Colleges. (2002). *The physician workforce: position statement- June 2002*. Washington, DC: Association of American Medical Colleges.

Association of American Medical Colleges Center for Workforce Studies. (2008). *The complexities of physician supply and demand: Projections through 2025*. Washington, DC: Association of American Medical Colleges.

Association of American Medical Colleges Center for Workforce Studies. (2010). *Help wanted: More US doctors*. Washington, DC: Association of American Medical Colleges.

Bindman, A. B., Grumbach, K., Osmond, D., Komaromy, M., Vranizan, K., & Lurie, N. et al. (1995). Preventable hospitalizations and access to health care. *Journal of the American Medical Association*, *274*(4), 305–311. doi:10.1001/jama.1995.03530040033037 PMID:7609259

Bodenheimer, T., Berenson, R. A., & Rudolf, P. (2007). The primary care-specialty income gap: Why it matters. *Annals of Internal Medicine*, *146*(4), 301–306. doi:10.7326/0003-4819-146-4-200702200-00011 PMID:17310054

Bodenheimer, T., & Pham, H. H. (2010). Primary care: Current problems and proposed solutions. *Health Affairs (Project Hope)*, *29*(5), 799–805. doi:10.1377/hlthaff.2010.0026 PMID:20439864

California Healthcare Foundation. (2006). *Overuse of emergency departments among insured Californians*. Oakland, CA: Issue Brief.

Casalino, L. P. (2010). A Martian's prescription for primary care: Overhaul the physician's workday. *Health Affairs*, *29*(5), 785–790. doi:10.1377/hlthaff.2010.0133 PMID:20439862

Center for Disease Control and Prevention. 2012. Retrieved April 17, 2013 from http://www.cdc.gov/obesity/index.html

Chen, C., Xierali, I., Piwnica-Worms, K., & Phillips, R. (2013). The Redistribution Of Graduate Medical Education Positions In 2005 Failed To Boost Primary Care Or Rural Training. *Health Affairs*, *32*(1), 102–110. doi:10.1377/hlthaff.2012.0032 PMID:23297277

Cherkin, D. C., Rosenblatt, R. A., Hart, L. G., Schneeweiss, R., & LoGerfo, J. (1987). The use of medical resources by residency- trained family physicians and general internists. Is there a difference? *Medical Care*, *25*(6), 455–469. doi:10.1097/00005650-198706000-00001 PMID:3695655

Cooper, R. A. (2001). Health care workforce for the twenty-first century: The impact of nonphysician clinicians. *Annual Review of Medicine*, *52*(1), 51–61. doi:10.1146/annurev.med.52.1.51 PMID:11160767

Cooper, R. A. (2004). Weighing the evidence for expanding physician supply. *Annals of Internal Medicine*, *141*(9), 705–714. doi:10.7326/0003-4819-141-9-200411020-00012 PMID:15520427

Council on Graduate Medical Education. (2007). *New paradigms for physician training for improving access to health care.* Eighteenth Report. Rockville, MD: COGME. Retrieved on March 24, 2010 from: http://www.cogme.gov/18thReport/default.htm

Donaldson, M. S., Yordy, K. D., Lohr, K. N., & Vanselow, N. A. (1996). *Primary care: America's health in a new era*. Washington, DC: National Academy Press.

Ferrer, R. L., Hambidge, S. J., & Maly, R. C. (2005). The essential role of generalists in health care systems. *Annals of Internal Medicine*, *142*(8), 691–699. doi:10.7326/0003-4819-142-8-200504190-00037 PMID:15838088

Fiscella, K., Meldrum, S., Franks, P., Shields, C. G., Duberstein, P., McDaniel, S. H., & Epstein, R. M. (2004). Patient Trust. *Medical Care*, *42*(11), 1049–1055. doi:10.1097/00005650-200411000-00003 PMID:15586831

Friedberg, M. W., Hussey, P. S., & Schneider, E. C. (2010). Primary care: A critical review of the evidence on quality and costs of health care. *Health Affairs (Project Hope)*, *29*(5), 766–772. doi:10.1377/hlthaff.2010.0025 PMID:20439859

Fronstin, P. (2011). Findings from the 2011 EBRI/MGA Consumer Engagement in Health Care Survey. *EBRI Issue Brief*, *365*, 1–26. PMID:22312794

Goldberg, G. A., & Newhouse, J. P. (1987). Effects of cost sharing on physiological health, health practices, and worry. *Health Services Research*, *22*, 279–306. PMID:3119520

Green, L. V., Savin, S., & Lu, Y. (2013). Primary care physician shortages could be eliminated through the use of teams, nonphysicians and electronic communication. *Health Affairs*, *32*(1), 11–19. doi:10.1377/hlthaff.2012.1086 PMID:23297266

Greenfield, S., Nelson, E. C., Zubkoff, M., Manning, W., Rogers, W., & Kravitz, R. L. et al. (1992). Variations in resource utilization among medical specialties and systems of care: Results from the Medical Outcomes Study. *Journal of the American Medical Association*, *267*(12), 1624–1630. doi:10.1001/jama.1992.03480120062034 PMID:1542172

Grundy, P., Hagan, K. R., Hansen, J. C., & Grumbach, K. (2010). The multistakeholder movement from primary care renewal and reform. *Health Affairs*, *29*(5), 791–798. doi:10.1377/hlthaff.2010.0084 PMID:20439863

Gulla, R. (2009, June 26). *MMS physician workforce study finds continued shortages in primary care*. Massachusetts Medical Society News Releases. Retrieved on February 22, 2010 from http://www.massmed.org/AM/Template.cfm?Section=MMS_News_Releases&CONTENTID=31507&TEMPLATE=/CM/ContentDisplay.cfm

Hansen-Turton, T., Ware, J., & McClellan, F. (2010). Nurse practitioners in primary care. *Temple Law Review*, *82*, 1235–1263.

Hauer, K. E., Durning, S. J., Keman, W. N., Fagan, M. J., Mintz, M., & O'Sullivan, P. S. et al. (2008). Factors associated with medical students' career choices regarding internal medicine. *Journal of the American Medical Association*, *300*(10), 1154–1164. doi:10.1001/jama.300.10.1154 PMID:18780844

Health Resources and Services Administration. (n.d.). *Health Center Program Terms and Definitions*. Retrieved April 12, 2013, from http://www.hrsa.gov/grants/apply/assistance/buckets/definitions.pdf

Hochheiser, L. I., Woodward, K., & Charney, E. (1971). Effect of the neighborhood health center on the use of pediatric emergency departments in Rochester, New York. *The New England Journal of Medicine*, *285*(3), 148–152. doi:10.1056/NEJM197107152850305 PMID:5087704

Hofer, A. N., Abraham, J. M., & Moscovice, I. (2011). Expansion of coverage under the Patient Protection and Affordable Care Act and primary care utilization. *The Milbank Quarterly*, *89*(1), 69–89. doi:10.1111/j.1468-0009.2011.00620.x PMID:21418313

Huang, E. S., & Finegold, K. (2013). Seven millions Americans live in areas where demand for primary care may exceed supply by more than 10 percent. *Health Affairs*, *32*(3), 614–621. doi:10.1377/hlthaff.2012.0913 PMID:23426931

Hurley, R. E., Freund, D. A., & Taylor, D. E. (1989). Emergency room use and primary care case management: Evidence from four Medicaid demonstration programs. *American Journal of Public Health*, *79*(7), 843–846. doi:10.2105/AJPH.79.7.843 PMID:2660603

Jerant, A., Bertakis, K. D., Fenton, J. J., & Franks, P. (2012). Extended office hours and health care expenditures: A national study. *Annals of Family Medicine*, *10*(5), 388–395. doi:10.1370/afm.1382 PMID:22966101

Kirch, D. G., Henderson, M. K., & Dill, M. J. (2012). Physician workforce projections in an era of reform. *Annual Review of Medicine*, *63*(1), 435–445. doi:10.1146/annurev-med-050310-134634 PMID:21888514

Ku, L., Jones, K., Shin, P., Bruen, B., & Hayes, K. (2011). The states' next challenge-securing primary care for expanded Medicaid populations. *The New England Journal of Medicine*, *364*(6), 493–495. doi:10.1056/NEJMp1011623 PMID:21268720

Leigh, J. P., Tancredi, D., Jerant, A., Romano, P. S., & Kravitz, R. L. (2012). Lifetime earnings for physicians across specialties. *Medical Care*, *50*(12), 1093–1101. doi:10.1097/MLR.0b013e318268ac0c PMID:22922430

Lohr, K. N., Brook, R., Kamberg, C., Goldberg, G. A., Leibowitz, A., & Keesey, J. et al. (1986). Use of medical care in the RAND Health Insurance Experiment: diagnosis- and service-specific analyses in a randomized controlled trial. *Medical Care*, *24*, S1–S87. PMID:3093785

Margolius, D., & Bodenheimer, T. (2010). Transforming primary care: From past practice to the practice of the future. *Health Affairs*, *29*(5), 779–784. doi:10.1377/hlthaff.2010.0045 PMID:20439861

Marx, J. (2010). *Rosen's emergency medicine: Concepts and clinical practice* (7th ed.). Philadelphia, PA: Mosby/Elsevier.

Massachusetts Medical Society. (2008). *2008 Physician workforce study*. Waltham, MA: Massachusetts Medical Society.

National Association of Community Health Centers. (2008). Access transformed: Building a primary care workforce for the 21st century. Bethesda, MD: Author.

National Association of Community Health Centers. (2009). Primary care access: An essential building block of health reform. Bethesda, MD: Author.

National Association of Community Health Centers. (20213). *A sketchbook of community health centers*. Retrieved April 19, 2013 from http://www.nachc.com/client// Chartbook2013.pdf

National Institute on Health Care Reform. (2011). *Matching Supply to Demand: Addressing the U.S. Primary Care Workforce Shortage*. NIHCR Policy Analysis No. 7. Retrieved on April 24, 2013 from http://www.nihcr.org/PCP_Workforce

National Residency Matching Program. (2008). *Results and Data: 2008 main residency match*. Retrieved on April 27, 2012 from: http://www.nrmp.org/data/resultsanddata2008.pdf

O'Malley, A. S. (2013). After-hours access to primary care practices linked with lower emergency department use and less unmet medical need. *Health Affairs*, *32*(1), 175–183. doi:10.1377/hlthaff.2012.0494 PMID:23242631

O'Malley, A. S., Samuel, D., Bond, A. M., & Carrier, E. (2012). After-hours care and its coordination with primary care in the U.S. *Journal of General Internal Medicine*, *27*(11), 1406–1415. doi:10.1007/s11606-012-2087-4 PMID:22653379

Palmeri, M., Pipas, C., Wadsworth, E., & Zubkoff, M. (2010). Economic Impact of a primary care career: A harsh reality for medical student and the nation. *Academic Medicine*, *85*(11), 1692–1697. doi:10.1097/ACM.0b013e3181f5b754 PMID:20881829

Parchman, M. L., & Culler, S. (1994). Primary care physicians and avoidable hospitalization. *The Journal of Family Practice*, *39*, 123–128. PMID:8057062

Petterson, S. M., Liaw, W. R., Phillips, R. L., Rabin, D., Meyers, D., & Bazemore, A. W. (2012). Projecting US primary care workforce needs: 2010-2025. *Annals of Family Medicine*, *10*(6), 503–509. doi:10.1370/afm.1431 PMID:23149526

Pugno, P. A., Schmittling, G. T., Fetter, G. T. Jr, & Kahn, N. B. Jr. (2005). Results of the 2005 national resident matching program: Family medicine. *Family Medicine*, *37*, 555–564. PMID:16145633

Reed, M., Graetz, I., Wang, H., Fung, V., Newhouse, J. P., & Hsu, J. (2012). Consumer-directed health plans with health savings accounts: Whose skin is in the game and how do costs affect care seeking? *Medical Care*, *50*(7), 585–590. doi:10.1097/MLR.0b013e3182495cb3 PMID:22322099

Rieselbach, R. E., Crouse, B. J., & Frohna, J. G. (2010). Teaching primary care in community health centers: Addressing the workforce crisis for the underserved. *Annals of Internal Medicine*, *152*(2), 118–122. doi:10.7326/0003-4819-152-2-201001190-00186 PMID:20008743

Rust, G., Jiali, Y., Baltrus, P., Adesunloye, B., & Fryer, G. E. (2008). Practical barriers to timely primary care access. Impact on adult use of emergency department services. *Archives of Internal Medicine*, *168*(15), 1705–1710. doi:10.1001/archinte.168.15.1705 PMID:18695087

Sanders, B. (2013). *Primary care access- 30 million new patients and 11 months to go: Who will provide their primary care? Report from Chairman Bernard Sanders, Subcommittee on Primary Health and Aging*. U.S. Senate Committee on Health, Education, Labor & Pensions.

Schoen, C., Osborn, R., Doty, M. M., Bishop, M., Peugh, J., & Murukutla, N. (2007). Toward higher-performance health systems: Adults' health care experiences in seven countries, 2007. *Health Affairs (Project Hope)*, *26*(6), w717–w734. doi:10.1377/hlthaff.26.6.w717 PMID:17978360

Smith, S. R. (2011). A recipe for medical schools to produce primary care physicians. *The New England Journal of Medicine*, *364*(6), 496–497. doi:10.1056/NEJMp1012495 PMID:21306236

Starfield, B. (1994). Is primary care essential? *Lancet*, *344*(8930), 1129–1133. doi:10.1016/S0140-6736(94)90634-3 PMID:7934497

Starfield, B., Shi, L., & Macinko, J. (2005). Contributions of primary care to health systems and health. *The Milbank Quarterly*, *83*(3), 457–502. doi:10.1111/j.1468-0009.2005.00409.x PMID:16202000

The Commonwealth of Massachusetts. (2006). Retrieved on April 24, 2013 from http://www.malegislature.gov/Laws/SessionLaws/Acts/2006/Chapter58

The Henry J. Kaiser Family Foundation. (2010). *Focus on Health Reform- Summary of new health reform law*. Retrieved on April 24, 2013 from http://www.kff.org/healthreform/upload/8061.pdf

The Kaiser Family Foundation. (2012). *Massachusetts Health care reform: Six years later.* Retrieved on April 24 2013 from: http://www.kff.org/healthreform/upload/8311.pdf

The Patient Protection and Affordable Care Act. (n.d.). Retrieved on April 24, 2013 from http://www.healthcare .gov/law/full/index.html

United States Government Accountability Office. (2008). Primary care professionals: Recent supply trends, projections, and valuation of services. Washington, DC: Author.

US Department of Health and Human Services Council on Graduate Medical Education. (2005). *Physician workforce policy guidelines for 2000-2020*. Rockville, MD: COGME.

Vaughn, B. T., DeVrieze, S. R., Reed, S. D., & Schulman, K. A. (2010). Can we close the income gap between specialists and primary care physicians? *Health Affairs (Project Hope)*, *29*(5), 933–940. doi:10.1377/hlthaff.2009.0675 PMID:20439883

Wasson, J. H., Sauvigne, A. E., Mogielnicki, R. P., Frey, W. G., Sox, C. H., & Gaudette, C. et al. (1984). Continuity of outpatient medical care in elderly men: A randomized trial. *Journal of the American Medical Association*, *252*(17), 2413–2417. doi:10.1001/jama.1984.03350170015011 PMID:6481927

West, C. P., Popkave, C., Schultz, H. J., Weinberger, S. E., & Kolars, J. C. (2006). Changes in career decisions of internal medicine residents during training. *Annals of Internal Medicine*, *145*(10), 774–779. doi:10.7326/0003-4819-145-10-200611210-00010 PMID:17116922

KEY TERMS AND DEFINITIONS

Community Health Centers: Local, not-for-profit, community-owned centers that serve all patients without regard to ability to pay or insurance coverage.

Healthcare Reform: A common term referring to the provisions of the Patient Protection and Affordable Care Act signed into law in March of 2010.

Primary Care Physician Shortage: The difference between the number of physicians needed and the number of physicians available in the workforce.

Primary Care Physician: A generalist physician who provides definitive care to patients at the point of first contact and takes continuing responsibility for providing these patients' care.

Primary Care: Is the provision of integrated, accessible health care services by clinicians who are accountable for addressing a large majority of personal health care needs, developing a sustained partnership with patients, and practicing in the context of family and community.

Chapter 3
Non-Physician Providers

ABSTRACT

In this chapter, the role played by non-physician providers such as Nurse Practitioners (NPs) and Physician Assistants (PAs) is discussed in depth. These providers have delivered services in a variety of healthcare settings for a long time, but there is a recent urgency about the importance of the role that they can play in the healthcare system. The authors expound on research related to cost, quality, and satisfaction of patients receiving care from non-physician providers, and address barriers such as restrictive scope of practice and unjust payment policies. The use of other providers such as pharmacists and grand-aides is also addressed.

The NP workforce presents a potential answer to [these] pressures, but it has been largely overlooked by policy makers, the public, and other healthcare stakeholders. Fully integrating the contributions and skills of all primary care practitioners and, specifically, the contributions of nurse practitioners is a vital policy step toward achieving high-value healthcare.
—Naylor and Kurtzman, 2010, p. 898

INTRODUCTION

Nurse practitioners (NPs) and physician assistants (PAs) have delivered services in a variety of healthcare settings for a long time, but there is a recent urgency about the importance of the role that they can play in the healthcare system. In this chapter, we outline the roles, training and education of NPs and PAs, discuss their scope of practice, and review the literature on the quality and costs of the services that they provide. We also discuss the potential for other non-physician providers such as pharmacists and grand-aides. It is important to note that many labels have been commonly used to refer to these providers, such as "mid-level providers" (MLPs) or "physician extenders." We chose to use the more neutral "non-physician providers."

DOI: 10.4018/978-1-4666-6355-8.ch003

1. EDUCATION AND GROWTH OF NON-PHYSICIAN PROVIDERS

Definitions

Advanced Practice Registered Nurses (APRNs) are registered nurses (RNs) with a master's, post-master's or doctoral degrees that have passed national certification examinations (Brassard and Smolenski, 2011). They are certified by professional or specialty nursing organizations, and are licensed to provide services that are consistent with their areas of expertise and state-specific laws that govern nursing scope of practice (Naylor and Kurtzman, 2011). For example, they teach and counsel patients to understand their health conditions and ways to improve their health, coordinate care and advocate for patients, and refer patients to physicians (Brassard and Smolenski, 2011). There are four types of APRNs: Clinical Nurse Specialists (CNSs); Certified Registered Nurse Anesthetists (CRNAs); Certified Nurse Midwives (CNMs) and NPs. CNSs "provide advanced nursing care in hospitals and other clinical sites; provide acute and chronic care management; develop quality improvement programs; [and] serve as mentors, educators, researchers and consultants" (Brassard and Smolenski, 2011, p. 2). CRNAs administer anesthesia before and after surgical, therapeutic, diagnostic, and obstetrical procedures and provide pain management in settings such as operating rooms, outpatient surgical centers, and dental offices (Brassard and Smolenski, 2011). CNMs provide women-specific primary care services such as gynecological exams, contraceptives, prenatal care, management of low-risk labor and delivery, and neonatal care. They typically practice in hospitals, birthing centers, and community clinics (Brassard and Smolenski, 2011). NPs "take health histories and provide complete physical exams; diagnose and treat acute and chronic illnesses; prescribe and manage medications; order and interpret lab tests and X-rays;[and] provide health teaching and supportive counseling" (Brassard and Smolenski, 2011, p. 2).

Physician Assistants (PAs), on the other hand, are providers who practice medicine under physician supervision. They perform physical exams, diagnose and treat illnesses, order and read tests, provide preventative services, assist in surgery, and prescribe medications (United States Government Accountability Office, 2008).

History and Education

The evidence for nurses practicing independently from physicians dates back to the 19th century, especially in nurse midwifery and other fields that are outside mainstream medicine (Hansen-Turton, Ware, and McClellan, 2010). But it wasn't until after World War II that advanced nursing education and practice started to gain significant recognition, with military nurses granted federal funding to study in universities. Subsequently, nurses started to expand their reach and manage school-based clinics and home-based care (Hansen-Turton, et al., 2010). In the 1960s', the establishment of Medicare and Medicaid's public insurance programs for the elderly and the poor respectively, created new opportunities for growth for nurses in primary care. These new programs resulted in a physician shortage that prompted greater demand on the primary healthcare system.

The first formal NP educational program in the U.S. was offered by the University of Colorado in 1965. This was followed by several other nursing programs, which created an environment where NP curricula and roles started to flourish (Hansen-Turton, et al., 2010). These programs now require nurses with a bachelor's degree to complete a master's program in nursing to become an NP. They range in length between 18 and 24 months, and consist of classroom studies as well as clinical rotations (United States Government Accountability Office, 2008; Yee, Bokus, Cross and Samuel, 2013). Areas of specialization include acute care, adult health, child health, emergency care, geriatric care, neonatal health, occupational health, and oncology (United States Government Accountability Office, 2008). Some NPs earn doctoral degrees requiring an additional year of training and more clinical rotations. In fact, Doctorates of Nursing Practice are gaining some support in nursing, although they have "not been universally accepted or endorsed" (Hansen-Turton, et al., 2010, p. 1243).

Licensure and certification for NPs is different. Licensure gives a provider the right to engage in a profession and is usually based on the criteria of essential education and measure of competence, whereas certification assures that a professional has mastered a body of knowledge and acquired skills in a particular specialty or area. Credentialing includes licensure, certification, accreditation and recognition and is necessary to bill for reimbursement (discussed later in this chapter). In the United States, for the most part, recognition and practice as an NP requires national certification. The only exceptions are California, Kansas and Indiana which allow NP practice without a national board certification. In these states, NP licensure is awarded based on graduation from an accredited NP education program or completion of a specific amount of work experience. In all other states, certification examinations that are accredited by the National Commission for Certifying Agencies or the American Board of Nursing Specialties are recognized by nursing boards (Hellier and Ramponi, 2013). These boards exhibit great variability in specific regulations for NP practice, as will be discussed later. NP titles vary from state to state and include "nurse practitioner, certified registered nurse practitioner, licensed nurse practitioner, advanced practice nurse, certified nurse practitioner, advanced registered nurse practitioner, and advanced practice registered nurse" (Hellier and Ramponi, 2013, p. 1).

The creation of the PA profession also dates to the mid 1960's and the above-discussed PCP shortage. The main agent behind the PA movement was Eugene A. Stead Jr., a physician at the Duke University Medical Center. According to the Physician Assistant History Society (2013), Dr. Stead had developed with nurse educator Thelma Ingles an advanced nurse clinician program. But he grew disillusioned with organized nursing's rejection of the program, and therefore decided to create a program for the "physician's assistant" instead (Physician Assistant History Society, 2013). Dr. Stead put together the first class of PAs in 1965 mainly for former military corpsmen, and he modeled the relationship between MDs and PAs mainly on the well-known relationship between Amos N. Johnson, MD, and Henry Lee "Buddy" Treadwell, his assistant (American Academy of Physician Assistants, 2013). The first class of PAs graduated in 1967 and the concept "was lauded early on and gained acceptance and backing federally as early as the 1970s as a creative solution to physician shortages" (American Academy of Physician Assistants, 2013). Soon after, accreditation standards, national certification and standardized examinations, and continuing medical education requirements were created, mainly with support from the medical community.

Nowadays, applicants to PA programs need to have some college education, and most programs are 26 months in length. They consist of classroom education and clinical rotations in internal medicine, family medicine, surgery, pediatrics, obstetrics and gynecology, emergency medicine and geriatrics (United States Government Accountability Office, 2008).

Services and Practice

As mentioned above, NPs have the authority to provide many services such as to "obtain medical histories and perform physical examinations; diagnose and treat health problems; order and interpret laboratory tests and x-rays; prescribe medications and other treatments; prenatal care; well-child care; immunizations and family planning services; gynecological examinations and pap smears; health promotion, illness prevention, patient education about health risks; and case management and coordination of services" (Hansen-Turton et al., 2010, p. 1244). The ability to prescribe medications is one area that has become most uniform in NP practice in the last few years. APRNs, and more specifically NPs, can prescribe medications in all 50 states, and have the ability to prescribe controlled substances in 48 of them. NPs are trained to prescribe a medication regime, or change an existing medication of a patient, with 96% of NPs prescribing medications and averaging about 20 prescriptions per day (AARP Public Policy Institute, 2011).

The main difference between NPs and PAs is that NPs work with physicians, but have independent practice authority in many states, whereas PAs have to work under physician supervision. This allows NPs to provide a variety of services with minimal physician involvement (United States Government Accountability Office, 2008). Moreover, as a result of the difference in their training, NPs provide care according to the "nursing model" of care, whereas PAs (and physicians) practice under the "medical model" of care. The nursing model emphasizes a holistic approach where treatment includes the evaluation of the patient's total well-being within his/her environment, with special attention given to patient education (Hansen-Turton et al., 2010). The medical model, on the other hand, is geared more towards diagnosing and treating diseases in isolation.

Despite these differences, NPs and PAs tend to practice in similar settings such as PCP practices, hospitals, long-term care settings and specialty physician offices. Only 43% of NPs in the U.S. have hospital privileges, with half of them able to admit patients from an office or outpatient setting directly to the hospital (Goolsby, 2011). Moreover, NPs and PAs practice in retail clinics, urgent care centers, and other non-traditional settings discussed later in this book.

Workforce Supply and Growth

The current number of NPs practicing in the United States is about 155,000 (American Academy of Nurse Practitioners, 2011), the number of PAs is about 83,000 (American Academy of Physician Assistants, 2011), whereas the number of practicing PCPs is at 209,000 (AHRQ, 2011). These numbers reflect an accelerated growth in the numbers of non-physician providers in the last 20 years, compared to slow or stagnant growth in the PCP workforce. For example, the ratio of NPs to PCPs grew from 0.23 to 0.48 from 1995 to 2009, whereas the ratio of PAs to PCPs grew from 0.12 to 0.28 during that same time period (Stange and Sampson, 2010). In addition, the annual growth in the number of practicing NPs is about 9.5%, compared to 1.17% for practicing physicians, which led experts to suggest that "NP programs are educating three NPs to every one PCP" (Hansen-Turton et al., 2010, p. 1241). Non-physician providers are playing an increasingly important role in primary care, with NPs and PAs accounting for 19% and 7% of the U.S. primary care workforce, respectively (Green, Savin and Lu, 2013). In 2009, 49% of PCPs were in practices that had NPs, PAs or CNMs (Park, Cherry and Decker, 2011).

Despite the growth in the supply of the non-physician provider workforce, experts caution that there won't be enough of them to address the primary healthcare demands of the U.S. population. There is a well-documented nursing shortage in the United States currently, and it is expected to reach 260,000 registered nurses (RNs) by 2025, mainly due to the lack of qualified nursing faculty and training sites (Buerhaus, Auerbach, Staiger, 2009). Nurse practitioner numbers are directly affected by this crisis. Bodenheimer and Pham (2010) warn that "figures on the numbers of NPs and PAs graduating from training programs each year, and the proportion of those entering primary care rather than specialty careers, reveal that their numbers will not be sufficient to close the projected gap. Adding primary care physicians, NPs, and PAs together, the ratio of primary care practitioners to population is expected to fall 9 percent from 2005 to 2020" (p. 801). A contributing factor to the limited availability of non-physician providers, especially PAs, in primary care, is their increased specialization. Evidence suggests that more and more PAs are choosing procedure-driven specialties such as surgery, cardiology, and oncology, as well as emergency medicine, dermatology, and orthopedics (Hooker, Cawley and Leinweber, 2010, United States Government Accountability Office, 2008). While family medicine remains the largest single PA specialty, the net number of PAs leaving family medicine exceeds the net number of those moving into it every year since the late 1990s (Hooker, Cawley and Leinweber, 2010). Bennett and Phillips (2010) summarized the dangers: "With the current focus on expanding access to health insurance, the primary care workforce could become more strained as demand for care increases. Although advanced practice nurses, physician assistants, international medical graduates (IMGs), and osteopathic physicians have potential to reduce this gap, their valuable contributions will be inadequate. With the possible exception of nurse practitioners, all of these providers are specializing more, and their absolute numbers are small in comparison with the primary care shortage" (p. S81).

2. NURSE PRACTITIONERS

NPs constitute the single largest non-physician provider profession, and continue to play a vital role in the healthcare system. In this section, we focus on relevant NP-specific issues such as quality and cost of care, scope-of-practice laws, payment policies, and physician resistance.

Quality of Care

A strong body of empirical evidence suggests that NPs provide care that is of similar or better quality to care provided by PCPs for specific conditions and patient populations. In 1974, the first study comparing NPs and physicians' outcomes was conducted in Canada (Spitzer, Sackett, Sibley, Roberts, Gent, Kergin, et al., 1974). It concluded that patient outcomes including mortality; patient satisfaction; and physical, emotional and social functioning of patients seen by NPs were equivalent to those of patients seen by physicians. This was followed by two independent reviews of non-physician providers in the U.S. conducted by the congressional Office of Technology Assessment (OTA) (LeRoy and Solkowitz, 1980; U.S. Congress Office of Technology Assessment, 1986). The studies concluded that "within their areas of competence, nurse practitioners, physician's assistants, and certified nurse-midwives provide care whose quality is equivalent to that of care provided by physicians"(U.S. Congress Office of Technology Assessment, 1986, p. 5).

In the early 2000s, a landmark randomized trial compared patient outcomes, health status, and patient satisfaction of NP and physician practices, and found no differences after 6 months and after two years (Mundinger, Kane, Lenz, Totten, Tsai, Cleary, et al., 2000; Lenz, Mundinger, Kane, Hopkins and Lin, 2004). These findings were substantiated by two other systematic reviews published during the same time period. They showed that patients of NPs were more satisfied with no noticeable differences in outcomes (Horrocks, Anderson and Salisbury, 2002; Laurant, Reeves, Hermens, Braspenning, Grol and Sibbald, 2004). These reviews were followed by several individual studies that added further evidence that the care provided by NPs is equivalent to, and sometimes more effective on certain measures, than care provided by physicians (Dierick-van Daele, Metsemakers, Derckx, Spreeuwneberg, Vrijhoef, 2009; ter Bogt, Bemelmans, Beltman, Broer, Smit, van der Meer, 2009; Hopkins, Lenz, Pontes, Lin, Mundinger, 2005; Leese, Allgar, Heywood, Walker, Darr, Din et al., 2006; Ohman-Strickland, Orzano, Hudson, Solberg, DiCiccio-Bloom, O'Malley, et al., 2008; Running, Kip, Mercer, 2006; Seale, Anderson, Kinnersley, 2006; Wilson, Landon, Hirschhborn, McInnes, Din, Marsden, et al., 2005).

Cost of Care

The evidence related to cost of care provided by NPs compared to that of PCPs is equivocal. Two above-mentioned reviews found that patients of NPs had more tests but with no significant differences in resource use (Horrocks, Anderson and Salisbury, 2002; Laurant, Reeves, Hermens, Braspenning, Grol and Sibbald, 2004). Another study comparing insurance claims found lower costs associated with NP care (Roblin, Howard, Becker, Adams & Roberts, 2004). However, a recent systematic review of the literature has concluded that "the effects [of the use of non-physician clinicians] on healthcare costs is mixed, with savings dependent on the context of care and the specific nature of role revision" (Laurent, Harmsen, Wollersheim, Grol, Faber and Sibbald, 2009). For example, some studies have shown that nurse practitioners ordered significantly more tests and investigations than physicians, while others have found no difference or inconclusive evidence. Similar ambiguous results were found for length of hospitalizations and overall cost-effectiveness.

A recent policy analysis prepared by the Rand Corporation on behalf of the Commonwealth of Massachusetts provides specific cost estimates and potential cost savings of NP/PA visits compared to physician visits. The analysis estimated that the average cost of NP/PA visit is 20-35% lower than the average cost of a physician office-based visit.

For instance, if Massachusetts relied more on NPs/PAs for the period 2010-2020, it could save between $4.2 and $8.4 billion (Eibner, Hussey, Ridgeley, McGlynn, 2009).

Scope of Practice Laws

Scope of practice for a healthcare professional refers to the permissible boundaries of practice, i.e. the range of services that can be provided by that professional and the extent to which he/she can provide services independently (Yee, et al, 2013). In the United States, decisions about NP scope of practice are made at the state level. These are dictated in statutes, state codes, or in rules and regulations disseminated by medical and nursing boards (Hansen-Turton et al., 2010).

There is a wide variation in the degree of autonomy granted by the various states to NPs to treat and prescribe medications for patients without physician supervision or collaboration. Eighteen states (Washington, Oregon, Idaho, Montana, Wyoming, North Dakota, Utah, Colorado, New Mexico, Arizona, Iowa, Maine, New Hampshire, Vermont, Rhodes Island, Maryland, Alaska, and Hawaii), and the District of Columbia have granted NPs the right to diagnose, treat and prescribe without physician supervision. Seven states (Michigan, Indiana, Kentucky, Tennessee, West Virginia, Oklahoma and New Jersey) require physician oversight over NP prescribing of medication, but not over diagnosis and treatment. Twenty-five states (California, Nevada, South Dakota, Nebraska, Kansas, Texas, Minnesota, Wisconsin, Illinois, Missouri, Arkansas, Louisiana, Mississippi, Alabama, Georgia, Florida, South Carolina, North Carolina, Virginia, Ohio, Pennsylvania, New York, Massachusetts, Connecticut and Delaware) require physician supervision of NPs for diagnosis, treatment and prescribing (Yee et al., 2013). Because of these differences, NPs do not have the same consistency in scope-of-practice that physicians, physician assistants and registered nurses have (Kleinpell, Hudspeth, Scordo, and Madgic, 2011).

In states where physician supervision is required for prescribing only, or for prescribing, diagnosis and treatment, a "collaborative agreement" should be in place between physicians and NPs. According to Medicare, collaboration is defined as "a process in which a nurse practitioner . . . works with a physician to deliver healthcare services within the scope of the practitioner's professional expertise, with [physician] medical direction and appropriate supervision . . . as defined by the law of the State in which the services are performed." (Social Security Act, quoted in Hansen-Turton et al., 2010). In some of these states, collaborations ensure a means for consultation, referral, and review of provided care. In others, collaboration is coupled with a requirement for "detailed written guidelines or protocols that document the scope of practice functions NPs may follow". These protocols establish the procedures that NPs are able to perform, which in some case may be more limited in scope than what their training allows (National Governors Association, 2012).

A recent study by the National Institute for Healthcare Reform (2013) compared and contrasted six states with a wide range of scope of practice laws: Maryland and Arizona have no physician oversight requirements; Michigan and Indiana have collaborative agreements with physicians to prescribe; and Massachusetts and Arkansas have collaborative agreements with physician required to diagnose, treat and prescribe. Despite these major differences, there were surprisingly no significant differences across the states in terms of services delivered by NPs at the point-of-care. This is due to the fact that scope-of-practice laws generally do not specify the tasks that NPs can perform, but rather authorize a broad range of practice and define whether physician supervision for specific tasks is required or not (National Institute for Healthcare Reform, 2013). Moreover, physician supervision was more a function of the relationship between an individual physician and NP, rather than the corresponding state scope-of-practice law. For example, even in states with restrictive scope-of-practice, NPs "described having latitude to make clinical decisions, although with a greater level of documented supervision," and a more collaborative rather than supervisory relationship with physicians (National Institute for Healthcare Reform, 2013, p. 2). The level of autonomy enjoyed by NPs was mainly influenced by practice culture and individual practitioner traits, such as years at the organization or level of experience (National Institute for Healthcare Reform, 2013). For example, a physician practicing in Indiana relayed: "I have worked with and supervised many NPs, and for those that are just starting out, [chart review] is quite useful. For someone 20 years out? Not so much" (National Institute for Healthcare Reform, 2013, p. 2). The major impact of the regulations appears to be where and how NPs can practice. NPs practicing in physician oversight states "reported being more likely to have work delegated to them by physicians to satisfy supervision requirements" and "more often co-managing patient panels with physicians rather than acting as the sole, designated care provider" (National Institute for Healthcare Reform, 2013, p. 2). Collaborative agreements were viewed by most study respondents as a formality that does not stimulate meaningful interaction between NPs and physicians. A significant effect was in limiting the range of practice settings for NPs, especially in underserved rural communities. An NP in Arkansas explained: "We are tethered to physicians; we can't go farther out into rural communities than physicians are willing to go to provide care because of the collaborative practice agreement requirement. The collaborating physician has to be available and accessible, and I wouldn't want to collaborate with someone 200 miles away" (National Institute for Healthcare Reform, 2013, p. 3).

Another study examining NP-physician collaboration reported that despite several areas of agreements, physicians expected NPs to seek the collaboration (O'Brien, Martin, Heyworth, and Meyer, 2009). Physician's interpretation of collaboration was closer to supervision, as they believed that communication would improve if NPs heard and implemented their directions. NPs, on the other hand, believed that physicians did not listen to them (O'Brien, Martin, Heyworth, and Meyer, 2009).

The wide state-to-state variations in scope of practice have led NPs to migrate from more restrictive to less restrictive states. This has resulted in reduced access to patient care in the more restrictive states. According to the Pearson Report (2011), the ratio of NPs to state population is the lowest in the heavily regulated states. For example, Alabama has the fifth lowest ratio of NP to state population in the U.S. with 40 NPs per 100,000 population and scores an "F" according to the report's ranking system for NP scope of practice. New Hampshire, on the other hand, has the second highest ratio with 114 NPs per 100,000, and scores an "A+" with no restrictions on NP scope of practice (Pearson, 2011).

In states where NP scope of practice is still not well defined, there is a lack of clarity that leads to disputes about what a NP can and cannot legally do. This can be traced back to historical efforts by physician groups to reduce the scope of practice of NPs. Hansen-Turton et al. (2010) describe these efforts: "In the 1950s, physician groups introduced state-by-state legislation defining physician-only services, which included many things that nurses were already doing. In response, the American Nursing Association (ANA) created a model definition of nursing, which stated that nursing shall not be deemed to include any acts of diagnosis or prescription of therapeutic or corrective measures. Meanwhile, nurses continued to diagnose illness in the course of their practices. Nurse practitioners have since been slowly changing the legal definition of the practice of medicine to broaden their authority" (p. 1249).

To address the variations in regulations, the Consensus Model for Advanced Practice Registered Nurse (APRN) Regulation was created by the profession in 2008. The document aims to "resolve the issues of inconsistent APRN education, issues of certification, and issues of inconsistent licensure requirements across jurisdictions," and "states that the education, accreditation, certification, and licensure (LACE) of APRNs should be aligned in order to ensure patient safety while also expanding patient access to ARPN care and promoting a consistent SOP [scope-of-practice]" (Kleinpell et al., 2011, p. 12). The implementation date for the Consensus Model has been set for 2015. Meanwhile, professional associations and regulators are working to restructure educational programs to meet new accreditation requirements, refine certification exams, and modify nurse practice acts (Kleinpell et al., 2011).

Payment Policies

Payment policies may have an even stronger impact on where NPs practice and how they practice. In fact, the level of restrictiveness of state scope-of-practice laws is related to the level of autonomy enjoyed by NPs under public and private payer policies. Payers can determine the services for which NPs can be paid for, the payment rates, whether NPs can be paid directly and whether they can be designated as primary care providers. In areas with restrictive state-of-practice laws and payment policies, NPs may be limited to working as employees of physician practices and hospitals, and not in their own independent practice (Yee et al., 2013).

Under federal law, NPs are eligible to receive reimbursement from both Medicare and Medicaid. However, private managed care organizations that contract with the federal and local governments to administrate Medicare and Medicaid services are not required by law to include NPs as primary care providers. A 2006 survey of national insurance companies reported that only 33% of managed care organizations have a uniform policy allowing NPs to be credentialed as primary care providers, and of those only 52% of them reimburse them at the same rates as physicians. A large number of these organizations "appeared to have difficulty understanding how an NP could be even capable of acting as a PCP [primary care provider]" (Hansen-Turton, Ritter, Begun, Berkowitz, Rothman, and Valdez, 2006, p. 218.) A follow-up study in 2008 showed similar numbers: only 73% of insurers with Medicaid products, 33% of insurers with Medicare products, and 43% of insurers with commercial policies credentialed NPs are primary care providers (Hansen-Turton, Ritter and Torgan, 2008). It is important to note that in some states, payers impose additional restrictions that go beyond scope-of-practice laws. In Arkansas for example, NPs are not recognized as primary care providers by Medicaid, and Medicaid programs do not reimburse for streptococcal screens or influenza swabs performed by NPs. An examination of the state's scope-of-practice statutes reveals that they do not prohibit the performance of these tests by NPs (Yee et al., 2013).

Massachusetts provides an interesting example of a state with restrictive scope-of-practice laws, but where a new statute related to payment policies was passed in parallel with overall reform to provide universal insurance (Craven and Ober, 2009). The "Act Providing Consumer Choice of Nurse Practitioner Services" mandated the recognition of NPs as primary care providers. NPs are now formally accepted as primary care providers in provider networks, are listed in health plans directories, and are credentialed by the insurance carriers (Craven and Ober, 2009).

In most states, NPs are reimbursed only a portion of what physicians are reimbursed for the same services. Typically, NP reimbursement by Medicare, Medicaid and private insurance plans is at 75-85% of physician reimbursement. For example, under Medicare, if NPs bill under their own provider number, they can bill only 85% of the physician fee. However, if they bill under a physician provider number and are directly supervised by a physician, they can get 100% of a physician's bill (Naylor and Kurtzman, 2010). Medicaid variations among states are staggering. In Kentucky, for example, NPs are reimbursed at 75 percent of the physician's charge for the same service, whereas in Texas they are reimbursed at 92 percent and in Virginia, they are reimbursed at 100 percent of the physician's charge (National Governors Association, 2012). These disparate payment policies have been in place for a long time. A report by Medicare Advisory Commission (MedPAC) however found no analytic reasons for the disparities, and called for additional study of the issue (Naylor and Kurtzman, 2010).

Malpractice

Healthcare providers can be held liable for harm suffered by a patient for medication errors; inadequate patient monitoring; failure or delay in giving a diagnosis; committing an error in documentation or charting; failure to consult or refer; incorrect use of equipment; failure to obtain informed consent; failure to follow up; or exceeding legal scope of practice. NPs face potential tort liability under these same rules, with special focus on two unique issues: appropriate standard of care and expert witnesses (Hansen-Turton, 2010).

The first issue relates to the medical professional against whom the NP is compared when determining the appropriate standard of care in case of negligence. A healthcare provider is supposed to exercise care that a reasonable professional of the same medical specialty would use under similar circumstances. The question is whether the reasonableness of the NP's conduct should be judged by the conduct of another NP, or by the conduct of a physician who provides care for the same conditions. While there is considerable overlap in the services and treatments provided by NPs and physicians, the NPs approach and underlying philosophy is very different from that of physicians (Baker, 1992).

The second issue relates to who should testify as an expert witness to the NP standard of care. In general, to qualify for expert witness, the professional should possess "special education or training that will aid the court and/or jury in determining whether a deviation from the accepted standard has occurred, and whether any deviation has caused hard to the plaintiff" (Hansen-Turton et al., 2010, p. 1253). While some courts have allowed physician testimony on nursing standard of care, others have precluded them because medicine is a separate profession with separate licensing. The American Association of Nurse Attorneys (AANA) argues that "only nurses should be permitted to provide expert testimony as to the nursing standard of care in malpractice actions, because only the nursing profession has the right, duty and responsibility to determine the scope and nature of nursing practice including the standard of care for nurses" (Hansen-Turton et al., 2010, p. 1255).

It is important to note that medical malpractice claims against NPs rarely relate to allegations that they had exceeded their scope of practice. Rather, they mostly relate to claims of improper diagnosis and treatment. More specifically, diagnosis-related claims constitute 45% of all claims against NPs, whereas treatment-related claims constitute 25% of them (Hansen-Turton et al., 2010).

Physician Opposition

Despite the clear evidence that NPs provide high quality care in a variety of primary care settings, there is still very strong physician opposition to NPs replacing physicians in the delivery of needed services. In 2009, the American Medical Association (AMA), the oldest and largest organization of physicians and medical students, published a "Scope of Practice Data Series" to educate "policymakers on the qualifications of a particular non-physician healthcare profession, as well as on the qualifications [that] physicians possess [which] prepare them to accept the responsibility for full, unrestricted licensure to practice medicine in all its branches" (AMA, 2009, p. 4). In the report directly related to NPs, education and licensing is discussed and comparisons to physicians' longer training and more comprehensive testing for licensure are drawn (AMA, 2009).

Similarly, a 2012 report by the American Academy of Family Physicians (AAFPs) suggested that the only way to deal with the physician shortages was to transition to physician-lead team-based, and not to substitute physicians with NPs. The report stated: "The rationale behind most proposals to allow nurse practitioners to practice independently is that the nation is facing a primary care physician shortage. This is true. But substituting NPs for doctors cannot be the answer. Nurse practitioners are not doctors, and responsible leaders of nursing acknowledge this fact. Dr. Kathleen Potempa, the dean of the University of Michigan School of Nursing and president of the American Association of Colleges of Nursing told the New York Times that, "Nurses are very proud of the fact that they're nurses, and if nurses had wanted to be doctors, they would have gone to medical school." Dr. Potempa is right—nurse practitioners do not have the substance of doctor training or the length of clinical experience required to be doctors. For example, for licensure, NPs receive only 5.5-7 years of education compared with 11 years for a physician. The clinical experience that NPs receive within that education is only one-fifth of the clinical experience a physician receives" (AAFP, p. ii). It goes on to argue that "[g]ranting independent practice to nurse practitioners would be creating two classes of care: one run by a physician-led team and one run by less qualified health professionals. Americans should not be forced into this two-tier scenario. Everyone deserves to be under the care of a doctor. Nurse practitioners are a vital part of the healthcare team, but they cannot fulfill the need for a fully trained physician. A physician brings a broader and deeper expertise to the diagnosis and treatment of all health problems, ranging from strep throat to chronic obstructive pulmonary disease, from unsightly moles to cancer, from stress headaches to refractory multiple sclerosis. The family physician is trained to provide a complex differential diagnosis, develop a treatment plan that addresses multiple organ systems, and order and interpret tests within the context of the patient's overall health condition" (AAFP, p. 7-8).

Other Primary Care Providers

In addition to NPs and PAs, other non-physician providers such as pharmacists and "grand-aides" can play an important role in primary healthcare delivery. Given their education and training, pharmacists are "remarkably underutilized" in the American healthcare system (Giberson, Yoder, Lee, 2011, p. 10). The Social Security Act recognizes a number of healthcare professionals such as PA, NPs, certified nurse midwives, clinical social workers, clinical psychologists, and registered dieticians/nutrition professionals as healthcare "providers or practitioners" but omits pharmacists from this definition. A recent report by the chief pharmacist of the United States Public Health Service suggests that "pharmacists provide expertise and healthcare delivery in a number of ways from primary prevention, to counseling and adherence programs, to comprehensive medication and chronic disease management - and are not yet recognized in this important piece of legislation" and that "this omission is despite evidence that medications are involved in 80 percent of all treatments (and impact every aspect of a patient's life), and drug-related morbidity and mortality cost this country almost $200 billion annually" (Giberson, Yoder, Lee, 2011, p. 8). It suggests that recognizing expanded roles of pharmacists increases the potential for patients to benefit from improved access to quality primary care services. Pharmacists can "perform patient assessment (subjective and objective data including physical assessment); have prescriptive authority (initiate, adjust, or discontinue treatment) to manage disease through medication use and deliver collaborative drug therapy or medication management; order, interpret and monitor laboratory tests; formulate clinical assessments and develop therapeutic plans; provide care coordination and other health services for wellness and prevention of disease; and develop partnerships with patients for ongoing (follow-up) care" (Giberson, Yoder, Lee, 2011, p. 8). Empirical evidence supports these claims. A recent systematic review suggests that integrating pharmacists has positive effects on direct patient care such as improving outcomes, increasing access to care, shifting time for physicians to focus on more critically ill patients, improving patient and provider satisfaction, assuring patient safety and enhancing cost-effectiveness (Chisholm-Burns, Kim, Spivey, 2010). The report concludes that "[p] harmacists' formal education appropriately prepares them to successfully perform clinical services related to the prevention and control of disease through medications. Pharmacists are also well-positioned (through accessibility, expertise and experience) to play a much larger primary care role in the U.S. healthcare system to meet these demands and improve healthcare delivery (and the health) of the nation" (Giberson, Yoder, Lee, 2011, p. 12).

"Grand-Aides" are a new type of healthcare providers that operate under the direct supervision of nurses, and "who are trained and equipped to conduct telephone consultations or make primary care home visits to patients who might otherwise be seen in emergency departments and clinics" (Garson, Green, Rodriguez, Beech, Nye, 2012, p. 1016). The term was coined in recent years when Arthur Garson Jr. created the "grandparent corps" in response to the idea that grandparents have been doing simple primary care for centuries. Later, the term was expanded to include local community members, not just grandparents, "who are wise and nurturing, have cared for others, and generate respect and trust in patients" (Garson, Green, Rodriguez, Beech, Nye, 2012, p. 1016). Recent pilot tests of the use of grand-aides in Texas and Virginia estimated that they averted 64% of drop-in visit clinics and 74% of emergency room visits. Significant cost-savings were also apparent as the cost of an encounter with a grand-aide was $16.88 compared to $200 for a clinic visit, and $175 for an emergency room visit (Garson, Green, Rodriguez, Beech, Nye, 2012). However, given the recency of this concept, more evidence is needed regarding the effectiveness of these providers in delivering high quality primary care services. Similarly, so-called "primary care technicians," based on the model of emergency medical services, can "dramatically expand the impact and reach of patient-centered medical homes by providing basic preventive, minor illness, and stable chronic disease care in rural and resource-deprived communities" (Kellerman, Saultz, Mehrotra, et al., 2013).

3. CONCLUSION

Non-physician providers, especially NPs, have overcome many challenges to play an increasingly important role in primary care. While there is strong evidence that care provided by NPs (and other providers) is of high quality and leads to patient satisfaction, questions remain about potential cost savings. Despite a boom in the numbers of providers, their supply will likely be insufficient to meet the healthcare demands. Barriers such as restrictive scope of practice and unjust payment policies have stifled progress, and physician opposition is still a major factor in some states. Opportunities exist in some state and federal legislation to expand the scope of practice and revamp payment policies, while the recently enacted PPACA can provide some relief towards improving the pipeline of some non-physician providers. Figure 1 summarizes the strengths, weaknesses, opportunities and threats that face the NP profession.

Figure 1. Nurse practitioner profession: Strengths, weaknesses, opportunities, and threats

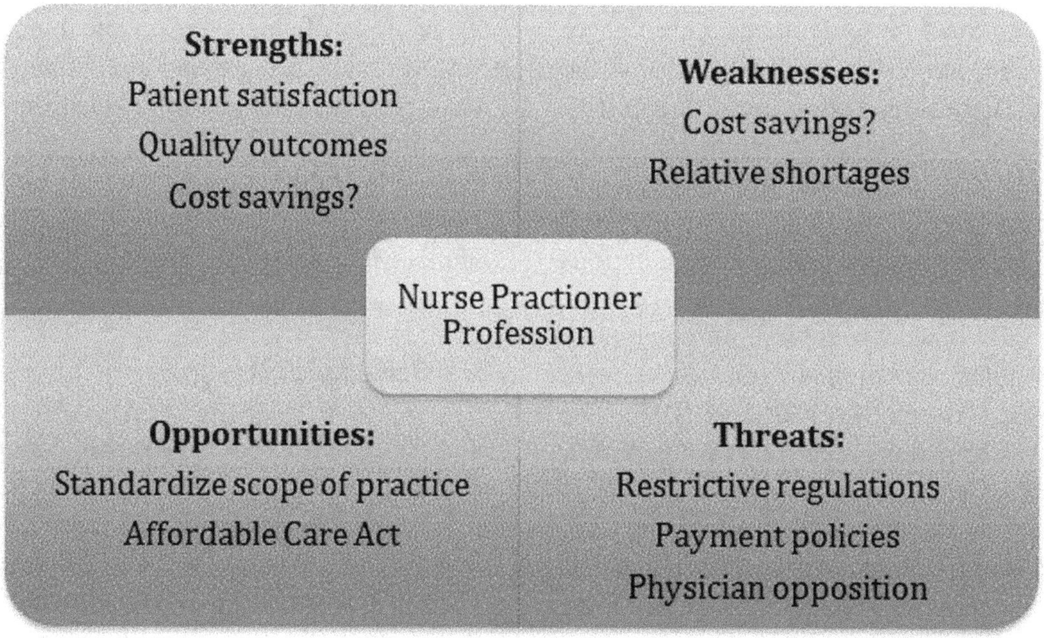

REFERENCES

Agency for Healthcare Research and Quality. (2011). *The Number of Practicing Primary Care Physicians in the United States*. Retrieved on May 6 2013 from http://www.ahrq.gov/research/findings/factsheets/primary/pcwork1/index.html

American Academy of Family Physicians. (2012). *Primary care for the 21st century: Ensuring a quality physician-led team for every patient*. Leawood, KS: Author.

American Academy of Nurse Practitioners. (2011). *Nurse Practitioner Facts*. Retrieved on May 6 2013 from http://www.aanp.org/images/documents/research/2010-2011np%20facts2012.pdf

American Academy of Physician Assistants. (2013). Retrieved on May 6, 2013 from http://www.aapa.org/the_pa_profession/history.aspx

American Medical Association. (2009). *Scope of practice data series: Nurse practitioners*. Chicago: AMA.

Baker, S. E. (1992). The nurse practitioner in malpractice actions: Standards of care and theory of liability. *Health Matrix*, *2*, 325–355. PMID:10124882

Bennett, K. L., & Phillips, J. P. (2010). Finding, recruiting, and sustaining the future primary care physician workforce: A new theoretical model of specialty choice process. *Academic Medicine*, *85*(10), S81–S88. doi:10.1097/ACM.0b013e3181ed4bae PMID:20881711

Bodenheimer, T., & Pham, H. H. (2010). Primary care: Current problems and proposed solutions. *Health Affairs (Project Hope)*, *29*(5), 799–805. doi:10.1377/hlthaff.2010.0026 PMID:20439864

Brassard, A., & Smolenski, M. (2011). Removing barriers to advanced practice registered nurse care: Hospital privileges. *AARP Public Policy Institute Insight on the Issues*, *55*, 1–12.

Buerhaus, P. I., Auerbach, D. I., & Staiger, D. O. (2009). The recent surge in nurse employment: Causes and implications. *Health Affairs*, *28*(4), w657–w668. doi:10.1377/hlthaff.28.4.w657 PMID:19525286

Chisholm-Burns, M. A., Kim Lee, J., Spivey, C. A., Slack, M., Herrier, R. N., & Hall-Lipsy, E. et al. (2010). US pharmacists' effect as team members on patient care: Systematic review and meta-analyses. *Medical Care*, *48*(10), 923–933. doi:10.1097/MLR.0b013e3181e57962 PMID:20720510

Craven, G., & Ober, S. (2009). Massachusetts nurse practitioners step up as one solution to the primary care access problem. A political success story. *Policy, Politics & Nursing Practice*, *10*(2), 94–100. doi:10.1177/1527154409344627 PMID:19783534

Dierick-van Daele, A. T., Metsemakers, J. F., Derckx, E. W., Spreeuwenberg, C., & Vrijhoef, H. J. (2009). Nurse practitioners substituting for general practitioners: Randomized controlled trial. *Journal of Advanced Nursing*, *65*(2), 391–401. doi:10.1111/j.1365-2648.2008.04888.x PMID:19191937

Eibner, C. E., Hussey, P. S., Ridgeley, M. S., & McGlynn, E. A. (2009). *Controlling healthcare spending in Massachusetts, an analysis of options*. Rand Health.

Garson, A. Jr, Green, D. M., Rodriguez, L., Beech, R., & Nye, C. (2012). A new corps of trained grand-aides has the potential to increase the reach of primary care workforce and save money. *Health Affairs*, *31*(5), 1016–1021. doi:10.1377/hlthaff.2011.0859 PMID:22566441

Giberson, S., Yoder, S., & Lee, M. P. (2011). *Improving patient and health system outcomes through advanced pharmacy practice. A Report to the U.S. Surgeon General.Office of the Chief Pharmacist*. Public Health Service.

Goolsby, M. J. (2011). 2009-2010 AANP national nurse practitioner sample survey: An overview. *Journal of the American Academy of Nurse Practitioners*, *23*(5), 266–268. doi:10.1111/j.1745-7599.2011.00611.x PMID:21518075

Green, L. V., Savin, S., & Lu, Y. (2013). Primary care physician shortages could be eliminated through the use of teams, nonphysicians and electronic communication. *Health Affairs*, *32*(1), 11–19. doi:10.1377/hlthaff.2012.1086 PMID:23297266

Hansen-Turton, T., Ritter, A., Begun, H., Berkowitz, S. L., Rothman, N., & Valdez, B. (2006). Insurers' contracting policies on nurse practitioners are primary care providers: The current landscape and what needs to change. *Policy, Politics & Nursing Practice*, *7*(3), 216–226. doi:10.1177/1527154406294339 PMID:17071708

Hansen-Turton, T., Ritter, A., & Torgan, R. (2008). Insurers' contracting policies on nurse practitioners are primary care providers: Two year later. *Policy, Politics & Nursing Practice*, *9*(4), 241–248. doi:10.1177/1527154408319450 PMID:18562764

Hansen-Turton, T., Ware, J., & McClellan, F. (2010). Nurse practitioners in primary care. *Temple Law Review*, *82*, 1235–1263.

Hooker, R. S., Cawley, J. F., & Leinweber, W. (2010). Career flexibility of physician assistants and the potential for more primary care. *Health Affairs*, *29*(5), 880–886. doi:10.1377/hlthaff.2009.0884 PMID:20439875

Hopkins, S. C., Lenz, E. R., Pontes, N. M., Lin, S. X., & Mundinger, M. O. (2005). Context of care or provider training: The impact on preventive screening practices. *Preventive Medicine*, *40*(6), 718–724. doi:10.1016/j.ypmed.2004.09.013 PMID:15850870

Horrocks, S., Anderson, E., & Salisbury, C. (2002). Systematic review of whether nurse practitioners working in primary care can provide equivalent care to doctors. *BMJ (Clinical Research Ed.)*, *324*(7341), 819–823. doi:10.1136/bmj.324.7341.819 PMID:11934775

Kellermann, A. L., Saultz, J., Mehrotra, A., Jones, S. S., & Dalal, S. (2013). Primary care technicians: A solution to the primary care workforce gap. *Health Affairs (Project Hope)*, *32*(11), 1893–1898. doi:10.1377/hlthaff.2013.0481 PMID:24191077

Laurant, M., Reeves, D., Hermens, R., Braspenning, J., Grol, R., & Sibbald, B. (2005). Substitution of doctors by nurses in primary care. *Cochrane Database of Systematic Reviews*, (2): CD001271. PMID:15846614

Leese, B., Allgar, V., Heywood, P., Walker, R., Darr, A., Din, I., & West, R. O. B. E. R. T. M. (2006). A new role for nurses as primary care cancer lead clinicians in Primary Care Trusts in England. *Journal of Nursing Management*, *14*(6), 462–471. doi:10.1111/j.1365-2934.2006.00644.x PMID:16919124

Lenz, E. R., Mundinger, M., Kane, R., Hopkins, S., & Lin, S. (2004). Primary care outcomes in patients treated by nurse practitioners or physicians: Two-year follow-up. *Medical Care Research and Review, 61*(3), 332–351. doi:10.1177/1077558704266821 PMID:15358970

Lenz, E. R., Mundinger, M. O., Hopkins, S. C., Lin, S. X., & Smolowitz, J. L. (2002). Diabetes care processes and outcomes in patients treated by nurse practitioners or physicians. *The Diabetes Educator, 28*(4), 590–598. doi:10.1177/014572170202800413 PMID:12224199

LeRoy, L., & Solkowitz, S. (1980). The costs and effectiveness of nurse practitioners, prepared for the Office of Technology Assessment, U.S. Congress. Washington, DC: U.S. Government Printing Office. Health Technology Case Study no. 16, Pub. no. OTA-HCS-16.

Margolius, D., & Bodenheimer, T. (2010). Transforming primary care: From past practice to the practice of the future. *Health Affairs, 29*(5), 779–784. doi:10.1377/hlthaff.2010.0045 PMID:20439861

Mundinger, M. O., Kane, R. L., Lenz, E. R., Totten, A. M., Tsai, W. Y., & Cleary, P. D. et al. (2000). Primary care outcomes in patients treated by nurse practitioners or physicians: A randomized trial. *Journal of the American Medical Association, 283*(1), 59–68. doi:10.1001/jama.283.1.59 PMID:10632281

Naylor, M. D., & Kurtzman, E. T. (2010). The role of nurse practitioners in reinventing primary care. *Health Affairs, 29*(5), 893–899. doi:10.1377/hlthaff.2010.0440 PMID:20439877

O'Brien, J. L., Martin, D. R., Heyworth, J. A., & Meyer, N. A. (2009). A phenomenological perspective on advanced practice nurse-physician collaboration within an interdisciplinary healthcare team. *Journal of the American Academy of Nurse Practitioners, 21*(8), 444–453. doi:10.1111/j.1745-7599.2009.00428.x PMID:19689441

Ohman-Strickland, P. A., Orzano, A. J., Hudson, S. V., Solberg, L. I., DiCiccio-Bloom, B., & O'Malley, D. et al. (2008). Quality of diabetes care in family medicine practices: Influence of nurse-practitioners and physician's assistants. *Annals of Family Medicine, 6*(1), 14–22. doi:10.1370/afm.758 PMID:18195310

Park, M., Cherry, D., & Decker, S. L. (2011). Nurse practitioners, certified nurse midwives, and physician assistants in physician offices. *NCHS Data Brief, 69*, 1–8. PMID:22142469

Pearson, L. J. The Pearson Report 2011. Retrieved on May 9 2012 from http://www.pearsonreport.com/

Pearson, L. J. (2012). *The 2012 Pearson Report: A nation overview of nurse practitioner legislation and healthcare issues*. Monroe Township, N.J.: NP Communication, LLC.

Physician Assistant History Society. (2013). Retrieved on May 6, 2013 from http://www.pahx.org/period02.html

Roblin, D. W., Howard, D. H., Becker, E. R., Kathleen Adams, E., & Roberts, M. H. (2004, June). (22004). Use of midlevel practitioners to achieve labor cost savings in the primary care practice of an MCO. *Health Services Research, 39*(3), 607–626. doi:10.1111/j.1475-6773.2004.00247.x PMID:15149481

Running, A., Kipp, C., & Mercer, V. (2006). Prescriptive patterns of nurse practitioners and physicians. *Journal of the American Academy of Nurse Practitioners, 18*(5), 228–233. doi:10.1111/j.1745-7599.2006.00120.x PMID:16681710

Sackett, D. L. (2009). A landmark randomized healthcare trial: The Burlington trial of the nurse practitioner. *Journal of Clinical Epidemiology, 62*(6), 567–570. doi:10.1016/j.jclinepi.2009.01.001 PMID:19356898

Seale, C., Anderson, E., & Kinnersley, P. (2006). Treatment advice in primary care: A comparative study of nurse practitioners and general practitioners. *Journal of Advanced Nursing, 54*(5), 534–541. doi:10.1111/j.1365-2648.2006.03865.x PMID:16722950

Spitzer, W. O., Sackett, D. L., Sibley, J. C., Roberts, R. S., Gent, M., & Kergin, D. J. et al. (1974). The Burlington randomized trial of the nurse practitioner. *The New England Journal of Medicine, 290*(5), 251–256. doi:10.1056/NEJM197401312900506 PMID:4808929

ter Bogt, N. C., Bemelmans, W. J., Beltman, F. W., Broer, J., Smit, A. J., & van der Meer, K. (2009). Preventing weight gain: One-year results of a randomized lifestyle intervention. *American Journal of Preventive Medicine, 37*(4), 270–277. doi:10.1016/j.amepre.2009.06.011 PMID:19765497

United States Government Accountability Office. (2008). Primary care professionals: Recent supply trends, projections, and valuation of services. Washington, DC: Author.

U.S. Congress, Office of Technology Assessment. (1986). Nurse practitioners, physician assistants, and certified nurse-midwives: a policy analysis. Washington, DC: U.S. Government Printing Office. Health Technology Case Study no. 37, Pub. no. OTA-HCS-37.

Wilson, I. B., Landon, B. E., Hirschhorn, L. R., McInnes, K., Ding, L., & Marsden, P. V. et al. (2005). Quality of HIV care provided by nurse practitioners, physician assistants, and physicians. *Annals of Internal Medicine, 143*(10), 729–736. doi:10.7326/0003-4819-143-10-200511150-00010 PMID:16287794

Yee, T., Boukus, E., Cross, D., & Samuel, D. (2013). Primary care workforce shortages: Nurse practitioner scope-of-practice-laws and payment policies. *National Institute for Healthcare Reform Research Brief, 13*, 1–7.

KEY TERMS AND DEFINITIONS

Nurse Practitioner: A nurse who is qualified to treat certain medical conditions without the direct supervision of a doctor.

Physician Assistant: Healthcare professional licensed to practice medicine with supervision by a licensed physician.

Scope of Practice: A terminology used by national and state/provincial licensing boards for various professions that define the procedures, actions, and processes that are permitted for the licensed individual.

Section 2

New Trends in Healthcare Delivery

Chapter 4
Convenient Care Trends

ABSTRACT

In this chapter, the author introduces several alternatives to traditional care provided in the physician office during regular business hours. While the settings where the care is delivered are different, the common characteristics among these alternatives are to have non-physician providers deliver care that is more convenient and less costly than that delivered in regular physician offices. Convenient care alternatives such as urgent care centers, retail clinics, worksite clinics, house call services, and virtual/online services are highlighted. These services are described as "disruptive innovations," or powerful changes in which a larger population of less-skilled providers can provide care in more convenient, less expensive settings that historically was only provided by expensive specialists in centralized, inconvenient locations. Given the myriad of problems faced by the American healthcare systems, the authors argue that these innovations are well positioned to change the way healthcare is delivered for generations to come.

We can't look at health in isolation. It's not just in the doctor's office. It's got to be where we live, we work, we play, we pray— Dr. Regina Benjamin, U.S. Surgeon General, 2011

INTRODUCTION

As discussed in the first section of this book, primary care in the United States is in a deepening crisis as physician shortages and reduced patient access loom. The Patient Protection and Affordable Care Act (PPACA) will improve the coverage for uninsured and underinsured people, but will not solve the primary care access conundrum, especially with 32 million people expected to be added to the realm of the insured by the year 2019. As healthcare costs continue to rise, patients continue to deal with an inconvenient system where access to after-hours care is very limited. With the availability of non-physician providers to treat limited-scope conditions, several alternatives to traditional care provided in the physician office during regular business hours have started to surface in the

DOI: 10.4018/978-1-4666-6355-8.ch004

last decade. While the settings where the care is delivered are different, the common characteristics among these alternatives are to have non-physician providers deliver care that is more convenient and less costly than that delivered in regular physician offices. These alternatives include urgent care centers, retail clinics, worksite clinics, house call services and online services, among others. We group these types of services under the label "convenient care." In this chapter, we describe the factors that have contributed to the proliferation of these new models, and discuss an overall framework that can help better understand them. In chapters 5-8, we cover each one of them separately.

1. CONVENIENCE

Since its inception, the American healthcare delivery system has been designed according to the preferences of the providers, not the consumers/patients. Consumers and patients face a myriad of hassles as they attempt to access healthcare services for themselves and their families (Fottler & Malvey, 2010). First, there are problems in getting appointments. In addition to provider shortages, some providers do not accept the patient's specific insurance plan or may be considered out of his/her network. Some providers overbook their schedules to minimize the impact of patients who don't show up. As a result, many patients can't see a provider when they need it. Second, there are long waits for services. Patients who manage to get an appointment find that they must spend a considerable amount in waiting areas to see a physician, to get a diagnostic procedure performed or to pick up a prescription. Third, many providers spend little time with patients. Pressures on providers' time have increased as reimbursement rates have continuously decreased while documentation requirements and paperwork have heightened. Fourth, administrative paperwork has also affected patients as the number of forms to be filled constantly increase due to requirements by insurance companies, government agencies, accrediting bodies and risk managers. Patients are often confused about what information to include, and many fill up the same forms when seeing multiple providers in different settings. Fifth, many physician offices and hospitals are located in overcrowded medical centers where parking is unavailable, inaccessible and expensive. Sixth, for many patients, providers are located far from their home or their work, and physician offices are not in proximity to diagnostic or laboratory services which forces patients to travel long distances to receive different services. Seventh, and as discussed in Chapter 1, many physician offices are open only during normal business hours. As a result, some patients requiring medical care and on weeknights and weekends may decide to go the hospital emergency room, self-diagnose, or delay/forego necessary care. Eighth, out-of-pockets costs (such as co-payments) keep increasing, and high-deductible plan make patients more sensitive to price of medical services. Schleiter (2010) described an important aspect of this trend: "Consumers are paying more of their own healthcare costs in the form of higher premiums and deductibles, and are increasingly making decisions about how, when and where they receive medical services. Copayments are expected to rise for all insurance plans. The purchase of health insurance that requires subscribers to pay for much or most out-of-pocket medical costs has been prompted by a new tax shelter for Health Savings Accounts (HSA). These HSAs are designed to induce patients to shop like consumers for quality medical care at a low cost. As a result, patients, rather than physicians, insurers or the government, are often in the driver's seat for medical spending decisions" (p. 540). Ninth, most medical facilities, especially physician offices, do not have electronic medical records, which causes breakdowns in communication between provider-patient and provider-provider. Patients requiring care from multiple providers, find themselves giving redundant information or undergoing duplicate tests. Tenth, care is not coordinated among various providers. There are few facilities that provide a one-stop shop where the patient can be diagnosed and treated, undergo a laboratory tests or a diagnostic procedure, and obtain his/her prescription medication in the same location. In the backdrop of such hassles in traditional care settings, disruptive innovations started appearing on the healthcare scene.

2. DISRUPTIVE INNOVATIONS

To better understand the factors that led to the emergence of convenient care, the theory of disruptive innovations provides insight and examples from inside and outside the healthcare industry. In the "Innovator's Dilemma" and the "Innovator's Solution," Clayton Christensen, a Harvard Business School professor and influential business thinker, described the concept of disruptive innovations. These are powerful changes in which a larger population of less-skilled providers can provide care in more convenient, less expensive settings that historically was only provided by expensive specialists in centralized, inconvenient locations (Christensen, 1997).

When introduced to a market, the performance of a product or service gradually improves over time. But there are two types of trajectories of performance improvement: sustaining innovations and disruptive innovations. Companies typically introduce innovations through small and incremental or dramatic breakthroughs. Sustaining innovations, as the label suggests, sustain the existing trajectory of performance improvement. These are products and services of the highest quality that are sold to the best and most sophisticated customers at higher profits. However, sustaining innovations not only meet the demands of these customers, but almost always overshoot their needs and their ability to absorb it. This happens when companies upgrade their products with features much more quickly than customers can utilize them.

When sustaining innovations overshoot customer needs by packing in more functionality than they deem essential or desirable, the potential for disruptive innovations emerges. Initially, disruptive innovation products and services do not appeal to many customers, because they are considered inferior to what customers are used to. However, since the new product or service is typically cheaper, simpler and more convenient, it attracts a new type of customers who were previously unable to participate due to price and convenience barriers. Typically, these customers are least demanding, and are least attractive to market leaders offering expensive and sophisticated sustaining innovations. While these companies continue to focus on "higher-paying, performance-hungry" customers (Huang & Christensen, 2008, p. 1330), disruptive innovation companies attract low demand-customers and convert non-customers. These companies tend to be new entrants to the market rather than dominant incumbents, and are therefore not initially perceived as serious threats. However, as they start to establish their products and services, their performance improves, and begins to meet the needs of more and more customers, including those of the sustaining innovations. Before long, the majority of the market will prefer the disruptive innovation, and the sustaining one will fail or cease to exist. As Christensen, Bohmer, and Kennagy (2000) explain: "Disruptive technologies have caused many of history's best companies to plunge into crisis and ultimately fail" (p. 2).

In summary, disruptive innovations in any industry tend to sneak in from below. The major dominant companies continue to improve and force products and services that average consumers don't even need, and while doing that miss the opportunity to provide simpler, more convenient and less expensive innovations. These are typically introduced by newer and smaller companies that gradually improve their products and services until they finally meet the demands of the vast majority of users and drive the dominant companies out. Numerous examples illustrate this phenomenon. In the 1960's, people who needed help computing took their punched cards to the corporate mainframe computer center and waited in line for data-processing specialists to perform the job for them. These large and outrageously expensive computers represented the sustained innovations that were so sophisticated that they could only be operated by highly-skilled specialists in inconvenient centralized locations. However, these products overshot the needs of the majority of less-skilled people who needed to perform simple computing tasks. Minicomputers and personal computers represented the disruptive innovation: they were first introduced by smaller companies, and because of their lack of sophistication, were originally dismissed by the dominant companies producing the mainframe computers. However, as more and more people started buying mini and personal computers at low prices to use in the convenience of their homes and offices, the market began to shift towards the disruptive innovation (Christensen, 1997).

Other examples of disruptive innovations include small photocopy machines replacing professional printers, portable transistor radios replacing analog big furniture radios, pocket calculators replacing desktop calculators, and mini-mills replacing integrated steel mills, etc. (Sandstrom, 2010). In the last ten or fifteen years, cases of disruptive innovations started emerging in some pockets within the healthcare industry. For example, patients with diabetes need to monitor and control their blood glucose levels on a continuous and periodic basis. The sustained innovation was urine tests or blood tests that could only be conducted in physician offices using expensive laboratory equipment. A disruptive technology appeared in the 1980's in the shape of miniature blood glucose meters that allowed patients to manage their blood glucose levels anywhere they were. This resulted in a cheaper, more convenient, and high quality product that eventually drove large laboratory blood-glucose testers out of the market (Christensen et al., 2000).

The case of patients with coronary artery disease provides another example. For this condition, the sustained innovation for treatment was bypass surgery: a complex, technologically sophisticated procedure that was performed by multiple expensive specialists using advanced equipment. The surgery could only be performed in hospital operating rooms, was very costly, and resulted in a long recovery period for the patient. Angioplasty emerged in the early 1980's as the much simpler disruptive innovation in which a balloon is used to dilate narrowed arteries. The procedure was less expensive, could be performed by less specialized healthcare professionals in stand-alone cardiac centers, resulted in lower costs and less pain and disability. While initially used only in the easiest cases and deemed as ineffective by bypass surgeons, the innovation's performance continued to improve with increased skills and experience and technological advances such as stents, thus overtaking surgery as the treatment of choice for many patients (Christensen et al., 2000). A more recent example is represented by the advances in technology in LASIK (laser-assisted in situ keratomileusis) surgery, in which a previously complex and expensive surgery is now performed at a lower cost using automated and standardized procedures (Smith, 2007).

Applying the concept of disruptive innovations to healthcare, Christensen observes that there are three classes of medical problems. The first class relates to acute conditions that are amenable to precise diagnosis and rules-based therapy, such as simple infectious diseases. The second class relates to chronic diseases such as cancer and heart disease, while the third class relates to nonstandard complex cases such as multiple comorbidities. He believes that the first class and to a lesser extent the second class are amenable to disruptive innovations, whereas the third class is not (Smith, 2007). He notes that the major healthcare institutions such as hospitals, medical schools, specialist physicians and research organizations have historically overshot the level of care needed by most patients in the system. While the majority of patients need primary care for simple conditions, "medical schools and residency programs have churned out specialists and subspecialists with extraordinary capabilities" (Christensen et al., 2000, p. 2). Similarly, research organizations have focused on curing very complex diseases, while general hospitals have focused on a very small population of very sick patients (Christensen et al., 2000). Under these circumstances, the situation seemed ripe for new disruptive innovations to emerge and displace these sustained innovations. However, other than the examples mentioned above, these disruptive innovations were slow to come in healthcare, especially before the year 2000. The main reason is the strong resistance that has come mainly from hospitals and physician associations that see the alternatives as a threat to their livelihood. Christensen and his colleagues describe this situation by stating that "enabling less expensive people to do things that were previously unimaginable has been one of the fundamental engines of economic progress- and the established healthcare institutions have fought that engine tooth and nail" (Christensen et al., 2000, p. 6).

The case of nurse practitioners and physician assistants, discussed in depth in Chapter 3, is very telling. Advances in diagnostic and therapeutic technologies have enabled these non-physician providers nowadays to reliably diagnose and treat simple conditions and disorders that previously required the skills of a physician. However, many states consistently passed regulations limiting the scope of practice of nurse practitioners. Christensen et al. comment on the situation: "The flawed rationale behind such policies is that because nurse practitioners are not as highly trained as physicians, they are not capable of providing care of comparable quality. This is the same logic that minicomputer makers used to discredit the personal computer. When a physician diagnoses a simple infectious disease, the patient uses only that fraction of the physician's training that relates to simple infectious diseases. Studies have shown that nurse practitioners with comparable training in simple infectious diseases can provide care of comparable quality in that tier of the market-even though they lack training in more complex disorders. Some nearsighted advocates of patients' rights assert that nurse practitioners might not have the judgment to recognize when a disorder is beyond their expertise. But family practice doctors recognize when they can treat a disorder and when it merits referral to a specialist. Surely nurse practitioners, working at even simpler tiers of the market, can be equipped to do the same thing. The real reason for blocking such disruption, we suspect, is the predictable desire of physicians to preserve their traditional market hegemony. Instead of working to enable the natural upmarket migration that is an intrinsic part of economic progress, today's managed care organizations, insurers, and regulators have done just the opposite. They have forced highly trained physicians down-market to diagnose ear infections and bronchitis and have prevented nurse practitioners from doing things that technology enables them to do perfectly well. The result of this policy is perverse. To maintain their incomes, primary care physicians are forced to churn patients at an alarming rate-frequently spending only a few minutes with each patient. That reduces the quality and convenience of care"(Christensen et al., 2000, p. 6).

In addition to resistance from powerful institutions resulting in regulatory barriers, other obstacles have limited disruptive innovations in healthcare in the past. One of these is the argument that these innovations could possibly lead to fragmentation of care. Coordination of care is a crucial aspect of high-quality, cost-effective care, and any innovation channeling patients out of traditional care settings might disrupt that. Moreover, the healthcare industry lacks a retail market in which consumers have proper incentives to shop for products and services that best meet their needs (Huang & Christensen, 2008). True shopping behavior does not exist in healthcare, mainly due to relative lack of information on the patient's side, and the absence of financial incentives to choose cheaper alternatives for insured patients.

Several solutions were proposed in 2000 by Christensen and his colleagues to overcome these barriers and to allow disruptive innovations to flourish in healthcare. First, they suggested that a system where clinician's skill level is matched to the difficulty of the medical problem should be created and embraced (Christensen et al., 2000). The simplest tiers of medical problems (e.g. infectious diseases) where diagnosis is rule-based and where accurate data can lead to a certain diagnosis should be left to nurse practitioners and physician assistants. Physicians should instead focus on more serious problems (e.g. diabetes) where diagnosis occurs through pattern recognition, or on the most complex problems (e.g. multiple chronic conditions) where diagnosis and treatment requires the collective experience of a team of clinicians and that involve several rounds of testing and experimentation.

Second, they argued that the healthcare industry should spend more money on technologies that simplify complex problems, instead of spending more on high-end, complex technologies. The focus in healthcare investments has been on sustaining technologies that enable the most skilled providers to solve previously unresolved problems. However, Christensen et al. (2000) argue that these are not the technologies that will transform healthcare. Rather, it is technologies that allow simplification so that less skilled and less expensive professionals can provide care in more convenient settings that will allow that transformation to take place.

Third, they reasoned that new organizations should be created to do the disrupting. Traditional institutions such as hospitals and physician groups are not the answer, because rather than creating transformations, they have consistently tried to tighten controls on existing business model (Christensen et al., 2000). For example, hospitals have engaged in mergers, facility closing, worker lay-offs, buying group formation, and consultant hiring, while continuing to function in a fundamentally unchanged way. Christensen et al. (2000) posit that "if history is any guide, the healthcare system can be transformed only by creating new institutions that can capably deliver the vast majority of such care, rather than attempting a tortuous transformation of existing institutions that were designed for other purposes "(p. 8). Lastly, the healthcare industry should overcome the inertia of existing regulations that affect the scope of practice of non-physician providers. Regulators should detach themselves from the powerful lobbies of hospitals and physicians and enable disruptive innovations to emerge (Christensen et al., 2000).

Since the year 2000, but especially in the last few years, several disruptive innovations have surfaced in the healthcare industry. These innovations appear to have taken valuable lessons from the solutions discussed above. New types of organizations, such as urgent care centers, retail clinics, worksite clinics, online health services and house call services have appeared outside of traditional hospitals and physician clinics. In these organizations, non-serious medical problems are treated by less skilled providers such as physician assistants and nurse practitioners. New health information technologies have enabled clinical decision-making, standardized pathways to manage common problems, and ready storage and retrieval of health data, to provide care in decentralized and more convenient settings (Mulcahy et al., 2012).

3. CONVENIENT CARE MODELS

Urgent Care Centers first appeared in the United States in the early 1980's. Despite original optimism that this was a significant "innovative alternative method" that will likely replace emergency rooms (Goldsmith, 1980), the initial growth was followed by a decline that was mainly due to hospital systems acquiring urgent care centers and then closing them because of their inability to market them and operate them profitably (Weinick & Bentacourt, 2007). That was followed by another wave of growth in the mid 1990's that has continued till today. There are currently around 9,899 urgent care centers operating in the United States (Son, 2013). Urgent care is healthcare provided on a walk-in, no-appointment basis for acute illnesses or injuries that are not life-threatening (Urgent Care Association of America, 2011). Most urgent care centers provide primary care services, occupational medicine, routine immunizations and school physicals, and some of them provide lab tests, X-rays, fracture and laceration care, and intravenous fluids. They are typically open for extended hours including nights and weekends and can be owned by physicians, groups of physicians, hospitals and corporations. The centers are staffed with physicians, with approximately half also employing non-physician providers such as physician assistants and nurse practitioners (Urgent Care Association of America, 2011).

The first retail clinic in the United States appeared at a Target store in Minneapolis in 2000. By the beginning of 2006, there were only 63 clinics open (Deloitte Center for Health Solutions, 2008). The main growth occurred during the three-year period of 2006, 2007 and 2008 when about 1,000 new clinics opened nationwide. However, the following two years (2009 and 2010) witnessed a slow-down and even stagnation as the number of clinics opening barely surpassed the number of clinics closing (Kaissi & Charland, 2013). The main reasons for that slow-down can be attributed to the economic recession. Starting in 2011, with economic recovery on the horizon, another wave of growth started with a net increase of 125 clinics. The current number of clinics is at 1,623 (Merchant Medicine, 2014). Retail clinics are walk-in clinics located in grocery stores, drugstores and general merchandise retailers. In the United States, these clinics have surfaced in popular stores that are visited by customers several times per week, such as Wal-Mart, Target, CVS, Walgreens, etc. They offer a limited scope of diagnostic and treatment services for common medical conditions, as well as preventative and wellness services (Fottler & Malvey, 2010). Studies show that 90% of retail clinic visits are for simple conditions and services such as upper respiratory infections, urinary tract infections, sinusitis, bronchitis, pharyngitis, otitis media, otitis externa, conjunctivitis, immunizations, screening laboratory tests/ blood pressure checks (Mehrotra, Wang, Lave, Adams, & McGlynn, 2008). Care is delivered by a non-physician provider such as a nurse practitioner or physician assistant, and many clinics have up-front menu-style pricing, a feature that is unparalleled in the American healthcare system (Lin, 2008). The clinics operate on a walk-in basis with no appointments needed and very short wait times, and are open on evenings and weekends when most PCP offices are closed. They charge an average of $70 per visit and accept all types of insurance plans. It is important to note that some experts refer to retail clinics as "convenient care clinics." In fact, the professional trade association for retail clinics is called the Convenient Care Association. However, in this book, we will use the term "retail clinics" to refer to clinics located in grocery stores and pharmacy chains, and reserve the term "convenient care" organizations to refer to the overall trend of providing care outside the traditional physician office, including urgent care centers, retail clinics, and other types of services described in this chapter and discussed in detail in the next five chapters.

Worksite clinics are not a new phenomenon. Prior to the 1980s, many large employers operated onsite company clinics to treat work-related injuries. However, many of these clinics closed in the 1980s and 1990s because of the decline in heavy industry and manufacturing sectors and the reduction in workplace hazards. Recently, there has been a significant resurgence of worksite clinics. The new generation of clinics is markedly different in that their main focus is on primary care, health promotion and wellness rather than occupational injuries (Tu, Boukus, & Cohen, 2010). There are about 2,200 worksite clinics operating today. They are typically located on employers' campuses and dedicated to serving employees. The clinics serve on-campus employees (60%), employees' dependents (25%), and retirees (20%). They are staffed by a registered nurse (RN) or physician assistant (PA) that can address occupational health and safety issues, administer travel and influenza vaccinations, conduct new employee drug screenings, provide health and wellness education, and refer employees to in-network physicians. Clinics associated with larger employers employ full or part-time physicians and some operate on-site pharmacies and fitness centers (Fuld & Company, 2009).

Evidence for the first online healthcare services seem to appear in 2008, although it is hard to pinpoint an exact date or year (Hawn, 2009). In the last couple of years these services have proliferated significantly that it is almost impossible to determine the total number of organizations operating them. A variety of services are offered, with two main types: live interaction with a provider using video camera or online chatting, and "asynchronous" services where diagnosis and treatment is based on patient answers to a variety of questions on a website (Hawn, 2009; Courneya, Palattao, & Gallagher, 2013). House-call services are also a recent appearance on the healthcare scene and it is very hard to determine when the trend started and how many organizations are offering that service. The scope of service is very similar to that of retail clinics with nurse practitioners proving care for minor conditions in patients' home or work offices. Figure 1 provides a timeline for the convenient care services described in this section.

Analyzing the overall trend of convenient care services, it is obvious that these represent different stages of disruptive innovations. The sustained innovation is the care provided in traditional primary care offices. Urgent care centers appeared in the 1980s and resurfaced in the mid-1990s, whereas primary-care focused worksite clinics started growing in the mid-2000s. These organizations started taking away patients from the incumbent organizations. Retail clinics appeared in the early 2000s' and grew exponentially after 2006 by taking away patients from primary care physicians and urgent care centers. More recently, online services and house call services have started attracting patients from retail clinics and other forms of care. The growth of these different waves of disruptive innovations is illustrated in Figure 2.

Several drivers have contributed to these trends. Patients nowadays have instant care demands. While a 24-hour or 48-hour wait time before an appointment may be clinically acceptable, many patients expect quicker access. Low overhead costs allow many new models to provide care that is cheaper than that provided in traditional settings, and insurance companies are attracted by the potential to save money. The availability of published

Figure 1. Timeline of convenient care services

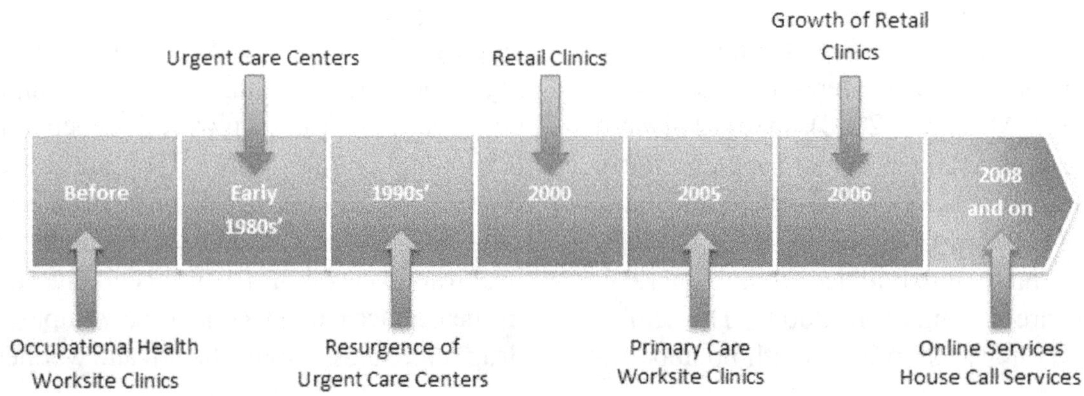

Figure 2. Convenient care services as disruptive innovations

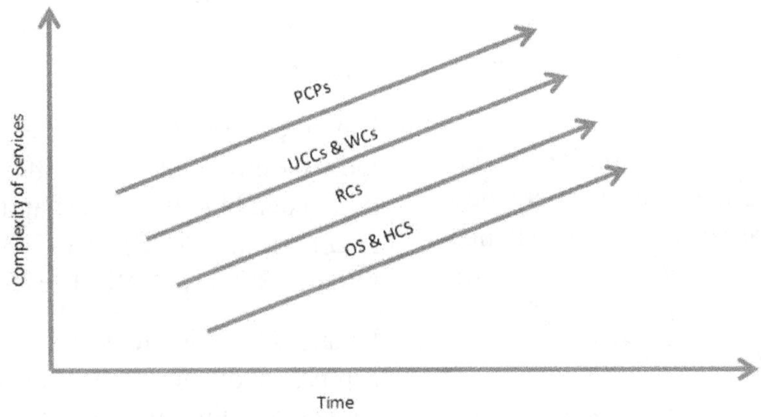

PCP: Primary Care Physicians
WCs: Worksite Clinics
UCCs: Urgent Care Centers
RCs: Retail Clinics
OS: Online services
HCS: House-call Services

guidelines and electronic medical records allow new models to provide consistent and standardized high quality that reduces the need for interaction with a physician. Mehrotra describes: "With automation and interoperable medical records, a patient may identify with a certain convenient care brand, rather than a specific physician. Just as a person who visits a Starbucks in Seattle or Boston expects similar-if not identical lattes, a patient can visit a TakeCare Clinic in Seattle and Boston and expect similar if not identical care" (Mehrotra, 2013, p. 35). And finally, the low-acuity market is a $5 billion per year market that has been traditionally neglected by hospitals and other care providers focusing on more complicated care. As a result, the opportunity exists for entrepreneurs and venture capitalists to invest in this growing market (Mehrotra, 2013).

4. CONCLUSION

Disruptive innovations offering convenient care services in settings that are easily accessible to patients and open after-hours represent a recent revolution in healthcare. Given the myriad of problems faced by the American healthcare systems, these innovations are well positioned to change the way healthcare is delivered for generations to come. In the next four chapters, we discuss specific issues, trends, and challenges related to urgent care centers, retail clinics, worksite clinics, online services and house calls services.

REFERENCES

Brown, E. (2011, March 13). Surgeon general discusses health and community. *Los Angeles Times*.

Carret, M. L., Fassa, A. C., & Domingues, M. R. (2009). Inappropriate use of emergency services: A systematic review of prevalence and associated factors. *Cadernos de Saude Publica, 25*(1), 7–28. doi:10.1590/S0102-311X2009000100002 PMID:19180283

Christensen, C. (1997). *The innovator's dilemma: When new technologies cause great firms to fail*. Boston: Harvard Business School Press.

Christensen, C. M., Bohmer, R., & Kenagy, J. (2000). Will disruptive innovations cure healthcare? *Harvard Business Review, 78*(5), 102–112. PMID:11143147

Courneya, P. T., Palattao, K. J., & Gallagher, J. M. (2013). HealthPartners' online clinic for simple conditions delivers savings of $88 per episode and high patient approval. *Health Affairs, 32*(2), 385–392. doi:10.1377/hlthaff.2012.1157 PMID:23381532

Deloitte Center for Health Solutions. (2008). *Retail clinics: Facts, trends and implications*. Author.

Fottler, M., & Malvey, D. (2010). *The retail revolution in healthcare*. Santa Barbara, CA: Praeger.

Fuld & Company. (2009). *The growth of on-site health clinics on-site clinics are expected to serve over 10% of the under 65s by 2015*. White Paper Press.

Goldsmith, J.C. (1980, September/October). The healthcare market: Can hospitals survive? *Harvard Business Review*, 100–112. PMID:10247957

Hawn, C. (2009). Take two aspirin and tweet me in the morning: How Twitter, Facebook and other social media are reshaping healthcare? *Health Affairs, 28*(2), 361–368. doi:10.1377/hlthaff.28.2.361 PMID:19275991

Huang, J., & Christensen, C. M. (2008). Disruptive innovation in healthcare delivery: A framework for business-model innovation. *Health Affairs, 27*(5), 1329–1335. doi:10.1377/hlthaff.27.5.1329 PMID:18780919

Jerant, A., Bertakis, K. D., Fenton, J. J., & Franks, P. (2012). Extended office hours and healthcare expenditures: A national study. *Annals of Family Medicine, 10*(5), 388–395. doi:10.1370/afm.1382 PMID:22966101

Kaissi, A., & Charland, T. (2013). The evolution of retail clinics in the United States, 2006-2012. *The Health Care Manager, 32*(4), 336–342. doi:10.1097/HCM.0b013e3182a9d73f PMID:24168869

Lin, D. Q. (2008). Convenient care clinics: Opposition, opportunity, and the path to system integration. *Frontiers of Health Services Management, 24*(3), 3–11. PMID:18435355

Margolius, D., & Bodenheimer, T. (2011). Redesigning after-hours care. *Annals of Internal Medicine, 155*(2), 131–132. doi:10.7326/0003-4819-155-2-201107190-00011 PMID:21768588

Mehrotra, A. (2013). The convenience revolution for treatment of low-acuity conditions. *Journal of the American Medical Association, 310*(1), 35–36. doi:10.1001/jama.2013.6825 PMID:23821082

Mehrotra, A., Wang, M. C., Lave, J. R., Adams, J. L., & McGlynn, E. A. (2008). Retail clinics, primary care physicians, and emergency departments: A comparison of patients' visits. *Health Affairs*, *27*(5), 1272–1282. doi:10.1377/hlthaff.27.5.1272 PMID:18780911

Mehrotra, A., Wang, M. C., Lave, J. R., Adams, J. L., & McGlynn, E. A. (2008). Retail clinics, primary care physicians, and emergency departments: A comparison of patients' visits. *Health Affairs*, *27*(5), 1272–1282. doi:10.1377/hlthaff.27.5.1272 PMID:18780911

Merchant Medicine. (2014). Retrieved from http://www.merchantmedicine.com

Mulcahy, A. W., Lowsky, D., Chari, R., Hussey, P. S., Vaiana, M. E., & Kellermann, A. L. (2012). *Flattening the trajectory of health-care spending: Facilitate high-value innovation* (RB-9690/5). Santa Monica, CA: Rand Corporation. Retrieved from http://www.rand.org/pubs/research_briefs/RB9690z5

Niska, R., Bhuiya, F., & Xu, J. (2010). *National hospital ambulatory medical care survey: 2007 emergency department summary. National health statistics reports; no 26.* Hyattsville, MD: National Center for Health Statistics.

O'Malley, A. S. (2013). After-hours access to primary care practices linked with lower emergency department use and less unmet medical need. *Health Affairs*, *32*(1), 175–183. doi:10.1377/hlthaff.2012.0494 PMID:23242631

Pitts, S. R., Carrier, E. R., Rich, E. C., & Kellermann, A. L. (2010). Where Americans get acute care: Increasingly, it's not at their doctor's office. *Health Affairs*, *29*(9), 1620–1629. doi:10.1377/hlthaff.2009.1026 PMID:20820017

Rust, G., Ye, J., Baltrus, P., Daniels, E., Adesunloye, B., & Fryer, G. E. (2008). Practical barriers to timely primary care access: Impact on adult use of emergency department services. *Archives of Internal Medicine*, *168*(15), 1705–1710. doi:10.1001/archinte.168.15.1705 PMID:18695087

Sandstrom, C. (2010). *5 Examples Of Disruptive Innovation*. Retrieved from http://disruptiveinnovation.se/

Schleiter, K.E. (2010). Retail medical clinics: Increasing access to low cost medical care amongst a developing legal environment. *Annals of Health Law*, *19*(3), 527–575. PMID:21456398

Schoen, C., Osborn, R., Doty, M., Squires, D., Peugh, J., & Applebaum, S. (2007). Toward higher-performance health systems: Adults' healthcare experiences in seven countries, 2007. *Health Affairs*, *26*(6), 717–734. doi:10.1377/hlthaff.26.6.w717 PMID:17978360

Smith, D. (2007). Disruptive innovation: Can healthcare learn from other industries? A conversation with Clayton Christensen. *Health Affairs*, *26*(3), 288–295. doi:10.1377/hlthaff.26.3.w288

Son, A. (2013). *IBISWorld Industry Report OD5458*. Urgent Care Centers in the US.

Tu, H. T., Boukus, E. R., & Cohen, G. R. (2010). *Workplace clinics: A sign of growing employer interest in wellness (Research Brief 17)*. Center for Studying Health System Change.

Urgent Care Association of America. (2011). *The Case for Urgent Care*. Naperville, IL: Author.

Weinick, R., & Betancourt, R. (2007). *No appointment needed: The resurgence of urgent care*. Oakland, CA: California HealthCare Foundation.

KEY TERMS AND DEFINITIONS

Disruptive Innovations: Powerful changes in which a larger population of less-skilled providers can provide care in more convenient, less expensive settings that historically was only provided by expensive specialists in centralized, inconvenient locations.

Online Services: Healthcare services provided electronically in real time (synchronous) or through "store & forward" (asynchronous) delivery via images, video and audio.

Retail Clinics: Small clinics located in general merchandise or drug stores and offering a limited scope of diagnostic and treatment services for common medical conditions.

Urgent Care: Healthcare provided on a walk-in, no-appointment basis for acute illnesses or injuries that are not life-threatening.

Worksite Clinics: Small clinics located on employers' campuses and dedicated to serving employees by providing primary care services, health promotion and wellness as well as care for occupational injuries.

Chapter 5
Urgent Care Centers

ABSTRACT

This chapter focuses on urgent care centers as a unique innovation that has been in the making for the last 30 years. Urgent care centers provide unscheduled or walk-in care, are open for extended hours on weeknights and weekends, and provide services that go beyond what primary care physicians provide, such as occupational medicine, laboratory tests, and fracture care such as splinting and casting, with some providing intravenous fluids, routine immunizations, and primary care services. This chapter describes in-depth the history and growth, operations, and stakeholders of urgent care centers, and overviews the research that relates to quality of care, costs, and patient satisfaction in these centers. Given the expanding industry, strong growth in company numbers, greater employment opportunities, and rising per-capita usage of urgent care centers, the author argues that the urgent care industry is in the growth phase of its life cycle.

With all the changes in medicine today and the increasing move toward value, urgent care is a definite and increasingly valuable part of the answer to decreasing cost and improving quality. Although predicting the future is difficult, it looks bright for the new specialty of Urgent Care Medicine.—Sean McNealy, 2012

INTRODUCTION

Urgent care centers represent a unique innovation that has been in the making for the last thirty years. As such, they are considered more "mainstream" than other innovations studied in this book. The urgent care industry has proven to be recession-proof by evolving tremendously in the last few years, and represents a serious contender in the primary care market. In this chapter, we examine the industry's history and growth, assess its major operational challenges and opportunities, discuss its major stakeholders, evaluate its outcomes, and forecast its future outlook.

Hospital emergency room overcrowding is a well-documented predicament in the American healthcare system (as discussed in depth in Chapter 1). The total number of hospital emergency rooms has decreased in the last decade, whereas the number of patients seeking to receive emergency care continues to soar. Long wait times, patient boarding,

DOI: 10.4018/978-1-4666-6355-8.ch005

patients leaving without being seen and ambulance diversions are common occurrences in the majority of emergency rooms across the nation. Due to primary care physician shortages and lack of access for after-hours care, many patients with minor and urgent but non-emergent healthcare needs present to emergency rooms that are forced to treat them at very high costs. Urgent care centers represent a value proposition for less expensive, more convenient, and high quality care provided for serious but non-life threatening conditions. A recent letter from an emergency room nurse is a cry for help for a greater role for urgent centers in primary care: "Imagine the following scenario: It is 4 o'clock on a Monday afternoon. There are no seats; people are standing as patients line the walls in wheelchairs. A daughter is trying to get the attention of the triage nurse about why her mother has not been seen yet. The triage nurse is managing the triage of a patient and attending to a screaming woman in labor. People are complaining and comparing their wait times, ranging from 4 to 5 hours. There are no open rooms, and the number of patients waiting to be seen continues to increase. Unfortunately, this has become the typical day in the emergency department waiting room. Overcrowding is a pandemic across the United States that needs immediate intervention. As an emergency nurse, I face this crisis every day alongside my patients. I continually wonder about a solution. Increasing the number and utilization of urgent care centers will decrease overcrowding by deferring patients from the emergency department" (Borkowski, 2012, p.116).

Urgent care centers provide walk-in care during evening and weekend hours for patients who are unable to schedule a timely appointment with their primary care physician, for patients whose primary care physician office hours are limited to weekdays, and for patients who do not have a primary care physician relationship to start with. As such, they fill an important access gap in a fragmented, inconvenient and short-staffed primary care system.

Definition

Although urgent care centers have been in existence for about thirty years and have grown exponentially in numbers and utilization, there is no widely agreed-on definition. While some people refer to it as a "doc-in-a-box," the scope of service is larger than that of a primary care physician office but narrower than that of a hospital emergency room. For example, a non-physician provider delivering care in small clinic with no laboratory or radiological capabilities can be labeled as "urgent care," while a large center with multiple board-certified and ACLS-trained (Advanced Clinical Life Support) physicians, X-ray, laboratory, and emergency room equipment is also labeled as "urgent care" (Weinick & Bentacourt, 2007). In a recent paper entitled "The search for the urgent care center", Weinick and colleagues highlighted the difficulty of defining what urgent care is. They suggested that physician offices that are located in strip malls and that advertise that "walk-ins" are welcome; and physician offices that have storefront locations, accept only cash payments and perform some procedures should not be considered urgent care (Weinick, Bristol, Marder, et al., 2009). They provided the following specific criteria for inclusion as an urgent care center:

- Provide care primarily on a walk-in basis
- Have evening office hours Monday to Friday
- Are open at least one day over the weekend

- Provide suturing for minor lacerations
- Provide X-rays at the center

At the minimum, an urgent care center provides unscheduled or walk-in care, is open for extended hours on weeknights and weekends, and provides services that go beyond what primary care physicians provide, such as diagnostic testing, laceration repairs and Intravenous (IV) fluids provision. The Urgent Care Association of America (UCAOA), a professional trade organization representing urgent care centers provides the following definition: "Urgent care is defined as the delivery of ambulatory medical care outside of a hospital emergency department on a walk-in basis, without a scheduled appointment. Urgent care centers treat many conditions that can be seen in a primary care physician's office, but urgent care centers offer some services that are generally not in primary care physician's office such as X-rays and minor trauma treatment" (UCAOA, 2013). A similar definition is provided by the National Association for Ambulatory Care (NAFAC), another trade organization representing the industry: "All Urgent Care Medicine is provided in an office based practice. Urgent Care Medicine specializes in the treatment of any disease, illness, and injury, which is presented by otherwise healthy consumers. Urgent Care Medicine provides services to 85% of the population who do not suffer from a long-term chronic disease, or require the services of a hospital" (NAFAC, 2012).

1. HISTORY AND GROWTH

Urgent care centers first emerged on the healthcare scene in the late 1970s and early 1980s. At the time, the United States was witnessing a surplus of physicians, and many experts predicted that urgent care represented a lucrative entrepreneurial opportunity for physicians (Trafford, 1983). When the concept appeared, it was first referred to as a "free-standing emergency room"(which is different from the free-standing emergency rooms nowadays). There were about 50 of those facilities in 1978. A Harvard Business Review paper published in 1980 described the context in which these centers appeared, which, not surprisingly, is very similar to the healthcare environment today: "Many patients who are not acutely ill but who have no physician or other means of getting care use emergency rooms. In many under-served areas, as many as two-thirds of the visits may be non-emergency cases. Emergency rooms are the health system's current answer to the need for episodic healthcare. For reasons of both high cost and potential substitution, hospital emergency rooms are vulnerable to replacement by innovative alternative methods such as the freestanding emergency room" (Goldsmith, 1980, p. 120). The original scope of practice is comparable to the scope of modern-day urgent care centers: "They can provide most of the services of a hospital-based emergency room except for full-scale surgery that requires general anesthesia. Most of them have their own laboratory and radiology facilities, though some contract with others for these services if rapid turnaround on tests is available nearby. They bill as if the either emergency rooms (if corporately linked hospital) or doctors' offices, usually at half or of the prevailing emergency room visit charge" (p.120). Dr. Bruce Irwin, who opened his first urgent care center 30 years ago, describes the similarities between the healthcare environment then and now: "I remember a group of us got together in Chicago back in the early

1980s, there was a lot of investor interest back then just like today, and there were people who said you should open as many clinics as fast as you can… [But] this isn't about the doctor. And this isn't about urgent care medicine. It's about focusing on what patients want. It was that way 30 years ago and it is that way today. Patients want convenient access to primary care"(Merchant Medicine, 2012).

At first, urgent care centers were independent and privately-owned by physicians. One of the first clinics is documented by Goldsmith (1980): "In the Chicago area, a fresh entry into this mark is the brainchild of a former partner of Arthur Young & Company, Dr. Bruce Flashner. Its name, the Doctor's Emergency Officenter, expresses cogently its hybrid private physician/emergency room nature. It is, however, reimbursed by Blue Shield as a doctor's office […] The Officenter operates on a no-appointment basis and, six months after opening, receives an average of 50 visits a day. Dr. Flashner encountered difficulties with anxious physicians in the Arlington Heights community, where the facility is located, until it became clear that he did not intend to buy a practice through the center. Instead, its physicians return patients to their family doctors for continued care or refer them to specialists for complex conditions. In addition to a single doctor per shift, the center has two paraprofessionals who are trained handle billing, laboratory and radiology work, and other matters" (p.120).

As the centers became popular, hospitals and their emergency rooms saw them as a competitive threat. Predictably, they wanted a share of the market, and many hospital systems opened their own centers or acquired existing ones. For example, "In Phoenix, the Samaritan Health Service, one the nation's most successful voluntary multihospital systems, established a captive free-stand emergency facility in the far eastern suburbs. The facility feeds the easternmost satellite hospital the Samaritan group with emergency cases requiring hospitalization. It was established in a developed area to provide Samaritan with a medical presence that could form the nucleus of a hospital if population growth were to continue at the current rate. Captive facilities give the hospital control over geographic origins of patients coming into its facility and a low-cost method of entering new or developing markets" (Goldsmith, 1980, p. 120). However, while the initial impact of hospital involvement was a positive one, eventually it proved to be catastrophic to many urgent care centers. The main reason was that hospitals operated them not as nimble businesses, but as regular departments with bureaucracy layers, large overheads, and union workers. In addition, hospitals did not spend enough effort and money promoting them to the general public. Unlike today, patients at the time did not know what the centers were and what services they offered. Many of the urgent care centers lost money, so hospitals eliminated them and moved on to other services (Weinick & Bentacourt, 2007).

Despite this original setback, urgent care centers made a come-back in the mid-1990s. The new growth was mainly fueled by increased awareness and acceptance among consumers, and by severe backlash from long wait times at primary care physician offices and hospital emergency rooms. This growth wave continued on a steady rate till the late mid and late 2000's where a new surge appears to be in the making. In 2005, new urgent care centers opened at the rate of two per week, resulting in about 9,000-10,000 centers in operations today, according to some estimates (Son, 2013; Yee, Lechner & Boukus, 2013). In a 2009 survey using health insurers' websites, Internet searches and the UCAOA mailing lists, 8,113 urgent care centers were identified, although the authors conducting the survey admitted that the numbers reflected significant undercounting and included many anonymous organizations that are not urgent care centers (Weinick et al., 2009). Other experts disagree with these calculations and put the current number of "true" urgent care centers at 5,000 (Merchant Medicine, 2013b). Regardless of the numbers, the latest wave of growth is driven by large operators such as private equity firms, hospital systems (once again), and even insurance companies opening new urgent care centers or acquiring existing ones from smaller operators and "mom-and-pop" shops (Merchant Medicine, 2013a). Between 2007 and 2012, industry revenue grew at an average annualized rate of 6.3% to an estimated $13.7 billion, and the number of centers grew at an average annualized rate of 4.4%. During that same time period, average per-center visits increased by 28 visits per month from 2008 to 2012 (Son, 2013). What makes these numbers even more remarkable is that the growth has coincided with the economic recession of 2008 and the decrease in insurance coverage among many people. The industry was described in 2012 as "hot" and in a state of "continued expansion and investment" (Son, 2013, p.1). A recent survey by Harris Interactive found that 17% of the population had used an urgent care center (not associated with a physician office or hospital) in the last 12 months (Richman, 2013). The Urgent Care Association of America estimated that between 71 million and 160 million patient visits to urgent care centers occur annually (UCAO, 2011).

2. OPERATIONS

Physical Set-Up, Staffing and Hours

Half of all urgent care centers are located in freestanding clinic buildings and the other half are in retail shopping centers, and all are conveniently located and easy to find and access. Average size varies between 3600 and 12,000 square feet depending on the types of services offered. Many centers have procedure rooms for lacerations and fractures, radiology services such as X-ray services, laboratory, and physical therapy (NAFAC, 2012). Many of the older urgent care centers' external and internal look are plain and industrial, but lately a focus on slick, modern facilities has been observed among some of the new operators. WellStreet, an Atlanta-based urgent care chain, has designed clinics that are modern and consumer-friendly. For example, flat-screen TVs throughout the clinic, custom wall reliefs, bright clean LED lighting and granite countertops are becoming the norm in some centers (Merchant Medicine, 2012).

A fundamental difference between the urgent care model and other innovations discussed in this book is that urgent care relies primarily on physicians being physically present at the site of care, whereas the other models rely on non-physician providers. Most urgent care centers are staffed by full time physicians, and at least one physician has to be present at the center all the time, although exceptions can be made in remote rural areas. About 70% of physicians in urgent care are board-certified in Family Practice or Emergency Medicine (NAFAC, 2012). A minor number undergo a fellowship in urgent care medicine, a small but growing discipline that includes primary care (family medicine; sport medicine and orthopedics), emergency medicine and occupational medicine (Lee

Resnick, personal interview, 2013). About 9.6% of urgent care centers have pediatricians on staff. A typical urgent care center has about 2.5 Full Time Equivalent (FTE) physicians, usually supported by a non-physician provider (nurse practitioner or physician assistant). The average physician salary is $158,845 per year (Weinick, Bristol, & DesRoches, 2009). According to Lee Resnick, Chief Medical Officer/Chief Operating Officer of WellStreet urgent care, "urgent care centers are already feeling the strains of competing for physicians. Physicians can ask for more money. As employees, physicians in urgent care make more money than physicians in primary care. They work 36-40 hours in actual clinical care. And the main attraction is they don't have to do paperwork, so they are not burnt out." Similarly, NAFAC (2012) maintains that "many physicians are moving into the UCC (urgent care center) practice. Physicians from traditional family practice, with all the demands to be on call, travel between an office, hospital, and nursing home, are looking for a change from this demanding schedule. Emergency room physicians, as well, sometimes experience "burn out" between the ages of 42-47 and are looking for a way to use their triage skills and reduce some of their stress. These physicians, both independent, and in concert with hospitals are opening new centers every day."

Other clinic staff include Registered Nurses (RNs), Licensed Practical Nurses (LPNs), Medical Assistants (MAs), Lab Technologists, X-ray Technologists and other medical support personnel, depending on state laws and other standards of care. In a recent survey, 52.9% of urgent care centers employed nurse practitioners or physician assistants, 47.9% employed registered nurses, and 80.5% employed medical assistants and other clinical staff (Weinick, et al., 2009). Most of the staff is cross-trained. For example, medical assistants can play multiple roles such as registering patients, processing billing claims, giving injections, and starting Intravenous (IV) fluids (Weinick & Bentacourt, 2007), while radiation technologists can be trained to staff the front office when no procedures are taking place (Tammy Mallow, personal interview, 2013). The staffing challenge is that "it should be appropriate to reduce wait times, and with the appropriate mix to be cost-effective" and "staff should be operating at the top of their license" (Lauren Cates, personal interview, 2013).

An important distinguishing factor for the staff of urgent care clinics as compared to that of physician offices or hospital emergency rooms is the importance of customer service. An industry consultant observes: "From an HR point of view, these are not only highly skilled individuals, they tend to be high-need individual. [...] They have to have very strong clinical knowledge, but they also have to have extremely good bedside manner. You are now operating in a retail environment and consumers have high expectations"(Merchant Medicine, 2011)

Most urgent care centers are open for about 80 hours per week. In terms of opening times, only 18.9% are open before 8:00 am on weekdays, and very few on Saturdays and Sundays. As for closing times, most centers close between 7:00 and 9:00 pm (49.5%) on weekdays and after 9:00 pm (41.1%) on weekdays. On Saturdays and Sundays, centers typically close between 5:00 and 7:00 pm (29.8% and 31.7% respectively) or after 7:00 pm (40.9% and 34.1% respectively) (Weinick, et al., 2009). These hours are especially convenient since most physician offices open at 9:00 am and close at 5:00 pm on weekdays, and are typically closed on Saturdays and Sundays.

Geographic Locations

Urgent care centers tend be located in high-density urban areas and states with larger populations. In 2013, most centers were in the Southeast (29.6%); the West (18.7%) and Mid-Atlantic (13.3%). The states with the largest numbers of centers are California (12.0%); Florida (8.7%) and Texas (8.0%) (Son, 2013).

A study of urgent care centers in six metropolitan areas, (Detroit, Michigan; Jacksonville, Florida; Minneapolis, Minnesota; Phoenix, Arizona; Raleigh-Durham, North Carolina.; and San Francisco, California), revealed that they are typically in more populous, higher-income regions. Operators strategically locate them in areas with a lot of vehicle or foot traffic and that are visible from major roads, usually in fast-growing suburbs where young people with high household incomes and private insurance coverage live (Yee, Lechner & Boukus, 2013). The ideal location is within 3 miles of 50,000 people, with demographics ranging between 18-44 years of age, in a shopping center next to "anchor stores" such as Target or PetSmart, and with traffic of about 20,000 cars per day (Ayers, 2013). An industry executive suggested that "urgent care is a volume-driven model, so a certain population density must be present for the UCC to capture sufficient volume to breakeven. That's a big reason you see UCCs in the suburbs of larger metro areas" (Yee, et al., 2013, p.2).

The latest surveys show that 55% of urgent care centers are located in suburban areas, with only 25% in urban areas and 20% in rural ones (Urgent Care Association of America, 2011). Borkowski (2009) maintains that the geographic distribution is not appropriate and suggests that "urban areas are most affected by [emergency room] overcrowding and therefore should be housing the majority of urgent care centers. There should be a joint effort between healthcare providers and state and federal officials to allocate funding for the development of more urgent care centers in urban settings" (p.17). Moreover, there is a strong need for urgent care in rural areas, especially in areas with no physicians and where most care is delivered by nurse practitioners (Ryan & Rahman, 2010). Son (2013) explains that "... many urgent care centers are expanding into rural areas. The growth rates and distribution of urban and rural urgent care centers suggest that urban markets may be becoming saturated while rural markets are growing. This also shows an increase in the desire to set up urgent care centers in rural communities. Needs in these areas are not met as often, providing operators with an opportunity to dominate a local market" (p.18).

Scope of Services

Services provided in urgent care centers are summarized in Table 1. Most centers provide occupational medicine, laboratory tests and fracture care such as splinting and casting, and sport and school physicals. More than half provide intravenous fluids, routine immunizations and primary care services (Weinick, et al., 2009). In addition to point-of-care testing such as urinanalysis, pregnancy tests and hemoglobin tests, some centers now provide complex tests such as troponins for chest pains, which historically were done only in hospital emergency rooms (Weinick & Bentacourt, 2007). Table 2 summarizes the different levels of urgent care.

The majority of urgent care centers provide services to patients of all ages. However, some specialize in pediatric care and tend

Table 1. Services provided in urgent care centers (Weinick, et al., 2009)

Services	Percent of Urgent Care Centers Providing the Service
Occupational Medicine	
Any occupational medicine services	92.6%
Employment physicals	74.0%
Employment-related drug testing	69.3%
Treatment of workplace illness or injury	89.8%
Case management and evaluation	37.2%
Lab Tests Processed Onsite	
Any lab tests processed onsite	93.3%
Lab tests waived under CLIA*	87.2%
Lab tests designated as moderate under CLIA	37.0%
Tests requiring full laboratory certification	21.4%
Other Diagnostic Tests Performed Onsite	
CT scans	14.0%
Ultrasound	18.6%
Orthopedic-Related Services	
Fracture care, including splinting and casting	80.7%
Physical therapy and rehabilitation	20.7%
Medications	
Prepackaged pharmaceuticals	48.6%
Pain management	37.2%
Other Treatments and Services	
Intravenous fluids	70.9%
Primary care	54.4%
Routine immunizations	63.5%
Travel medicine services	32.6%
Sports and school physicals	79.3%

*Clinical Laboratory Improvement Amendments

Table 2. Levels of urgent care (Boyle &Kirkpatrick 2012)

Urgent Care Level	Services Provided
Basic level urgent care	Limited waive testing; hours 8-12, some weekend and afterhours component; may be cash clinic or retail; no x-ray
Moderate level urgent care	Expanded waive testing; hours 8-12, with some weekend and afterhours component; EKG, basic plain film x-ray
Advanced level urgent care	Expanded waive testing with point of care and on-site STAT lab (CBC, comprehensive metabolic, liver function tests); hours 16-24, open 7 days per week with afterhours component, EKG, radiology/ Imaging center (plain films, ultrasound, CT scan).

to complement local pediatricians' offices. As such, these tend to be open only when the physician offices are closed, such as on evenings, weekends and holidays. Similarly, some general urgent care centers function as after-hours primary care for limited procedures, while others provide a full spectrum of services including laceration repair, fracture care and response to some cardiac conditions (Weinick & Bentacourt, 2007). For patients who have used the clinics for minor conditions, 38% used it for flu or cold-like symptoms, 16% because they thought that had sprained a joint or broken a bone, 15% because they needed a prescription, 11% because they needed a general check-up or a check-up for a chronic condition like diabetes or asthma, and 10% because they had a cut or a wound (Richman, 2013).

A large share of the services provided by urgent care centers is occupational health, which includes employer-paid services and workers' compensation. The former are done under contractual arrangement with local employers and include employment-related physicals, drug screening tests, workplace evaluations and other services. Most of these tests can be performed by a medical assistant and require little or no supervision from a physician. Workers' compensation services include treatment for on-the-job injuries that are covered by the employers. In that respect, urgent care centers are much more attractive than physicians' offices because no appointments are needed, and they are cheaper than hospital emergency rooms. From the center's perspective, these services are provided during midday hours, a typically slow time for urgent care (Weinick & Bentacourt, 2007). According to one industry consultant: "the first client you go for is the city municipality- teachers, firemen, et cetera. They're usually the largest employer in the city and have the most clout. They're the decision makers. They're the client you need to get everybody else [on board as your client]. Let's say they have 500 employees in small city, which translates to 1,500 patients because they have families. The city will do their best to steer their employees to you because you're going to show them what you do on their workers' comp. When that happens, the employees will start to use you for other needs, colds, et cetera, and that's where you make your money" (Weinick & Bentacourt, 2007, p.15).

All urgent care centers provide X-ray services, while some are able to perform electrocardiograms (EKG), magnetic resource images (MRI), electromyography (EMG), computed tomography (CT) scans and other types of testing. Urgent care centers also provide HIV, STD (Sexually Transmitted Diseases), pregnancy, preoperative and alcohol breath testing, as well as laboratory processing such as complete blood count and necessary screenings for different illnesses (Son, 2013).

Another important service provided by some urgent care centers is point-of-care dispensing, in which medications come in pre-filled tamper-proof packages and are sold as they are to the patients. These services tend to be very profitable, and provide the convenience of one-stop shopping to patients (Weinick & Bentacourt, 2007). They allow patients to receive their prescriptions before leaving the center, and those that are too sick or uncomfortable do not have to go to a pharmacy to pick up their prescription. Most urgent care centers contract with a point-of-care dispensing company for this service and some only dispense to their own patients, unlike pharmacies that can dispense to any patient with a medication prescription. Point-of-care dispensing is expected to make up about 15% of urgent care centers' revenue in 2013 (Son, 2013). Obviously, scope of care in an urgent care center is much narrower than that in hospital emergency rooms. In recent analyses comparing injuries presenting to an urgent care centers and those presenting to pediatric emergency rooms, the former were less serious with fewer open wounds, and more superficial contusions/abrasions and sprains/strains (Yard & Comstock, 2009).

Financials

Urgent care centers are reimbursed by third party payers on a fee-for-service basis. They usually accept most health plans such as managed care patients, traditional insurance, and private pay. Co-pays are comparable to those at primary care physician offices and average between \$25-\$50, although some plans have higher co-pays for urgent care (NAFAC, 2012). For instance, some payers have a three-tiered co-pay system, with lower co-pays for primary care physician offices, higher co-pay for hospital emergency rooms, and urgent care co-pays falling somewhere in the middle (Weinick & Bentacourt, 2007). Payer mix distribution is 50.8% private pay, 14.5% Medicare, 9.9% Medicaid or other public coverage, 12.1% self-pay or uninsured and 12.7% occupational medicine (Weinick, et al., 2009). Stephen Jones, Vice President of the Carolinas HealthCare System Medical Group, suggests that "if you have a reasonable payer mix with a good percentage of commercial insurance, you can be financially profitable as a stand-alone business. But if you have a high percentage of government-pay, it is difficult. One way you can reduce costs is by adopting the mid-level provider model with MD oversight, which allows for a lower expense per visit than the MD-run model" (Stephen Jones, personal interview, 2013).

Most urgent care centers use the same billing codes used by primary care, in addition to a flat rate code, which reimburses the center a flat fee regardless of services provided. While managed care plans prefer to use the flat fee, some urgent care centers find that these fees are not financially feasible, especially when the services provided are too complex. Therefore, some centers use a two-tiered or three-tiered system depending on the severity of the condition, whereas others negotiate carve-out with insurance plans to accept additional payments for X-rays and other procedures on top of the flat fee. Unlike hospital emergency rooms, urgent care centers are not authorized by insurance companies to receive a facility fee, which is typically a payment made to cover additional resource use that occur in addition to services and procedures provided by the physicians (Weinick & Bentacourt, 2007).

Some of the more recent financial challenges faced by urgent care centers include reduced reimbursement rates. For example, "lower reimbursement from health plans in the last 18 months, and restriction on benefits covered by the health plan. Some of the rates paid are lower than Medicare. It is a supply-demand issue. As more and more urgent care centers open, the large centers have to accept the contracts with the lower rates, and the small centers can't survive" (Tammy Mallow, personal interview, 2013).

Quality Assurance

The Urgent Care Association of America (UCAOA) has put in place specific criteria for urgent care centers. Moreover, it established a Certified Urgent Care Center (CUC) designation, which means that the approved urgent care center has the correct specific scope of service, hours of operation, and staffing requirements (Song, 2013). UCAOA also has a partnership with the Joint Commission (JC) to accredit urgent care centers. Under its ambulatory accreditation program, the JC accredits urgent care centers the same way it accredits community health centers and other ambulatory care providers (Weinick & Bentacourt, 2007). Other organizations that accredit urgent care centers are the Accreditation Association for Ambulatory Healthcare (AAAHC, 2013), as well as NAFAC which has created a specific program that accredits and certifies Urgent Care Centers (NAFAC, 2013).

In addition, the recently formed Urgent Care Foundation has launched several quality initiatives. According to Jeff Collins, chair of Foundation: "The initial goal is to look at urgent care educational programs and fellowships to make sure our providers coming out have the right clinical skills and knowledge base. [...] The next stage will be to fund research around quality, looking at benchmarks and best practices. There have been few clinical benchmark studies in urgent care; there is a huge void. We need to provide funding for these studies as the industry continues to grow"(Merchant Medicine, 2012b).

At the clinic level, quality is addressed in various ways. For example, one chain of urgent care centers "address[es] quality on two layers: first, education and latest guidelines, every physician that comes in has to get the training, regardless of his/her experience, and second, audits/chart audits. We have a chief quality officer, compliance officer, and logs to track labs and tests" (Lee Resnick, personal interview, 2013).

Marketing

Despite recent growth and increased visibility of urgent care centers, many consumers still don't have a clear awareness of what the clinics are and what services they provide. Compared to their more direct competitors, urgent care centers, especially small "mom-and-pop" ones, do not have the referral relationships that primary care physicians have, the brand awareness that hospital emergency rooms, and the deeper pockets that retail clinic operators have. Therefore, marketing is crucial for survival. Borkowski (2012) notes that "[m] any people do not know what an urgent care center is or what services it has to offer. If people cannot be seen at their primary care physician's practice, they either are referred to the emergency department by their primary clinician or believe that the emergency department is their only option for care. In addition to increasing the number of urgent care centers, funding must be allocated to educating the public and advertising the resources of urgent care centers. If urgent care centers are readily available to communities and people understand their role and advantages, patients will use this resource and defer the cost and long wait times in the emergency department" (p.117). Similarly, Vic Schmerbeck, managing director of corporate finance for FirstSouthwest which provides marketing support to some centers suggests: "You have to remember, this is a very retail-oriented business. [...] You can provide the best quality care, the best efficiency and the best patient experience, but you have to get them in the door first" (Merchant Medicine, 2012a).

Traditionally, urgent care centers, especially hospital-owned ones, have used mainstream advertising such as newsprint, direct mail and billboards. The focus is on educating patients to identify the severity of their conditions and "self-triage" into an urgent care center if their condition is urgent but not emergent. Some centers also advertise to local primary care physician office by emphasizing the non-competitive and complementary nature of their services on weeknights and weekends (Weinick & Bentacourt, 2007). When asked how they have heard about the center, more than half of patients state it was through word-of-mouth, which underscores the importance of providing a superior experience for existing patients (Merchant Medicine, 2012b).

More recently, some centers have used more innovative marketing tactics. In an effort to better understand their existing patient base, clinics have contracted with marketing firms to conduct market segmentation studies that allow them to see their patients in the context of specific household attributes. Another important source of patient awareness is clinic location and signage. Where to locate the clinic, its visibility in relation to traffic patterns, the external signage and the building itself are important factors to consider. For example PatientFirst urgent care in Pennsylvania, Maryland and Virginia has standalone structures with a unique green metallic roof. For such centers with visible buildings and unique structure, about 60% of patients know about the clinic not through word-of-mouth, but by seeing it while driving on adjacent streets (Merchant Medicine, 2012b). However, it is important to note that some states such as Illinois and New Jersey prohibit the centers from using the term "urgent" in their name or promotional material, so as not to confuse consumers about the difference and similarities with hospital emergency rooms (Stern, 2005).

Regulations

Urgent care centers that are owned by physicians are licensed as physician offices. Those that are owned by hospitals are licensed as hospital-based clinics and have to follow CMS (Center for Medicare & Medicaid) licensure. Regardless of ownership, urgent care facilities must comply with the U.S. Department of Human Services regulations, such as those relating to type of facility, equipment, personnel, standard of medical care and hygiene, compliance with all state and local laws and regulations, among other things. Moreover, they should abide by general federal laws such as anti-kick back statutes, Stark laws and HIPAA (Health Insurance Portability and Accountability Act). Employees working in urgent care centers must obtain appropriate state licenses to practice medicine or nursing. Urgent care centers that treat Medicare or Medicaid patients must also comply with the regulations pertaining to these programs (Son, 2013). Some states, such as California and Texas have "corporate practice of medicine" laws that prohibit employment of physicians by healthcare organizations, except if the organization is owned by physicians. Since more urgent care centers are owned by physicians, the law has not substantially affected the industry. However, some urgent care centers are owned by health systems, therefore contracts are signed with a physician group organization that employs the physicians to staff the centers (Weinick & Bentacourt, 2007).

Other legal issues specific to urgent care centers relate to medical malpractice. Malpractice risk in this setting falls between the higher levels of hospital emergency rooms and the lower levels of primary care physician practices. Factors that may lead to increased errors and risk are the episodic nature of care, the lack of a long-term relationship with the patient, the absence of clear discharge directions for patients, and the possibility of underdiagnosis by physicians and other providers (Weinick & Bentacourt, 2007).

Another legal issue resulting from the lack of an established relationship between providers and patients is the possibility of some patients to seek the urgent care center to satisfy drug addictions. Patrice Pash of National Med Network describes the situation: "Drug seekers know they can go in there, to the urgent care doctors. [...] Think about how easy it is to fake a hurt back. It is easy for a "narc hunter" to go into different urgent care centers to get drugs. It takes a very perceptive doctor to find about it" (Weinick & Bentacourt, 2007, p. 21). Given the large amount of pain-killer and narcotics scores, especially with centers providing point-of-care dispensing, the risk of robberies is also very large.

3. STAKEHOLDERS

Urgent care centers can compete with hospital emergency rooms for non-emergent, urgent patients and conditions, can compete with retail clinics for minor patients and conditions, and can compete or complement the services of primary care physicians, depending on their services and hours of operations. Consumers appreciate the convenience of walk-in, extended hours, while physicians and other providers see them as an opportunity to practice medicine in a more controlled environment. The owners of retail clinics are large organizations, health systems and individual physicians, operating in a highly fragmented industry. Two "rival" trade associations represent some of the urgent care centers and provide different accreditation and lobbying services.

Consumers

As previously discussed, consumers of urgent care centers are most likely to be younger families with children living in suburban areas with middle-to-high income levels and private insurance coverage. The main reason why consumers visit an urgent care center is that it is open when the physician's office is closed (54%). Other reasons include that no appointment is needed (44%), insurance is accepted (35%), the location is more convenient (32%), the short wait times (27%), the care not being expensive (22%), not having a regular physician (16%), and being more pleasant than a physician's office (11%) (Richman, 2013).

Owners

The urgent care industry is a highly fragmented one. One estimate suggests that the top 10 owners operate only 20% of the centers, and another one suggests that the largest four players account for only 1% of the industry's revenue (Merchant Medicine, 2013; Son, 2013). Table 3 highlights the top operators by number of centers in operation. A recent national survey found that 35% of the centers are owned by physicians or physician groups, 30% are owned by corporations, and 25% are owned by hospital systems, while another 7% are owned by non-physician individuals or franchisors (UCAOA, 2012).

The market is dominated by "owner-operators." These are individual family practice and emergency medicine physicians, or business people who have partnered with physicians. The centers are run as a business and as the personal source of income. These types of centers, as well as centers owned by small chains, have found themselves to be the target of larger chains looking for expansion and acquisition opportunities (Merchant Medicine, 2011). More recently, the following scenarios were predicted:

Smaller players will agree to be acquired either by hospital systems looking to enter the urgent care market locally or expand their service area.

Smaller players will agree to be acquired by large operators looking to expand their national footprint.

Smaller players will seek a price that larger players are unwilling to meet, causing the larger players to open de-novo sites in close proximity to those smaller player sites (Merchant Medicine, 2013)

Other centers are owned by private multispecialty group practices that consist of two or more physicians. Under this arrangement,

Table 3. Urgent care operators by numbers, as of December, 2013 (Merchant Medicine, 2013)

Operator	Number of Centers	Region	Funding/Ownership
Concentra*	296	Multistate	Humana
US HealthWorks*	145	Multistate	Dignity
MedExpress	121		Sequoia Capital; General Atlantic
American Family Care DRX	108	AL & TN	Private
NextCare	92	NextCare	Enhanced Equity Fund; Goldman Sachs
FastMed	62	NC & AZ	Comvest Partners
Doctors Care	52	SC and TN	Private
CareSpot	48	FL & TN	Welsh Carson, JVs
Patient First	47	PA/MD/DC/VA	Private
Physicians Immediate Care	31	IL/OK/NE	LLR Partners; Wellpoint

patients are captured from nearby providers and healthcare facilities that do not provide expanded hours and they have access to other specialties after an urgent care event, which guarantees continuity of care. Some of the urgent care corporations operate hundreds of centers, whereas others are small and operate only a few in specific markets or geographic locations. They tend to consolidate costs over multiple physician practices across a region. Also, having multiple locations can help in negotiating contracts for occupational medicine and can help generate brand recognition among consumers. An interesting model is that of franchise companies that support urgent care operators to open quickly by following a standardized plan. The urgent care operator pays an up-front franchise fee and a percentage of revenue. However, experts do not believe this is a sustainable model since urgent care centers are not very lucrative, so the franchise fee could result in very slim profits for the operators (Merhcant Medicine, 2011).

Another interesting and relatively recent trend is that of large insurance companies' involvement in urgent care chains. For example, Humana recently acquired Concentra; WellPoint invested in Physicians Immediate Care; and Blue Cross Blue Shield of North Carolina's (BCBSNC) invested in FastMed Urgent Care. The obvious reasons behind these strategies include reducing costs while providing health plan members with a convenient alternative to the hospital emergency room, but other factors may also be at play (Merchant Medicine, 2012c). A health plan executive explained the situation: "Everyone is trying to reduce medical expense while getting members to receive care in the most appropriate setting. [I would say that] 30 percent of patients that go to the ED could receive care in a less acute setting. If we can't get a member to engage with their primary care physician, [our urgent care centers are] probably the next best step" (Yee, et al., 2013, p.5).

Primary Care Physicians

Urgent care centers offer walk-in care and can provide an attractive alternative for patients who do not want to wait to see their physicians. Therefore, it is expected that many existing primary care physicians view urgent care centers as competition. However, since physicians themselves are involved in the ownership and delivery of care in urgent care centers, there hasn't been a strong opposition from the medical community to urgent care centers, and certainly not at the level of opposition to retail clinics (discussed in the next chapter). Many urgent care centers explicitly state that they do not directly compete with physician's offices, and that they do not intend to take patients away from their existing physicians. Many of them invest in communicating with physicians and working collaboratively with them. For example, some send reports to physicians describing the care their patients have received at the urgent care center, while other send "thank-you" notes to physicians for allowing them to participate in the patient's care. Collaboration can reach even more advanced levels when some physicians leave a message on their answering machines referring patients to urgent care centers when they call after hours and on weekends. As such, the centers can relieve physicians from night and weekend call. However, some other physicians prefer head-to-head competition over collaboration. As soon as urgent care centers open in some areas, many physician offices are forced to start thinking in more consumer-oriented way and offering evening and weekend hours. It is also important to note that, unlike retail clinics, urgent care centers have not expanded their services to include chronic disease management. According to an urgent care center operator: "[Patients] can't have chronic illnesses for us to continue to see them. If they need a physical or have an earache, we'll see them. But if [patients are] diabetic or hypertensive, we have to refer them to primary care because we do not follow that"(Yee, et al., 2013). As a result, physicians are less threatened by urgent care centers' capturing that portion of their patients.

Hospital Systems

Feeling some competition threat from large urgent care center operators directing emergency room patients to their new-built clinics, and feeling the need to better position themselves for future strategic and regulatory challenges, many hospital systems have started operating their urgent care centers, or entering into partnerships with existing operators. Table 4 highlights the top hospital urgent care operators. According to Phil Powell, a senior executive with Bayfront Health System and a long-time urgent care operator: "Hospital facilities are in it predominately for the downstream revenue. [...] The facilities serve to build market share and serve as a referral source to the hospital and/or its affiliated providers"(Merchant Medicine, 2011). For some hospital systems, the urgent care facility represents a separate service-line, away from the main core business, while for others, the urgent care center is on-site, typically adjacent to the emergency room to capture overflows of patients.

Partnerships range from simple co-branding schemes to equity-based joint ventures. For example TriStar, a division of HCA (Hospital Corporation of America) in Nashville, has entered a joint venture with CareSpot, to open 15 urgent care centers in Middle Tennessee in 2013, with others centers subsequently planned in other markets (Merchant Medicine, 2013).

Retail Clinics and Emergency Rooms

The minor primary care conditions treated by urgent care centers can overlap with services offered at retail clinics, which lead to a potential for competition. For example, among patients who visit retail clinics, 18% would have gone to an urgent care center if the retail clinic

Table 4. Top hospital urgent care operators, as of February 2013 (Merchant Medicine, 2013)

Hospital Operator	Number of Centers	State
Aurora Urgent Care	37	WI
Intermountain InstaCare	25	UT
Carolinas HealthCare	22	NC
CentraCare	20	FL
St. John Providence	18	MI
Norton Immediate Care	12	KY
Health Partners	13	MN
Advocate Health	11	IL
Marshfield Clinic	10	WI
Primary Health	10	ID
University of Pittsburgh Medical Center	8	PA

was not available (Wang, Ryan, McGlynn & Mehrotra, 2010). However, the potential for collaboration is also there. Many companies own urgent care centers and retail clinics, and some tend to locate them in adjacent locations so that patients who present to a retail clinic with an urgent condition can be channeled directly to urgent care centers, while patients who present with minor conditions to urgent care centers during peak times are referred to retail clinics with shorter wait times.

In addition, many of the non-life threatening conditions treated in hospital emergency rooms can be taken care of in urgent care centers. Weinick, Burns and Mehrotra (2010) estimated that 13.4% of emergency room visits could take place at an urgent care centers (8.9% if the hours are restricted to when urgent care centers are typically open). The authors noted that "[d]iverting these patients to alternative care sites could decrease the time spent waiting to be seen by a clinician, since many patients spend extended periods in emergency department waiting rooms. Diversion also could generate potential savings" (p.1634).

Professional Organizations

The original trade association that historically represented urgent care centers in the National Association for Ambulatory Care (NAFAC). Founded in 1973, NAFAC is "…committed to helping its members open new facilities, become nationally certified and thrive in the changing world of ambulatory healthcare. Members are predominantly physicians and clinic operators from a range of healthcare provider organizations. The association publishes the well-known "Bill's Book: Developing Urgent Care Centers," and is offers national certification in Urgent and Convenience care" (NAFAC, 2013). In 2004, due to political differences, a new professional trade organization branched out of NAFAC, and the Urgent Care Association of America (UCAOA) was formed. UCAOA is a professional trade association, representing urgent care centers and their operators. Members are mostly located in the United States but some are across the world. It offers educational and professional development resources as well as resources for developing a new urgent care center and provision of high quality care in urgent care centers (UCAOA, 2013). It has grown to about 4,000 members and some consider it today the "largest and only truly representative of urgent care" (Lee Resnick personal interview, 2013). The UCAOA publishes the "Journal of Urgent Care Medicine".

In its early days, the UCAOA was acting as a trade organization and physician organization for providers in urgent care. Recently, though, with support from UCAOA, the Urgent Care College of physicians (UCCOP) was formed to "allow leadership and members to advance the specialty further by focusing physician representation and efforts in the areas of academics, research, continuing education, and advocacy" (UCCOP, 2013). In addition, the American

Board of Urgent Care Medicine (ABUCM), established in 1997, serves as an independent certifying body for qualified urgent care physicians. Its purpose "is to define the domain of knowledge and clinical skills expected of the urgent care physician, to provide a valid assessment of knowledge demonstrated by the urgent care medicine physician, to encourage continued professional development in the field of urgent care medicine, and to serve the public by encouraging quality patient care" (ABUCM, 2013). Although the certification is not recognized by the American Board of Medical Specialties, more than 900 physicians have passed the ABUCM exam.

Moreover, physicians can complete a fellowship in urgent care medicine through a program developed in collaboration with UCAOA. The curriculum, modeled after the Accreditation Council for Graduate Medical Education (ACGME) training model, graduates five physicians every year (Lee Resnick, personal interview, 2013). The competencies include adult emergencies, pediatric emergencies, would and injury evaluation and treatment, occupational medicine, urgent care procedures, and business aspects of urgent care. More recently, the Institute for Urgent Care Medicine offers a mini-fellowship 60-hour online training program (Lee Resnick, personal interview, 2013).

4. OUTCOMES

Urgent care centers can prove to be a major player in the primary care and urgent care fields if patients are satisfied with the care they receive, quality of care provided is as good or better and costs of care are significantly lower than the alternatives. In this section, we review the evidence on urgent care centers' outcomes.

Patient Satisfaction

Patient satisfaction with care provided in urgent care centers is directly related to wait times. According to the UCAOA "Urgent Care Benchmarking Report," about 65% of patients wait less than 20 minutes to see a provider in an urgent care center, while less than 5% wait as long as 90 minutes. These data suggest a decrease in wait times as compared to 2008. It is also important to note that wait times vary by time of the day: shorter wait times are observed during the mid-day hours, while patients face longer wait times in the morning and evening hours (UCAOA, 2011). These numbers are telling, especially when compared to hospital emergency rooms where the average wait time is 58 minutes (Hing & Bhuiya, 2012). In addition, patients spend an average of four hours and seven minutes from the moment they walk into a hospital emergency room until the time they are discharged (Press Ganey, 2010).

Surprisingly, research relating to patient satisfaction in urgent care centers is rare. In a 2002 study by Press Ganey, patients gave urgent care centers a rating of 83/100, but 49% did not recommend the center to others, possibly due to long and unexplained waiting times (Miceli & Van Remortel, 2003). When comparing patients presenting with headaches in urgent care centers and hospital emergency rooms, those in urgent care centers were more likely to report waiting less than one hour to see the physician, having a provider who was polite and respectful, having the diagnosis clearly explained, having received effective treatment, and having been provided with clear discharge directions (National Headache Foundation, 2006). More recently, a study found high levels of satisfaction with care provided in rural urgent care centers by nurse practitioners (Ryan & Rahman, 2012).

Quality of Care

The evidence on the quality of care delivered in urgent care center is also scarce. The notable exception is a study by Mehrotra and his colleagues in 2009. The researchers examined three minor conditions treated in various settings: otitis media (ear infection); pharyngitis and urinary tract infections. Based on several quality indicators, they created an aggregate quality score for all conditions and measured whether patients received specific preventative services in the three months following their visits. Overall, aggregate quality scores were similar at urgent care centers (62.6%), retail clinics (63.6%) and physician offices (61.0%) but were lower for emergency rooms (55.1%). Compared to hospital emergency rooms, urgent care centers scored better on almost every indicator. For example, for otitis media, the pass rate for urgent care on "duration of therapy is at least 10 days" was 93.4% compared to 89.1% in emergency rooms. In treatment of pharyngitis for children, urgent care scored 72.7% on "culture or rapid strep test was obtained in diagnosis of GABH (Group A ß-hemolytic streptococcal)" while emergency rooms scored 52.4%. In treatment of urinary tract infections, urgent care scored 58.1% on "urine culture obtained for all high risk patients," while emergency rooms scored 54.8%. When comparing receipt of preventive services, urgent care centers scored significantly higher than emergency rooms (13.7% vs. 10.7%) but lower than retail clinics (14.5%) and physician offices (14.2%)(Mehrotra, Liu, Adam, et al., 2009).

Costs of Care

Urgent care centers can reduce the costs of care by diverting patients from expensive hospital emergency rooms, but may also increase costs if they divert a substantial number of patients from less expensive primary care physician offices. An executive at a health plan that contracts with urgent care center summarized: "The original model for urgent care was to keep people out of the ER. The more we started looking at that and reviewing the data, it was kind of a wash. Were we keeping them out of the ER? Or were we keeping them out of the primary care office and making it easy for folks to go someplace and get something taken care of that a PCP could've done?"(Yee, et al., 2013, p.5).

In terms of costs per episode of care for minor conditions, urgent care centers are actually much cheaper than hospital emergency rooms and slightly cheaper than physician offices. The above-mentioned study comparing episodes of treatment for three minor conditions concluded that the cost per episode at urgent care centers was $156, compared with $570 in hospital emergency rooms and $166 in physician offices (Mehrotra, Liu, Adam, et al., 2010). Claim analyses from Medica Choice Network, a system of more than 4,000 medical offices, clinics and hospitals across four Midwestern states reveals the following cost comparisons between urgent care centers and hospital emergency rooms (Debt.org, 2013):

- **Allergies:** $97 in urgent care vs. $345 in hospital emergency rooms
- **Acute bronchitis:** $127 in urgent care vs. $595 in hospital emergency rooms
- **Earache:** $110 in urgent care vs. $400 in hospital emergency rooms
- **Sore throat:** $94 in urgent care vs. $525 in hospital emergency rooms
- **Pink eye:** $102 in urgent care vs. $370 in hospital emergency rooms
- **Sinusitis:** $112 in urgent care vs. $617 in hospital emergency rooms

- **Strep throat:** $111 in urgent care vs. $531 in hospital emergency rooms
- **Upper respiratory infection:** $111 in urgent care vs. $486 in hospital emergency rooms
- **Urinary tract infection:** $110 in urgent care vs. $665 in hospital emergency rooms

Anthem Blue Cross and Blue Shield in Virginia (a health plan that is part of WellPoint), reviewed visit data and estimated that more than 60% of member hospital emergency rooms visits could have been treated in urgent care centers. Therefore, Anthem launched an educational campaign to promote the use of urgent care centers and other alternatives among its members, and saw a 14% drop in hospital emergency room visits. The UCAO estimates that if these numbers are applied to the approximately 70 million (out of the 116.8 million) emergency room visits that are for non-emergency care, the possible savings of using urgent care centers are between 15 and 40 billion dollars annually (UCAOA, 2011).

5. CONCLUSION

The problems associated with hospital emergency rooms' overcrowding do not appear to be resolved any time soon. Given the expected primary care physician shortages, the difficulty that patients encounter when trying to find timely appointments, and the expected increase in the number of insured populations as a result of the patient Protection and Affordable Care Act (PPACA), urgent care is well positioned for growth and expansion in the next few years. Given the expanding industry, strong growth in company numbers, greater employment opportunities and rising per capita usage of urgent care centers, the urgent care industry is in the growth phase of its life cycle. Some estimates suggest that the number of urgent care centers will continue to increase at an annualized rate of 4.4% over the next five years and will reach 12,299 centers by 2018 (Son, 2013).

In addition to growth in numbers and utilization, some experts predict new types of services to be offered by urgent care center. For example, "sports medicine has tremendous synergies with urgent care and occupational medicine. Sports injuries often require imaging and physical therapy. They also represent potential repeat visits to track progress, and pull from a wide age range of commercially insured patients. Chief among this demographic is the recent burst of interest by more active middle-aged and older adults in distance running, triathlons, mountain biking and climbing, where new forms of exertion result in sports injuries. Other new services [that are expected] to grow in 2013 are weight loss, skin care and corporate wellness" (Merchant Medicine, February 2013). Others suggest that urgent care centers could play a larger role in case of natural disasters. For example, if hospitals are overwhelmed with serious injuries, urgent care centers could be designated as treatment sites for less critical and non-emergency patients. Unlike traditional physician offices, urgent care centers are accustomed to managing an unscheduled, walk-in population (UCAOA, 2011).

REFERENCES

Accreditation Association for Ambulatory Healthcare. (2013). *Accreditation*. Retrieved from http://www.aaahc.org/accreditation/

American Board of Urgent Care Medicine (ABUCM). (2013). Available at http://aaucm.org/professionals/boardcertifications/default.aspx

Ayers, A. (2013). *Judges' Debriefing*. University of Alabama at Birmingham, Annual healthcare administration case competition.

Borkowski, S. (2012). Solutions for ED Overcrowding: Increasing Urgent Care Centers. *Journal of emergency nursing: JEN: official publication of the Emergency Department Nurses Association, 38*(2), 116–117. doi:10.1016/j.jen.2011.12.009 PMID:22401611

Goldsmith, J.C. (1980). The Healthcare Market: Can hospitals survive? *Harvard Business Review, 58*, 100–112. PMID:10247957

Hing, E., & Bhuiya, F. (2012). *Wait time for treatment in hospital emergency departments: 2009. NCHS data brief, no 102*. Hyattsville, MD: National Center for Health Statistics.

Kirkpatrick, B. (2012). *The Healthcare Executive's Guide to Urgent Care Centers and Freestanding EDs*. HealthLeaders Media.

McNeeley, S. (2012). Urgent Care Centers: An Overview. *The American Journal of Chinese Medicine, 9*(2), 80–81.

Medicine, M. (2011). *ConvUrgentCare Report, 4*(6), 1–6.

Medicine, M. (2012a). *ConvUrgentCare Report, 5*(6), 1–6.

Medicine, M. (2012b). *ConvUrgentCare Report, 5*(10), 1–7.

Medicine, M. (2012c). *ConvUrgentCare Report, 5*(11), 1–5.

Medicine, M. (2013). *ConvUrgentCare Report, 6*(2), 1–4.

Medicine, M. (2013a). *ConvUrgentCare Report, 6*(1), 1–5.

Medicine, M. (2013b). *ConvUrgentCare Report, 6*(2), 1–6.

Miceli, P. J., & Van Remortel, D. (2003). *Fostering patient loyalty in urgent care settings*. AACN Viewpoint, November/December.

National Association for Ambulatory Care. (2012). Available at http://www.urgentcare.org/

National Association for Ambulatory Care (NAFAC). (2013). *National Urgent Care Practice Standards Certification*. Retrieved from http://www.urgentcare.org/CertificationStandards/tabid/134/Default.aspx

National Headache Foundation. (2006). Emergency room vs. urgent care, a headache sufferer's dilemma. Chicago, IL: Author.

Press Ganey. (2010). *ED Pulse Report*. South Bend, IN: Author.

Richman, D. (2013, May 14). *Consumer trends in retail medicine*. Paper presented at the Retail Clinician Education Congress. New York, NY.

Ryan, K., & Rahman, A. (2012). Examining factors influencing patient satisfaction with nurse practitioners in rural urgent care centers. *Journal of the American Academy of Nurse Practitioners, 24*(2), 77–81. doi:10.1111/j.1745-7599.2011.00688.x PMID:22324862

Son, A. (2013). *IBISWorld Industry Report OD5458*. Urgent Care Centers in the US.

Stern, David. (2005). Status of Urgent Care in the U.S. *Business Briefing: Emergency Medicine Review*.

Trafford, A. (1983, December 19). For doctors, too, it is a surplus. *U.S. News & World Report*, 62–64. PMID:10264129

Urgent Care Association of America. (2011). (2010). Urgent Care Benchmarking Survey Results. *Structure (London, England)*.

Urgent Care Association of America. (2011). *The case for urgent care*. Naperville, IL: Author.

Urgent Care Association of America. (2013). Available at http://www.ucaoa.org/

Urgent Care College of Physicians. (2013). Available at http://www.uccop.org/

Wang, M. C., Ryan, G., McGlynn, E. A., & Mehrotra, A. (2010). Why Do Patients Seek Care at Retail Clinics and What Alternatives Did They Consider. *American Journal of Medical Quality*, *25*(2), 128–134. doi:10.1177/1062860609353201 PMID:20142442

Weinick, R., & Bentacourt, R. M. (2007). *No appointment needed- The resurgence of urgent care centers in the United States*. California Healthcare Foundation.

Weinick, R. M., Bristol, S. J., & DesRoches, C. M. (2009). Urgent care centers in the U.S.: Findings from a national survey. *BMC Health Services Research*, *9*(79), 1–9. PMID:19445656

Weinick, R. M., Bristol, S. J., Marder, J. E., & DesRoches, C. M. (2009). The Search for the Urgent Care Center. *The Journal of Urgent Care Medicine*, *3*, 438–440. http://jucm.com/2009-jan/ucupdate2.shtml

Weinick, R. M., Burns, R. M., & Mehrotra, A. (2010). Many Emergency Department Visits Could Be Managed At Urgent Care Centers And retail clinics. *Health Affairs*, *29*(9), 1630–1636. doi:10.1377/hlthaff.2009.0748 PMID:20820018

Yard, E. E., & Comstock, R. D. (2009). An epidemiologic comparison of injuries presenting to a pediatric emergency department and local urgent care facilities. *Journal of Safety Research*, *40*(1), 63–69. doi:10.1016/j.jsr.2008.12.004 PMID:19285588

Yee, T., Lechner, A. E., & Boukus, E. R. (2013). *The Surge in Urgent Care Centers: Emergency Department Alternative or Costly Convenience? (Research Brief 26)*. Center for Studying Health System Change.

KEY TERMS AND DEFINITIONS

Cost of Care: The amount in dollars spent on healthcare services within a certain healthcare system.

Patient Satisfaction: Patient expectation and attitudes regarding the quality of healthcare services received.

Quality of Care: The extent to which healthcare services provided to individuals and patient populations improve desired health outcomes.

Urgent Care: Healthcare provided on a walk-in, no-appointment basis for acute illnesses or injuries that are not life-threatening.

APPENDIX 1: TOM PASCUZZI, M.D, AN URGENT CARE ENTREPRENEUR

Dr. Tom Pascuzzi founded "MD Urgent Care" in New Mexico in 2009. He started with one clinic, opened another one in 2011, and then sold the clinics to Presbyterian Health System in 2012. Dr. Pascuzzi went to medical school at Wayne State University in Michigan. He served in the military in New Mexico in flight medicine. Then he did emergency medicine at Wilford Hall in San Antonio, transferred to Albuquerque, and became the director of 27 Emergency Rooms. Afterwards, he went to Santa Fe to work in emergency care and ran a group of private ER physicians. They created a "fast-track" in ER, and saw about 60-80 people per day. He then worked at Presbyterian Health System in Albuquerque in inpatient care from 1997-2006. He left in 2009 to start his own urgent care center. In 2011, he opened his second clinic, because of very high demand from patients.

He describes his experience in urgent care:

"In the past, most physicians used to go into private practice. Today it is less than 10%. So when I decided to go back to private practice and build my own urgent care center, it was not the trend. It was very scary as I had to buy a building, hire staff, the capital needs were $500-$700K, the biggest expense is X-ray. My town is very Managed Care-oriented, so I had to negotiate contracts. Presbyterian has a health plan, so they did not want to contract with me. I had to think of ways to get 35 patients per day breakeven. It took 8-10 months for start-up, a local community bank gave me a loan. I had 7 physicians and 2 PAs in both clinics, all emergency-trained, working 32 hours/week. It was called "MD Urgent Care", operating under the physician model. We did a survey and 99% of our patients said they didn't mind seeing a PA. They said they will see whoever will see them! Presbyterian realized that I was taking more of their patients, so they asked me to come back and bought my clinics in 2012. Now Presbyterian has 5 urgent care centers, plus my two, operating under a "Convenient Care Division", which also operates workplace centers at Intel and mobile units. I think urgent care will explode under the Affordable Care Act. New Mexico will set up exchanges, and will have Medicaid Managed Care. People over the age of 11 years do not go to a doctor anymore. However, Medicaid will pay less, that is why I sold my practices. Presbyterian will tighten their network to be ready for episodic contracting and bundled payments. It is going to get worse for the physicians because of reduced reimbursement. New Mexico will have 60% of people under Medicare/Medicaid, it is going to be a risk."

APPENDIX 2: A PROFILE OF TOP URGENT CARE OPERATORS (BY REVENUE)- ADOPTED FROM SON (2013)

NextCare Urgent Care Inc. (Estimated Market Share: 0.7%)

National urgent healthcare corporation NextCare is the largest provider of urgent care in the United States, as measured by annual revenue. The company benefits from its partnerships with doctors and hospitals. Since its inception in 1993, the company has grown to include 58 establishments in the United States. In 2012, the company is expected to generate $95.0 million in revenue, giving NextCare an estimated market share of 0.7%. To attract more customers, NextCare launched a NextCareAdvantage discount program in December 2011, which serves as an alternative to health insurance. Small- to medium-size companies can partner with NextCare, allowing employees to visit any of NextCare's urgent care clinics for $35. This significant cost savings for consumers is expected to attract more customers and serve as a competitive edge for the company.

Concentra Inc. (Estimated Market Share: 0.3%)

Concentra is the nation's second-largest urgent care medical practice. Since the company's inception in 1979, it has grown to include 320 establishments across the nation – the largest of any operator in this industry. After a period of operating as a public company, Concentra went private in 1999. The company's urgent care segment was launched in 2007. In December 2010, Humana Inc. (a publicly traded company) acquired Concentra for $804.7 million. According to the latest financial information released, Concentra generated 0.1% of Humana's consolidated revenue for the 2010 calendar year, at $36.6 million. Healthcare services rendered at Concentra's urgent care facilities generated about $42.8 million in 2012 revenue.

FastMed Inc. (Estimated Market Share: 0.2%)

FastMed, founded in 2001 and initially called Urgent Cares of America, has since grown to include 40 establishments in 2012. This growth was partially due to a phase of mergers and acquisitions. In November 2010, the Comvest Group acquired Urgent Cares of America. Soon after in February 2011, Urgent Cares of America acquired Tri-City Express Care, an Arizona-based company with five urgent care facilities. In April of 2011, United Cares of America announced a name change to FastMed. Given that the company is privately owned, there is limited financial information available. Based on IBISWorld estimates, the company is expected to generate about 0.2% of industry revenue in 2012, or $27.4 million.

Chapter 6
Retail Clinics

ABSTRACT

This chapter addresses the poster-child of convenient care models, namely retail clinics. Retail clinics are walk-in clinics located in grocery stores, drugstores, and general merchandise retailers such as Wal-Mart, Target, CVS, Walgreens, etc. They offer a limited scope of diagnostic and treatment services for common medical conditions, as well as preventative and wellness services. Most retail clinic visits are for simple conditions and services such as upper respiratory infections, urinary tract infections, immunizations, and tests. Care is delivered by a nurse practitioner or physician assistant, and many clinics have up-front menu-style pricing, a feature that is unparalleled in the American healthcare system. The clinics operate on a walk-in basis with no appointments needed and very short wait times, and are open on evenings and weekends when most physician offices are closed. The chapter discusses the evolution, operations, and stakeholders of retail clinics, and highlights the research related to their outcomes, such as cost, quality, continuity of care, and patient satisfaction. The author describes how some operators are expanding the scope of services to include management and treatment of chronic conditions and conclude that the future of retail clinics in terms of numbers and usage rates looks very bright.

An interesting thing happens when discussing retail medical clinics: individuals cease to be referred to as 'patients,' and begin to be referred to as 'consumers.' Retail clinics have placed patients in a role of medical consumer within the era of consumer-driven healthcare. —Schleiter, 2010

INTRODUCTION

Retail clinics represent a major revolution in healthcare in the last decade (Fottler & Malvey, 2010). Never before has a delivery option epitomized such a value proposition: convenient locations, walk-in care, short waiting times and affordable prices. Scott was first to address this value proposition in a report to the California Healthcare Foundation in 2006: "Most efforts to address escalating healthcare costs attempt to innovate within the insurance system but don't tackle the underlying structural costs of delivering healthcare. Labor overhead and technology expenses in the U.S. healthcare system are often assumed as givens,

DOI: 10.4018/978-1-4666-6355-8.ch006

even as health insurance benefits are cut to the point that neither the scope of benefits nor the expectations of what consumers will pay provide a compelling value proposition. As the trend in health insurance shifts more costs to consumers, the public has indicated that they are willing to approach at least their basic, routine, and elective healthcare needs with an eye towards price and value" (Scott, 2006, p. 3). In one of the first major media stories reporting on the topic, the Wall-Street Journal exclaimed: "With catchy slogans like "You're Sick! We're Quick!" retail health clinics are spreading fast in supermarkets, drugstores and big-box chains across the country, luring patients with walk-in treatment for minor ailments like strep throat - at about half the cost of a typical doctor visit" (Landro, 2006, p. 1). The concept was so foreign to healthcare delivery that Bohmer likened it in 2007 to the fast-food industry: "The originators based their design on the McDonald's hamburger chain, in which customers select items from a limited menu. The services listed are highly standardized interventions and require no physician evaluation. Diagnoses are made by using a simple binary test (such as for a streptococcal throat infection) or by applying a rigid, protocol-based decision rule. In some cases, no diagnosis is required (such as for a hepatitis vaccination). In addition, the conditions treated and therapies offered require no or minimal follow-up (for instance, clinics offer diabetes screening but not treatment), and decisions can be guided by highly specified protocols. More important, the conditions can be diagnosed and treated quickly" (Bohmer, 2007, p. 766-767). Healthcare strategy expert Preston Gee commented in 2007: "There's a hassle factor. Filling out forms and sitting in an office and feeling kind of intimidated by the whole medical milieu -we don't like that. You can go to a [retail clinic] you're comfortable with and buy a beach ball while you're waiting" (Callahan, 2007, p.1).

Physicians felt threatened and intrigued by the new trend. Douglas Kamerow, former U.S. assistant surgeon general wrote in the British Medical Journal in 2007: "These clinics clearly work for people who have an acute, limited problem or need an immunization or other offered service, as long as they also have the means or insurance to pay for it. Perfect for the recurrent ear infection on Sunday for a child or an assessment of dysuria in the evening. Quick examination, diagnosis, treatment, and the prescription can be filled without moving your car. Or if you're on vacation and develop conjunctivitis or a sinus infection, nothing could be more convenient. [...] Certainly the retail health clinics are a threat. But they are providing a useful service, from which conventional practitioners could learn a thing or two. In that sense they provide additional impetus for medicine to reinvent itself to become more patient focused and responsive" (Kamerow, 2007, p. 21). Since these early days, retail clinics have been extensively studied with special attention to usage rates, quality, cost, and savings, but the most enthralling argument about them remains their value proposition. Fottler and Malvey (2010) described them as "a concept that is new to healthcare: *no frills* healthcare that is offered at bargain prices. The care is provided by a physician substitute such as a nurse practitioner at a much lower cost to the consumer. The clinics are located within retail stores, pharmacies, and supermarkets. Patients spend little time waiting to be seen, and prescriptions are filled before they leave the premise. This is a walk-in business, with no appointments to schedule" (Fottler & Malvey, 2010, p. 3).

Different terms have been used to refer to retail clinics, such as retail health clinics, retail medical clinics, retail-based clinics, in-store clinics, mini clinics or convenient care clinics. In this book, we use the more common term "retail clinics" and borrow the definition used by Scott (2006): A retail clinic is "a medical clinic located within a larger operation that offers general medical services (as opposed to specialty clinics such as eye care) to the public on an ongoing (rather than one-time or seasonal) basis. These clinics differ from both urgent care clinics or the "Doc in a Box" concept in several ways: a limited service offering (increasing speed), co-location with a pharmacy (increasing convenience), and lower cost structure (reducing prices)" (Scott, 2006, p. 9).

1. EVOLUTION

Retail clinics first appeared on the healthcare scene in 2000. Since then, there have been periods of slow growth, exponential growth, relative stagnation and more measured growth. The total number of retail clinics at the time of the writing of this book was 1,623 clinics (Merchant Medicine, 2014).

History

The first retail clinic appeared in the Cub Foods grocery store in the Minneapolis-St Paul metropolitan area and was operated by a company called QuickMedx (Appendix A). The clinics were about 120-square feet in size, treated seven common medical conditions (strep throat, mono, flu, pregnancy testing and bladder, ear and sinus infections), and operated on a cash-only basis with a $35 per visit fee (Bohmer & Groberg, 2002; Martin, 2003; MinuteClinic, 2013). While the original strategy not to accept insurance was a deliberate choice to compete on a purely retail level, the clinics soon started to contract with insurance companies such as Blue Cross Blue Shield of Minnesota and Medica (Martin, 2003). As the company began to grow, it changed its name in 2003 to MinuteClinic (MinuteClinic, 2013). In 2006, CVS acquired MinuteClinic, and meanwhile, other retail clinic companies such as the Little Clinic and the Clinic at Target were formed and the field started to grow.

Growth

Retail clinics grew at a slim annual rate of about ten per year between 2000 and 2003 (Taylor, 2008). In the next three years, faster yet still modest growth occurred, bringing the total number of clinics to 130 nationwide by the beginning of 2006 (Kaissi & Charland, 2013a). Industry analysts agree that 2006 was the year when retail clinics finally took off as a new business model, as about 152 new clinics opened in that year. This was followed by two years of exponential growth with 554 and 426 new clinics in 2007 and 2008 respectively. In this three-year period (2006-2008), the net growth of clinics was 999. However, the following two years (2009 and 2010) witnessed a slow-down and even stagnation as the number of clinics opening barely surpassed the number of clinics closing. Another wave of growth seems to have started in 2011 with a net increase of 128 new clinics, followed by 63 new clinics in 2012 and 156 clinics in 2013 (Merchant Medicine, 2013). In a previous paper, we discussed these trends in details:

"The growth period of 2006-2008 can be traced to what was referred to at the time as a 'land grab,' in which competing operators were seeking to be the first to open in new markets regardless of anticipated financial performance. In 2008, with the start of the general economic recession, numerous clinics shut down during the slow spring and summer months and others closed all together, which led some industry experts to predict that the market may be reaching overcapacity and saturation, and that the trend is a bubble that is about to burst. The main reasons behind the slowdown included low profitability and low consumer demand. At the time, studies showed that only 13% of consumers had used a retail clinic in the preceding 12 months. Others disagreed that the trend was slowing permanently and suggested that while the first wave of growth was over, the industry was at an inflection point that will be followed by a fresh wave of growth characterized by new business models. This prediction seems to be coming true based on some encouraging 2011 numbers, although it is too early to predict whether this new growth will be sustainable. Regardless of the yearly changes, however, the results show that 503 clinics have closed in the last six years, pointing to the many challenges that clinics face. These challenges include but are not limited to negative cash flow, people's perceptions of retail clinics, and the newness of the business model. Previous research has shown that it is difficult for retail clinics to be profitable, and many clinics operate below capacity. Many consumers are simply not used to the idea of seeking healthcare at a retail pharmacy or grocery store; they continue to prefer the traditional physician office setting. And while in place for about 12 years, the retail clinic model is still relatively unknown to some owners and there is no template to follow. Some companies have been offering consulting services (Merchant Medicine, Bellin Health/Fast Care) but the model is still not as well understood as other healthcare delivery models. Therefore, clinics that closed during the time period covered by the study have barely survived more than two years on average"(Kaissi & Charland, 2013a, p. 339).

While the growth of retail clinics has been a remarkable phenomenon to observe, the current number of clinics has failed to match past forecasts. For example, in 2006, Peter Miller, chief executive officer of Take Care Health which operates retail clinics at Walgreens drugstores, predicted that the number of clinics would grow to 10,000 by the end of the decade (Landro, 2006). Other forecasts predicted 5,000 clinics by 2010 (Miller, 2007) and 6,000 by 2012 (Scott, 2006), whereas the Deloitte Center for Health Solutions estimated that "those numbers are unattainable in that timeframe" (p. 5) and thus provided a more "conservative" estimate of 2,500 clinics by 2013 (Deloitte Center for Health Solutions, 2009). Those predictions were based partly on wrong assumptions that retail clinics would be easy to operate and turn profits, as well as on the total number of stores owned by retailers operating those clinics such as CVS, Walgreens and Target. These giant organizations operate more than 7,000 stores each, and yet have less than 700 clinics at best, making it a very small clinics-to-store ratio (Merchant Medicine, 2011b). As discussed above, the major obstacle has proven to be a financial one. Tom Ryan, CVS Caremark's chairman, best summarized this: "We took a step back in 2010 to make sure we understood the economics, [MinuteClinic] is off the charts from a customer service standpoint. It's got convenience; it's got accessibility; it's got quality; and it's got low price. The issue is can we get the economics to work"(Merchant Medicine, 2011a, p. 1).

The growth in the number of clinics has been complemented by a growth in usage rates. Numerous studies and surveys have measured usage, often with conflicting results. Early surveys by Harris Interactive suggested that 5% of respondents and their immediate family members in 2007 had used retail clinics (Harris Interactive, 2007). A study by C.S. Mott Children's Hospital in 2007 reported that 11% of adults and 10% of children have visited the clinics (C.S. Mott Children's Hospital, 2007). The Deloitte Center for Health Solutions reported in 2008 that a staggering 16% of consumers had used retail clinics in the last 24 months. However, the most accurate numbers seem to come from the Health Tracking Household Survey conducted by the Center for Studying Health System Change and involving 18,000 people in 9,400 families in 2007. The survey concluded that only 1.2% of American families reported that they had visited retail clinics during the past 12 months while an additional 1.1% reported having visited retail clinics prior to the past 12 months, for a total of 2.3% having ever used a retail clinic (Tu & Cohen, 2008). A follow-up survey involving 17,000 people in 2010 by the same Center found that these rates have grown to 2.9% for usage in the past year, and 2% for usage prior to the last year, bringing the total percentage of people that have ever used a retail clinic to 4.8% (Tu & Boukus, 2013). Despite this growth, the authors noted that retail clinic use remains "modest." More recently, a Harris Interactive/HealthDay online poll of 3,000 adults showed that about 19% have used a retail clinic in 2011-2012 (Gardner, 2013), whereas a research by Kalorama has shown that 21.3% of 2,000 adults have visited a retail clinic in 2012 (Kalorama Information, 2012). In the most recent survey by the Health Research Institute at PwC (2013), 23% of the respondents indicated that they or someone in their household have sought treatment at a retail clinic. Of those, 73% said that they, or the member of their household, would go to retail clinic again in the future.

Other studies have focused on total number of visits. In a national sample, Mehrotra and Lave found that there were 1.48 million retail clinics in 2007. That number increased to 3.52 million visits in 2008 and 5.97 million visits in 2009 (Mehrotra & Lave, 2012). However, when compared to overall outpatient visits, retail clinic visits' share remains low as visits to physician offices annually top 577 million. As insurance coverage became more accepted among retail clinics, Ashwood and his colleagues studied usage among commercially insured patients between 2007 and 2009 (Ashwood et al., 2011). They found that the monthly rate of visits jumped from 0.3 per 1,000 enrollees in January of 2007 to 2.7 per 1,000 enrollees in December of 2009. Given that the majority of visits are for cold-related conditions and infections, it is not surprising to note that usage follows "a clear seasonal pattern with spikes in the winter months and troughs in the summer months" (Ashwood et al., 2011, p. 3). In fact, evidence suggests that many clinics shut down or reduce their operations during the slow spring and summer months (Rubenstein, 2009; Merchant Medicine, 2010).

2. OPERATIONS

Physical Set-Up

Retail clinics are located in small physical areas in grocery stores and drugstore. Early on, the clinics ranged between 200 and 500 square feet, and were often in spaces that generate low income per square feet, such as those typically used for video game arcades, vending machines, or waiting areas near pharmacies (Scott, 2006). They included a reception desk and one or two exam rooms. Many clinics didn't have sinks, toilets or private rooms, which resulted in a "plumbing and privacy" paradigm that forced clinics to focus on non-invasive procedures that don't require disrobing or fluid samples (Scott, 2006). However, more recently, clinics have grown in size to about 400-600 square feet and now typically consist of a small reception desk or kiosk for registration, a waiting area, a couple of exam rooms, a lab area, and a restroom. In large grocery stores, they tend to be located in prime spots such as at the front of the store next to the main cash registers. More attention to design is apparent, as "the clinics need to be a mix of retail and hospitality design with both visibility and curb appeal" (Horwitz-Bennett, 2013, p. 2). The main characteristics of a well-designed clinic include "an open, airy, and friendly environment; achieving HIPAA and code compliance; and designing for privacy, functional efficiency, and comfort, [leading to] patient access and comfort; efficient workspaces for staff; and easy, clear patient flow through the clinic" (Horwitz-Bennett, 2013, p. 2).

Staffing

Retail clinics are primarily staffed by nurse practitioners and physician assistants. These non-physician providers are typically supervised by an off-site physician that is available by phone for consultation. The physician acts as the medical director of the clinic. In this role, he/she provides quality oversight through periodic review of medical charts of patients seen in the clinic. Some clinics also employ a medical assistant/receptionist to take care of patient registration and other administrative issues (Scott, 2006; Hansen-Turton, Ryan, Miller, Counts, & Nash, 2007; Scott, 2013). An exception to this staffing model is the DR Walk-in medical clinics at Duane Read stores in New York which are staffed by licensed physicians (DR Walk-in Medical Clinics, 2013).

In a previous study of hospital-owned and hospital-affiliated retail clinics, we found that staffing was one of the major operational challenges faced by the operators (Kaissi, 2010a). The difficulty in attracting and retaining nurse practitioners that are willing to "sit in a box for ten hours" every day was stressed by the health system executives interviewed in the study. The clinics are open for long hours and their scope of practice is very limited, which can make the work of the clinicians seem unchallenging and repetitive. Hospital operators attempted to recruit and retain non-physician providers by providing higher salaries than those provided in other settings "to compensate them for their boredom and the fact that they are there all by themselves and they do everything for the patient" (Kaissi, 2010a, p. 333). Other systems rotated their providers between retail clinics and other primary care physician clinics on a weekly basis so they can be exposed to other potentially more challenging patients and conditions.

This issue has been addressed by other experts. Tom Charland, CEO of Merchant Medicine, a consulting firm for the convenient care industry, recently noted: "To most who are involved in the retail clinic industry, the match of a nurse practitioner (NP) or physician assistant (PA) and a retail clinic seems a perfect fit. But to the early providers who started practicing in that setting and their peers who did not, the fit was hardly perfect"

(Merchant Medicine, 2012d). In the early days of retail clinics, many non-physician providers did not take pride in their work at the retail clinics as it was viewed negatively by fellow non-physician providers and physicians. These attitudes seem to be changing in recent years. A survey conducted by Merchant Medicine and "Advance for NPs & PAs" found that about 70% of these providers view retail clinics positively, and that about 60% would be interested in working in retail clinics. However, the survey revealed that some providers have still not embraced the concept as can be seen from the following comments (Advance Healthcare Network for NPs and PAs, 2012):

Working at McDonald's is nicer than working at a retail clinic. At least you get support while you work as a team.

As the client based has increased, retail health owners have failed to meet the requirements of the NP.

They rob the patient of the advantages of continuity and a medical home, putting them at risk of inadequate care of their chronic problems.

I am interested in working in a retail clinic but would miss the relationship that is formed in primary care practice

Technology

The Convenient Care Association (CCA), the professional trade group that regulates retail clinics (discussed later in this chapter), mandates all clinics to use an electronic health record (EHR). Some clinics have purchased commercial EHRs, while others have created their own software to allow providers in the clinics to follow evidence-based treatment protocols (Hansen-Turton, Ridgway, Ryan, & Nash, 2009; Schleiter, 2010). These systems ensure consistent decision-making among providers and across clinics, and improve the quality by limiting the scope of practice of the clinics. When a patient presents to the clinic, a provider takes a full oral history and conducts the appropriate exams. All pertinent information is entered into the EHR using a computer located in the exam room. That information is matched to a knowledge base, and the software calculates the appropriate care algorithms for that specific patient. Therefore, if the patient presented with a condition that is outside the scope of practice of the retail clinic or that is potentially emergent or unusual, the software presents a red flag that requires the provider to direct the patient to an emergency room, urgent care center, or primary care physician (PCP) office. While the EHR prompts appropriate diagnosis and treatment, it also allows for the clinical judgment of the provider who ultimately selects the diagnosis code and treatment. Ideally, the EHR is linked to systems used by local physician offices. If a patient already has a primary care physician, their record from the retail clinic visit could be sent to his/her physician's office. Information systems are also used to enhance customer service. In some clinics, electronic check-in through a touch-screen kiosk is available for patients outside the exam room. Similar to airport check-in, the patient can log in and pull out their EHR (if they have used the clinic before) before even seeing a clinician. Other services may include online check-in, online search for locations with the shortest wait time, a magnetic card system to streamline check-in, access to personal health records, and payment. It is also common that the EHRs used by a certain clinic can be accessed from a different clinic site that belongs to the same retailer (Hansen-Turton et al., 2009; Schleiter, 2010).

In a previous study of hospital-owned retail clinics, we found that there was a wide variation in use of computers and electronic systems. Most of the clinics did not have on-line registration but the majority had the capacity to transmit patient encounters electronically by fax, e-mail or shared EHR to the primary care provider. They also had computers in their clinics used for diagnosis/procedure coding; billing management; tracking patient demographics; medical records; payroll management; prescription ordering and lab management, as well as inventory management (Kaissi & Charland, 2013b). Other technological advancements used in retail clinics include compact-diagnostic services. For examples, tests such as those enabling rapid and accurate assessment of blood pressure, glucose, cholesterol, strep throat, urinary tract infections and pregnancy are approved by the FDA as waived by CLIA (Clinical Laboratory Improvement Amendments). Other miniature devices such as ultrasounds that are the size of a laptop also provide affordable technology for retail clinics (Scott, 2006).

More recently, some retail clinics are considering evolving into new care formats via technology relying on telemedicine. In this model, staffing will be provided by a trained medical attendant with diagnostic equipment and an electronic connection to an offsite physician, who would make the diagnosis and treatment. Another "potential innovation is the use of interactive patient-interview software that obtains relevant information from the patient, asks appropriate follow-up questions using a branching logic system, and then creates a summary of relevant information for the clinician before he or she meets the patient" (Weinick, Pollack, Fisher, Gillen, & Mehrotra, 2010, p. 41). Similar models using telemedicine are discussed in Chapter 8.

Geographical Locations

The first study examining the geographic location of retail clinics revealed that, in 2008, they were mostly located in urban areas (88.2%) (Rudavsky, Pollack, & Mehrotra, 2009). At the time, 29.9 million of the U.S. population (10.6%) lived within a 5-minute driving distance to a retail clinic, and 80.7 million (28.7%) lived within a 10-minute driving distance. By 2010, 15.7% of the population lived within a 5-minute driving distance to a retail clinic, and 34.9% lived within a 10-minute driving distance (Tu & Boukus, 2013).

The top five cities in terms of population proximity to retail clinics in 2008 were Nashville (57% within a 5-minute distance, 94% within a 10-minute distance), Minneapolis-St Paul (51%, 96%), Las Vegas (51%, 96%), Milwaukee (44%, 89%), and Miami (43%, 85%) (Rudavsky, Pollack & Mehrotra, 2009). A follow-up study showed that only 12.5% of retail clinics were located in areas that are designated as Health Professional Shortage Areas (HPSA), whereas 20.9% of Americans live in these areas (Rudavsky & Mehrotra, 2010). It also concluded that retail clinics tend to be located in zip codes with higher incomes.

Retail clinics have opened in 40 states across the United States. When the clinics first emerged, nearly half of them were concentrated in five states: Florida, California, Texas, Minnesota and Illinois (Rudavsky et al., 2009). As of 2012, 12 states had at least 50 clinics, with Illinois, Florida and Texas still with the highest numbers. These states tend to have the largest population centers, where retail clinic operators prefer to open clinics. States with low population density, such as Wyoming, Montana, Iowa and Vermont had no retail clinics at the time of writing of this book (Kaissi & Charland, 2013a). Surprisingly, other more populous states such as Washington, Oregon, New Mexico, Arkansas and Alabama do not have any retail clinics either. Table 1 shows the state-by-state location of retail clinics that were in operation in 2012.

Financials

One of the main contributions of retail clinics to healthcare delivery is the provision of a menu-style pricing system that is displayed

Table 1. Clinics still open by state (2012) (Kaissi & Charland, 2013)

State	Clinics still open n (%)
Illinois	119 (8.8%)
Florida	108 (7.9%)
Texas	89 (6.5%)
Ohio	79 (5.8%)
Tennessee	78 (5.7%)
Minnesota	70(5.1%)
Arizona	64(4.7%)
Georgia	62(4.6%)
California	60 (4.4%)
Kentucky	57 (4.2%)
Missouri	54 (4.0%)
Pennsylvania	54 (4.0%)
Indiana	49 (3.6%)
North Carolina	37 (2.7%)
Wisconsin	36 (2.6%)
Maryland	33 (2.4%)
New Jersey	32 (2.4%)
Massachusetts	31 (2.3%)
Colorado	30 (2.2%)
Nevada	28 (2.1%)
Virginia	27 (2.0%)
Kansas	25 (1.8%)
South Carolina	22 (1.6%)
All other states*	116 (8.5%)
Total	1360 (100%)

*all states with less than 20 clinics each

in most sites and on the operators' websites. For example, at CVS' MinuteClinic, minor illness exams, minor injury exams and skin condition exams prices range between $79 and $89 (Table 2). Screenings and physical exams and health condition monitoring range between $59 and $79, whereas vaccinations range between $31.99 and $229.99. Laboratory tests range between $79 and $89 with specific additional charges per test (MinuteClinic, 2013). Similar prices are listed for Take Care clinics at Walgreens (Walgreens, 2013) and RediClinic (RediClinic, 2013). Patients with insurance coverage have a co-pay that is similar or less than their primary care physician co-pay, depending on their individual plan (Ashwood et al., 2011).

In their early days, retail clinics were cash-only businesses. Clinic operators did not initially accept insurance due to concerns that the claims process is inefficient and expensive. For example, for a typical physician office, billing-related expenses such as staffing, documentation, information technology, delays in accounts receivables and unpaid claims account for 30% of operations costs (Scott, 2006). Given the newness of the clinics, the operators could not support these overhead costs. However, as previously mentioned, MinuteClinic started negotiations with Blue Cross Blue Shield of Minnesota to design a radically different system that would not be as people and paper-intensive. The system they agreed on was extremely simple: 100% payment by the insurer for 100% of the claims within 10-14 days. Blue Cross Blue Shield agreed to a trial period, and once the model proved successful, it became the mainstream claims process for retail clinic operators (Scott, 2006). In 2006, 40% of retail clinics were accepting insurance. That rate increased to 85% in 2007, thus "enabling the clinics to

Table 2. Price menu at CVS' MinuteClinic (MinuteClinic, 2013)

Service	Price (Additional Charge)
Minor illness exam (Allergy symptoms -ages 2+; Bronchitis / cough; Earache / ear infection; Flu-like symptoms; Lice; Mononucleosis (mono); Motion sickness prevention; Sinus infection / congestion; Pink eye & styes; Sore throat / strep throat; Upper respiratory infection; Urinary tract / bladder infection-females ages 12+)	$79-$89
Minor injury exam (Blisters; Bug bites & stings; Deer tick bites; Jellyfish stings; Minor burns; Minor cuts & lacerations ; Minor wounds & abrasions; Splinter removal; Sprains / strains (ankle, knee); Suture & staple removal)	$79-$89
Skin condition exam (Acne; Athlete's foot; Chicken pox; Cold sores & canker sores; Impetigo; Lice ; Minor skin infections and rashes; Oral / mouth sores; Poison ivy / oak -ages 3+; Ringworm; Scabies; Shingles; Styes; Sunburn; Swimmer's itch ; Wart evaluation -ages 5+)	$79-$89
Screenings	
Basic health screening	$59
Cholesterol screening	$59
Comprehensive health screening	$69
Diabetes screening (glucose)	$69
Physical exams	
Administrative physicals	$69
Camp physical	$59
College physical	$69
DOT physical	$79
Sports physical	$59
Other Services	
Birth control injection	$20-$100
Ear wax removal	$79-$89
EpiPen refill	$59
Medication renewal (one time)	$59
Pregnancy evaluation	$59
Smoking cessation	$59
TB (tuberculosis) testing	$39
Vitamin B12 injection (prescription required)	$21
Weight loss program	$59-$69
Health Condition Monitoring	
A1c check	$59
Diabetes monitoring	$79
High blood pressure evaluation	$79
High cholesterol monitoring	$79
Vaccinations	
DTaP (diphtheria, tetanus, pertussis) $99.99	$99.99

Table 2. Continued

Service	Price (Additional Charge)
Flu – Seasonal (preservative-free available)	$31.99
Flu - High Dose (ages 65+)	$49.99
Flu – Intradermal (90% smaller needle)	$36.99
Hepatitis A (adult)	$139.99
Hepatitis A (child)	$112.99
Hepatitis B (adult) $139.99	$139.99
Hepatitis B (child) $112.99	$112.99
HPV (human papillomavirus) – Gardasil®	$229.99
IPV (polio)	$109.99
Meningitis	$144.99
MMR (measles, mumps, rubella)	$129.99
PPSV (pneumonia)	$79.99
Td (tetanus, diphtheria)	$89.99
Tdap (tetanus, diphtheria, pertussis)	$64.99
Labs and Tests	$79-$89
Blood sugar test	($19)
Flu test influenza A & B	($30 each)
HbA1c	($29)
Mononucleosis (mono) test	($20)
Cholesterol screen (Lipid panel)	($34)
Negative quick strep	($30)
Pregnancy test	($20)
Quick strep	($27)
Urine dip stick	($25)

enter the mainstream healthcare system with the benefit of inclusion in insurance coverage, the credibility conveyed by the carrier, and a price that consumers find affordable" (Laws & Scott, 2008, p. 1294). By 2008, 97% of the clinics were accepting private insurance, 93% were accepting Medicare fee-for-service, and 60% were accepting some form of Medicaid (Rudavsky et al., 2009). Nowadays, all clinics accept all types of insurance. A recent study found that for 28% of retail clinic patients insurance paid all the costs, for 39% insurance paid some of the costs and for 16% insurance paid none of the costs. Moreover, 11% of patients did not have health insurance, and 6% had health insurance but chose to pay with cash (Boehringer Ingelheim Pharmaceuticals, Inc., 2010).

Retail clinic operators and industry experts agree that the retail clinic business and economic model is extremely challenging. First, the cost of opening a retail medical clinic "includes the cost of design and construction of clinic space, including meeting building code requirements, infrastructure for electronic medical records systems, technology for practitioners to provide evidence-based care, marketing for the brand, and the cost of recruiting and training personnel" (Schleiter, 2010, p. 537-538). The physical retrofitting of the clinic space, often ranging between $25,000 and $145,000, is paid by the retailers. Once in operation, fixed costs such as labor, insurance, information technology, rent and corporate overhead account for 85% of the costs, whereas variable costs such as supplies and laboratory tests account for the rest. An average clinic has fixed costs of about $600,000 annually. Visits generate an average of $52, so in order to breakeven, clinics need to have 11,500 visits per year, which translates to more than 30 per day or 2-3 patients every hour (Scott, 2006). Therefore, clinics need between 18-36 months to recoup the investments for the retailers (Weinick et al., 2010). In a previous study, a clinic medical director that we interviewed summarized the issue: "The margin of profitability is very narrow, if you are seeing 25-30 patients per day then you need to hire a second clinician, which is very expensive. No one is going to make a lot of money from this business" (Kaissi, 2010, p. 332). Given these financial difficulties, it is not surprising that many clinics witness financial distress and close over the years. In fact, several operators such as CheckUps, QuickHealth, CornerCare, SmartCare, and WellnessExpress have gone out of business (Costello, 2008; Dolan, 2009; Mehrotra, Wang, Lave, Adams, & McGlynn, 2008). And while Wal-Mart had publicly announced in 2007 its desire to open thousands of clinics, it hosted less than 150 clinics in 2013, after a series of closings (Banjo, 2012). In a study of hospital-owned retail clinics, only 4 out of 19 hospital systems reported that their first owned retail clinic was operating at breakeven (Kaissi & Charland, 2013b).

It is important to note though that from the retailers' perspective, the clinics can bring in indirect revenue that go beyond what patients spend in the clinic or what their insurance claims amount to. Most clinics are located in stores that have an on-site pharmacy (Kaissi & Charland, 2013a). Therefore, retailers hope that while customers are in the store to be seen at the clinic, they might fill their prescription at the store's pharmacy, purchase over-the-counter medications, or otherwise buy miscellaneous items from the store, thus "expanding their basket" (Scott, 2006, p. 19). For example, MinuteClinics see about 25-30 patients per day. About 70% of these patients become new pharmacy visits, 38% buy an over-the-counter product, and 80% buy general items from the store during their visit (Eder, 2005). At the Clinic at Target, 95% of patients get their prescription filled at the same store, and pharmacy sales in some stores increased 15% within a year of opening the clinic. About 90% of patients end up buying something from the store, even though the original reason for their visit was to receive care and not to shop (Salganik, 2004).

In general, experts suggest that for "a clinic to be viable, a drugstore should receive at least 8,000 weekly shopped visits, a grocery store 20,000 and mass merchandisers 40,000 or more" (Scott, 2013). However, retail clinic operators and researchers suggest that the search for the perfect business model and location is still proving to be elusive. For example, Web Golinkin, Chief Executive Officer of RediClinic, a chain of retail clinics located at HEB grocery stores across Texas stated: "The business model is still challenging. You have to process a lot of patients at a relatively low margin. So how do you turn it into a sustainable business? We are providing value; there is no question about that. But the question is how to create a sustainable, efficient model? So while the challenges in the past were external, todays' challenges are more internal in nature. We have invented a new business, and even though we have served about one million patients, we are still inventing the business every day" (Golinkin, personal interview, 2013). Similarly, Ateev Mehrotra, a retail clinic researcher at Rand Corporation suggested: "Starbucks can predict based on market factors and traffic and demographics where to locate a coffee shop that will be successful. Retail clinics operators have not figured that out yet. Otherwise, they would be exploding" (Mehrotra, personal interview, 2013). However, in a more recent correspondence, Dr. Mehrotra noted that "it appears that MinuteClinic now has a much better sense of the success of a clinic and is expanding quite rapidly" (Mehrotra, personal correspondence, 2014).

Scope of Services

By design, retail clinics offer a very limited scope of practice. In a review of 1.35 million clinic visits in 2008, Mehrotra and his colleagues found that 90.3% of the visits are for ten simple acute conditions and preventative care: upper respiratory infections, sinusitis, bronchitis, pharyngitis, immunizations, otitis media, otitis externa, conjunctivitis, urinary tract infections, and screening lab test or blood pressure check (Mehrotra et al., 2008). These conditions account for only 18% of all primary care physician office visits and 12% of all emergency room visits. A follow-up study in 2012 showed that the ten conditions still accounted for the majority of visits (Mehrotra & Lave, 2012).

Another review of 42 operators and 982 retail clinics showed that 100% of the clinics offered treatment of sore throats and coughs, 99.7% offered treatment for minor skin conditions, 98.9% offered immunizations, 96.2% offered routine preventative health examinations or screenings such as cholesterol testing or diabetes testing, 96.0% offered pregnancy testing, and 95.6% offered treatment of allergies (Rudavsky et al., 2009). Only 57.6% of the clinics offered smoking cessation counseling, 4.8% offered travel-related services, 3.0% offered HIV and/or sexually transmitted disease testing or counseling, 1.6% offered prescription refills, and 1.2% offered weight loss counseling (Rudavsky et al., 2009). According to the Center for Health System Change 2010 Health Tracking Household survey, 69.1% of all retail clinic users reported that the primary purpose of their most recent visit was the diagnosis and treatment of a new illness or symptom. About 25.8% reported that vaccination was the reason for their visit, whereas 21.0% visited the clinic to renew their prescriptions and 12.7% to receive a physical exam for school, camp or employment (Tu & Boukus, 2013).

An interesting development in the reason for patients' visits to retail clinics is the increase in vaccinations and other preventative services. A comparison between the 2000-2006 and 2007-2009 time periods showed that preventative care (vaccines and other services) jumped from 21.8% to 47.5%, whereas acute care decreased from 78.2% to 51.4% (Mehrotra & Lave, 2012). Vaccination appears to be the main service sought by older patients (65 + years), as three quarters of their visits to retail clinics are for immunizations (Mehrotra et al., 2008). More specifically, an examination of 8.9 million retail clinic visits between 2007 and 2009 showed that the number of visits in which one or more vaccinations were administered increased from about 470,000 in 2007 to 1.9 million in 2009 (Uscher-Pines, Harris, Burns, & Mehrotra, 2012). The percentage of visits that included a vaccination increased from 39.9% in 2007 to 42.0% in 2009. Injectable influenza vaccinations account for the lion's share of all vaccinations with 96.2% in 2007 and 94.1% in 2009. Other vaccines administered include pneumococcal, tetanus, meningitis, measles mumps and rubella, hepatitis A, hepatitis B, human pappilovirus and polio. These numbers hint that retail clinics are playing an increasingly important public health role in the communities in which they operate. However, despite the remarkable increase in number of vaccines given, the results also suggest that only 1% of all the influenza vaccine doses given in the United States in 2008 were administered at retail clinics. In addition, "it appears that the typical retail clinic patient who received one or more recommended vaccinations was not "outside the medical system" but perhaps chose vaccination at retail clinics rather than medical offices because of convenience or because a regular provider did not offer the full range of recommended vaccinations" (Uscher-Pines et al., 2012, p. 66).

Days, Hours of Operation, and Wait Times

One of the basic convenience premises for retail clinics is their availability after hours on weekday evenings and weekends, when primary care physician offices are typically closed for business. A random sample of 98 retail clinics in 2008 showed that all had weekday and weekend hours and 97% were open some weekday evening hours (such as after 6:00 pm) (Rudavsky et al., 2009). Day-by-day analyses of visits between 2007 and 2009 concluded that Monday is the most popular day (16.4% of visits) while Sunday is the least popular day (10.7% of visits). However, about 29% of all visits occurring Monday to Friday were after 5:00 pm, a time when physician offices are closed. In addition, 15.5% of visits occurred during the weekend, which amounts to 44.4% of retail clinic visits occurring when physicians are not available (Mehrotra & Lave, 2012). Another study by Walgreens confirmed these numbers and showed that 44.6% of all retail clinics encounters occurred on weekends and weekday evenings (Patwardhan, Davis, Murphy, & Ryan, 2012). More recently, a study by Athena Health compared retail clinic and primary care physician visits by day and time. For physician offices, 93% of visits were during the weekday peek-hours (between 8:00 am and 6:00 pm), while only 4% of visits occurred during weekday off-peak hours (after 6:00 pm) and only 3% occurred on weekends (Grossman, 2013). In contrast, 58% of retail clinic visits were during the weekday peek-hours, 26% occurred on weekends and 16% occurred during weekday off-peak hours. Our previous analyses of 1,864 retail clinics between 2006 and 2012 indicated that clinics are open an average of 11 hours during weekdays, 8.5 hours on Saturdays and 7 hours on Sundays (Kaissi & Charland, 2013a).

These results imply overall that retail clinic providers are acting as important extenders for physician practices and are providing an alternative for the treatment of minor conditions to expensive settings such as emergency rooms and to a lesser extent urgent care centers. More worrying for physicians, what the results also show is that some patients are trusting retail clinics for the treatment of non-emergent conditions even when physician offices are open (Patwardhan et al., 2012).

Another major convenience aspect of retail clinics is the walk-in aspect and the short wait times. Some clinics even use pagers, such as those used in restaurants, to alert patients that a provider is available, which allows the patient to wonder around the store instead of waiting in the clinic itself (Callahan, 2007). A study conducted by Saperstein Associates, a public opinion research firm in Columbus, Ohio and commissioned by Boehringer Ingelheim Pharmaceuticals, Inc. showed that in sample of 513 retail clinic users, 21% were seen immediately, 54% waited less than 15 minutes, 19% waited between 15 and 30 minutes, and only 7% waited more than 30 minutes. The overall average wait time was 15 minutes (Boehringer Ingelheim Pharmaceuticals, Inc, 2010). The Athena study mentioned above specified that in retail clinics, the average check-in time is 0.4 minutes, the average wait time is 12.4 minutes, the average exam time is 15.6 minutes, the average sign-off time is 0.9 minutes, and the average check-out time is 2.7 minutes, for a total average visit time of 32 minutes. On the other hand, for primary care physician visits for the same conditions, the average check-in time is 2.0 minutes, the average wait time is 13.0 minutes, the average exam time is 45.3 minutes, the average sign-off time is 8.1 minutes, and the average check-out time is 13.5 minutes, for a total average visit time of 81.9 minutes. Therefore, the "retail clinic advantage" is 61% lower total visit time, 7% lower wait time and 66% lower exam time (Grossman, 2013).

Quality Assurance

Retail clinics offer healthcare services in a non-traditional setting and delivered by non-traditional providers. Therefore, ensuring quality of care is of crucial importance to gain credibility and public trust. The evidence suggests that many quality assurance programs are in place and are enforced internally as well as by external bodies and agencies. The majority of retail clinics are members of the Convenient Care Association (CCA). The CCA requires member clinics to conform to its Quality and Safety Standards. These guidelines are rooted in evidence-based protocols published by the American Academy of Pediatrics (APA) and the American Association of Family physicians (AAFP) (Hansen-Turton et al., 2007). The enforcement of these standards is done by the Jefferson School of Population Health, which acts as a third party to develop and conduct reviews of clinics (Miller & Nash, 2013). The initial application process requires clinics to provide documentation of the following standards:

- "Credentialing of providers
- Ongoing quality monitoring
- Coordination of care with outside providers (copy of visit notes faxed to primary care provider if the patient requests
- Provision to the patient of a written visit record with clear discharge instructions
- Encouragements of patients to form relationships and follow-up with primary care physicians (PCPs) and making referrals as indicated
- Health promotion and preventative screening information
- Compliance with regulatory standards (such as HIPAA, OSHA, and CDC guidelines)
- Use of electronic health records (EHRs)
- Peer and collaborative physician chart review
- Maintenance of a safe, infection-free environment
- Mechanisms to empower patients to make informed choices
- Emergency response procedures"

Clinics found to have met the guidelines are granted CCC certification for two years. Recertification can be achieved if clinics show evidence of additional quality improvement strategies, such as waiting time reports, patient satisfaction surveys and evidence of appropriateness of care based on chart reviews. The clinics must submit action plans to address any deficiencies (Miller & Nash, 2013). Clinics also have the option to get accredited by the Joint Commission, the main agency that accredits hospitals and other healthcare organizations in the United States. Accreditation is granted based on the Comprehensive Accreditation Manual for Ambulatory Care (CAMAC), which applies to ambulatory care, ambulatory surgery centers, diagnostic imaging services, patient-centered medical homes and urgent care (Joint Commission, 2013).

In addition, many clinic operators have incorporated their own rigorous quality assessments. For example, MinuteClinic incorporates guidelines from the Institute for Clinical Systems Improvement (ICSI) in its homegrown Electronic Medical Record (EMR). ICSI is a nonprofit organization composed of health plans and physician groups, and has published a series of clinical guidelines. For example, the ICSI pharyngitis (sore throat) guideline that is incorporated into MinuteClinic's EMR consists of the following: "When a nurse practitioner sees a patient with a sore throat, the electronic health record protocol guides him or her through a standardized set of ISCI guideline clinical history questions and elements of the physical examination. For example, the guideline includes questions about the onset of the sore throat and about whether the patient has experienced a fever, abdominal pain, a runny nose, a cough, or vomiting. The physical exam includes checking, whether the tonsils have an exudate (a whitish coating) and whether the patient has a rash. This history and these physical elements are documented using a combination of electronic checkbox selections, drop-down menus, and free text. The protocol forces the provider to the next step in the guideline, for example presenting, in the case of pharyngitis, first-line antibiotic choices (if a prescription is indicated). If the provider chooses to provide care outside the protocol or if additional documentation is warranted, free-text fields can be used to capture this information"(Weinick, et al., 2010, p.35). To achieve this, MinuteClinic has dedicated clinicians who review the research literature and recommendations from groups such as ICSI, AAFP and AAP. A guideline committee consisting of physicians, practitioners and pharmacists then reviews the guidelines and approves them, before they are subject to a secondary review and approval by a governance committee, consisting of additional physicians and nurse practitioners (Merchant Medicine, 2012c).

RediClinic, a chain of clinics based in Houston, Texas, does not use ICSI guidelines and is not accredited by the Joint Commission, but instead has a thorough internal quality program in place. For example, RediClinic has 16 measures that are tracked on an ongoing basis:

1. "Appropriate treatment for children with URI and nonstrep pharyngitis
2. Appropriate testing for children with Pharyngitis
3. Avoidance of inappropriate antibiotic treatment in adults with URI and acute bronchitis
4. Adult and child BMI assessment and follow-up
5. Immunizations for adolescents

6. Influenza immunization for patients 50 years or older
7. Influenza immunization for high risk patients aged 18-64
8. Pneumonia vaccination for patients 65 years and older
9. Pneumonia vaccination for high risk (define, where?) patients aged 18-64
10. Inquiry regarding tobacco use
11. Advising smokers to quit
12. Adult patients screened for at-risk drinking
13. Tetanus immunization in past 10 years for patients 12 years or older
14. Use of appropriate medications for people with asthma
15. Asthma symptoms assessment
16. Documentation and verification of current medications in the medical record"

Web Golinkin, RediClinic's CEO summarizes his company's commitment to quality: "There are many layers to our commitment to high-quality care. It starts with the fact that our clinics are staffed with licensed nurse practitioners and physician assistants, supported by medical assistants. These clinicians are supervised by local physicians, who regularly review patient charts and are available to provide support 24/7 if necessary. Our clinicians use evidence-based protocols, and we have a corporate medical director who ensures that "standards of care" are followed in every clinic. In addition, we have a quality assurance program in which we evaluate our performance against key healthcare industry benchmarks. We also have strict protocols that govern when patients need to be referred to other providers for treatment of conditions that are outside of our scope of practice or who need ongoing care, and we use an electronic medical record system that, among other things, facilitates record sharing with other providers. We are founding members of the Convenient Care Association, and adhere to their Quality & Safety standards, and this is verified through a third-party certification process. The result of all this is that we have treated more than 1.4 million patients without any safety issues. We know that – while the convenience and affordability RediClinics offer is very appealing to consumers- quality is job #1. We also know that poor performance by any operator in this area can spoil it for everyone, which is why we have been very active in our industry association and helping to ensure that it has a strong quality focus" (Golinkin, personal interview, 2013).

Take Care Health clinics (operated by Walgreens), on the other hand, track and trend HEDIS (Healthcare Effectiveness Data and Information Set) scores against the national average for a variety of conditions such as streptococcal infections, bronchitis, and upper respiratory infections. HEDIS is a widely used set of performance measures developed and maintained by the National Committee for Quality Assurance (NCQA) and primarily used in the managed care industry (Takach & Witgert, 2009). HealthRite (operated by AtlantiCare Physician Group) mandates that all its nurse practitioners undergo a 30-day clinical practice guidelines "boot camp." The camp provides an intensive orientation at a full-scope primary care facility, thus exposing the providers to a wide range of patients, diagnoses and treatments. New providers' treatment files are also reviewed at 100% for the first 90 days, and then at 10% towards the end of their first year at the clinics (Takach & Witgert, 2009).

Despite these assurances, some experts have legitimately questioned whether physician professionalism and agency on behalf of the patient can be replaced. For example, Schleiter (2010) warned: "Physician-informed or based on their own research, and driven by their own financial interest, insured patients are increasingly expected to decide which healthcare services and goods are worth the cost at each point of purchase in the healthcare system. However, few can negotiate the healthcare market wisely, and missteps can destroy patients economically. Doctors or contracts rarely specify upfront fees for services provided. Though this is understandable-physicians deal with a number of insurers, each with fees negotiated in a market that regards prices as trade secrets-patients are left not knowing and unable to discover upfront what such things will cost. It is even harder to anticipate hospital charges. This consumer-driven model of healthcare may have its drawbacks. The model calls for a fundamental reordering of the patient-physician relationship wherein the physician is no longer the ultimate decision-maker. Increased reliance is placed on commercial ethics, and professional ethics is diminished as the guiding force for patient-physician interactions. [...] As patients continue to take medical decision-making into their own hands, the market must adapt to offer consumer protection and guidance for these important decisions" (p. 260).

Marketing

Consumer awareness and perception of retail clinics remains an important hurdle for retail clinic long-term success. While usage rates and visit numbers have increased over the years, a large majority of the American public still does not know what a retail clinic is and what conditions are treated. According to recent studies, between 80 and 95% of Americans have never set foot in a retail clinic (Tu & Boukus, 2013; Gardner, 2013; Kalorama Information, 2012). A recent survey of non-users of retail clinics have shown that many are not sure what services are offered (13%), are concerned about the quality of care (13%) and are not sure where a retail clinic is located near them (13%) (Boehringer Ingelheim Pharmaceuticals, Inc., 2010).

In a previous study on hospital-affiliated and hospital-owned retail clinic, a hospital system vice president we interviewed summarized the situation: "Some of the challenges that we faced was getting people to understand what the retail clinic does. To get lay people realize that they don't need to see a doctor and that is a different mind-set. People did not recognize that this clinic might be of the same caliber as an urgent care clinic, because this was located in a grocery store. Plus you had to rely on people coming to [the grocery store], people do not come the retail clinic as a destination of its own. If you have a headache or a bad cold, you would not come to [the grocery store] and then find out about the retail clinic" (Kaissi, 2010a, p. 332). He added: "the challenge for retail clinics is to do a better job marketing themselves and to have a robust model. So that the average person understands what they do, and for this to work, you need a significant revolution in people's thinking. And this is not going to happen overnight, if it is ever going to" (Kaissi, 2010b, p.332).

It is also important to note that retail clinics require consumers to significantly change their behavior. They have to accept care in a different location and from a different kind of provider. While the clinics are very convenient, change may come very slowly. For example, innovations in the banking sector took a long time to gain acceptance. The first ATM (Automated Teller Machine) was installed outside a bank in 1967 and ATMs became available in the 1980's. However, widespread acceptance and usage did not come till the early 1990's. Therefore, it won't be surprising if it takes about twenty years for the majority of patients accept and use retail clinics (Scott, 2006).

Appropriate and effective marketing of retail clinic services is crucial. In the past, the sole marketing effort was is in-store, and advertising was not part of the promotional mix (Deloitte Center for Health Solutions, 2009). Some operators also relied exclusively on word-of-mouth. However, recent evidence suggests that operators, especially hospital systems owning retail clinics, have invested in more aggressive marketing tactics. When asked about how they have heard about the retail clinic, the majority of patients report that it was by word of mouth (34.8%), print advertising (12.0%); and direct mail (7.9%). The approaches used by hospital systems to promote their clinics vary, but the most common media outlets include direct mail, Internet banner/website, print advertising, radio advertising, and sponsoring community events (Kaissi & Charland, 2013b). A case-in-point is Heartland Health which operates retail clinics at Wal-Mart. Heartland contracted with Truven Health Marketing Solutions to identify patients that are likely to use retail services, and used advanced, data-based segmentation to reach those patients (Truven Health Analytics, 2012).

Regulatory Issues

Many regulatory issues govern the ownership, operations and scope of practice of retail clinics. These include retail clinic-specific state laws, corporate practice of medicine laws, anti-trust laws and laws affecting independence and scope of practice of non-physician providers. State legislatures are required to support the public health and safety and ensure that basic structural requirements are in place in order for healthcare facilities to provide safe, quality care in their states. Since they are medical facilities, many states treat retail clinics as physician practices and regulate them through the state's medical board. To date, only the state of Massachusetts has passed specific regulations related to retail clinics. Other state policy makers seem to be in a "wait-and-see" mode to determine if retail clinics are here to stay and thus warrant their own specific regulations (National Conference of State Legislatures, 2012). Meanwhile, states can regulate "the buildings or the people who work in the buildings"(Takach & Witgert, 2009, p. 10).

The Commonwealth of Massachusetts passed retail clinic-specific legislation in 2008. The legislation focused on the establishment and operations of retail clinics and was the subject of intense debate, especially in relation to anticompetitive issues. In 2006, CVS' Minute Clinic requested permission to open clinics in Massachusetts. However, existing clinic regulations did not fit within the retail clinic model. For the state to license the clinics, multiple waivers needed to be granted and the scope of services offered by the clinics could not be limited. Moreover, regulations related to the physical space, potential for fragmentation of care, and concerns raised by physicians were lacking. Therefore, the Massachusetts Department of Public Health (MDPH) held public hearings and heard testimonies from the Federal Trade Commission (FTC), the Massachusetts Association of Family Physicians, and the Massachusetts

Medical Society. Issues raised related to corporate profits, fragmentation of care, tobacco sales, nurse practitioners practicing without supervision and related quality and safety issues. The legislation ultimately passed and MinuteClinic opened the first retail clinics in the state. The regulation was a pioneer especially that it was the first in the country to address ways to improve cooperation between retail clinics and primary care physicians. The law focused on credentialing of non-physician providers to ensure sufficient staffing, age and medical conditions treated, proper medical record keeping procedures, referral procedures, and treatment of repeat patients. And while it does not prohibit alcohol or tobacco sales outright, the law regulates the sale of tobacco products if the clinic is located in a retailer that sells such products (Takach & Witgert, 2009; Schleiter, 2010). Specific requirements of the regulation are listed below (RMCs refer to Retail Medical Clinics):

- "RMCs must make referrals to primary care providers including physicians, nurse practitioners and community health centers
- RMCs must develop a process to identify and limit, if necessary, the number of
- repeat encounters with individual patients
- RMCs must prominently post (a) a list of the services provided (b) a statement that indicates that the patient should seek care from his primary care practitioner or; emergency care provider for all other complaints or concerns ; and (c) a statement that indicates that the patient may purchase prescription medication at any location.
- With patient consent, RMCs will provide a copy of the visit encounter to the patient's primary care providers
- If the RMC is located within a retail location that sells tobacco products, the clinic must post information regarding tobacco usage.
- RMCs must provide a toll-free number that will enable the caller to speak w/a practitioner during off-hours
- RMCs are not required to provide a reception area.
- RMCs examination rooms must be at least 56 square feet.
- Each RMC must provide hand sanitizer outside examination rooms"(Massachusetts Department of Public Health, 2008)

The Massachusetts' legislation has served as a model law for other states to learn from or follow. Illinois and Oklahoma have attempted to pass retail clinic-specific regulations but with no success. In Illinois, retail clinics are classified as physician offices, and are not licensed or subject to oversight by the Illinois Department of Public Health (IDPH) and are not required to obtain certificate of need licensure. The legislation that did not pass was backed by the state's medical society and would have imposed a requirement for clinics to acquire a permit before they could open. Other states have taken different approaches. California and Texas have corporate practice of medicine laws and strict nurse practitioner supervision laws. Both states have tried to work around those regulations to allow greater access to retail clinics. New Jersey has allowed retail clinics to organize under a "captive physician" model, whereas Florida has strict control over retail clinic licensing through recent regulations relating to general healthcare clinics (Schleiter, 2010).

Corporate practice of medicine is a legal doctrine that prohibits people that are not a licensed medical providers from interfering with a physician's professional medical judgment and that bans organizations and corporations from directly employing physicians. These state laws are designed to ensure that physician professional medical judgment and treatment decisions are not influenced by managerial or other type of non-medical control. In relation to retail clinics, corporate practice of medicine laws make it very hard for the clinics to operate and control the quality or standard of care since they cannot employ physicians directly. Clinic operators in states with these kinds of laws have adopted different ownership arrangements. For example, under the "captive physician" model mentioned above, the retail clinic is legally owned by a physician or a group of physicians but is closely tied to a corporation by contractual and managerial agreements. However, corporate practice of medicine laws appear to be on the decline and many states are considering eliminating them. Therefore they are not likely to affect the future growth of retail clinics (Takach & Witgert, 2009; Schleiter, 2010).

Federal antitrust laws have a significant impact on retail clinics. These laws are enforced by the Federal Trade Commission (FTC) and aim to regulate commerce and prevent anticompetitive conduct that discourages competition in the market. Some of the states mentioned above have attempted to over-regulate retail clinics due to pressure from physician groups (Deloitte Center for Health Solutions, 2008; Schleiter, 2010). The FTC has investigated the effects of these proposed regulations and had sought to limit the anticompetitive and anti-consumer effects of unnecessary restrictions. For example, the Illinois bill discussed above was the subject of intense examination and criticism from the FTC. The bill intended to prohibit the sale of alcohol or tobacco products in stores with clinics, but the FTC argued that the bill "would put retail clinics at a competitive disadvantage without offering countervailing consumer benefits" for Illinois consumers. Moreover the bill sought to put advertising restrictions on retail clinics but the FTC interpreted the provisions as having the potential to prohibit consumer access to truthful and non-misleading information about prices for basic medical services. The Illinois bill also required that a physician be the medical director of no more than two clinics, but the FTC found the reasoning behind such a provision to be unclear. Moreover, the bill stated that retail clinics should charge insured customers the same co-payment, deductible, or coinsurance requirements that they would pay for a visit to a physician or non-physician provider. But the FTC reasoned that this requirement would limit the ability of clinic operators to negotiate favorable contracts with third-party payers which might result in higher prices. In summary, while the FTC "commended Illinois in its efforts to open new points of access to healthcare through new models of delivery," it expressed serious concerns that the bill may have "caused undue burden on retail clinics, thereby limiting their ability to compete" (Takach & Witgert, 2009, p. 13). The FTC's comments were considered a significant win for the retail clinic industry and a blow to various state-level physician organizations (Deloitte Center for Health Solutions, 2008).

Scope of practice laws governing the provision of healthcare services by non-physician providers were discussed in chapter 3. A recent study has concluded that these state-specific laws have significant effects on delivery of services in retail clinics. The review of insurance claims in 27 states found that when nurse practitioners are allowed to practice independently from physicians, the cost savings of retail clinic episodes were even greater than when they could not (Spetz, Parente, Town, & Bazarko, 2013).

In summary, the legal environment surrounding retail clinics has witnessed many push and pull forces from the medical societies, the FTC, the retail clinic operators and the general public. Much remains to be seen about whether a federal law governing retail clinics will be passed or whether states will continue to grapple separately with their own regulatory issues. As Schleiter notes: "… many legal questions relating to [retail clinics] remain unanswered" and "as the clinics continue to develop, so too will the laws that guide them" (Schleiter, 2010, p. 548).

3. STAKEHOLDERS

Many organizations, groups, associations and individual providers affect and are affected by retail clinics. In a 2006 article, Malvey and Fottler offered a stakeholder assessment that predicted the potential effects of retail clinics on a variety of players in the healthcare system. In the assessment (revised in a 2010 book), the main winners were considered to be insurance companies and third-party payers, hospital emergency departments, specialist physicians, non-physician providers, urgent care clinics, employers, patients, and policymakers. The main losers were thought to be primary care physicians and medical group practices, whereas hospital systems were classified as potential winners/losers, depending on their ability to collaborate with, become subcontractors for, and extend services of retail clinics (Figure 1)(Malvey & Fottler 2006; Fottler & Malvey, 2010). In this section, we assess the position of various stakeholders and review the research and evidence pertaining to their relationships with retail clinics.

Consumers and Patients

Traditional healthcare providers have always thought of patients as passive, inactive, noninformed and totally dependent on their physicians. Early on in the retail clinic experiment, many questions about consumer behavior were raised. Laws and Scott (2008) asked: "Would services at retail clinics replace visits to EDs or PCPs, or would they simply be additive? Would retail clinics disrupt the PCP relationship? Would consumers prove smart enough to shop for healthcare services and choose appropriate venues of care for their conditions and overall health? Would consumers prefer this venue, or would they consider it to be an inferior substitute choice of locations or providers? Would price transparency prove to be a powerful force in the market?"(p. 1295).

Consumer demographics have been well assessed and studied in the last eight years. It is widely thought that the profile of the typical retail clinic consumer is a middle aged male that has never visited a primary care physician. However, the data suggests that the picture is a bit more complex than that. An early study of MinuteClinic users found that there is an equal split between males and females, that 40% are non-white (vs. 18% for non-users), 28% have less than \$40,000 household income (vs. 16% for non-users), 30% are between the ages of 19-30 (vs. 17% for non-users), 28% do not have a primary physician (vs. 15% for

Figure 1. Stakeholder model for retail clinics (Kaissi, 2010a)

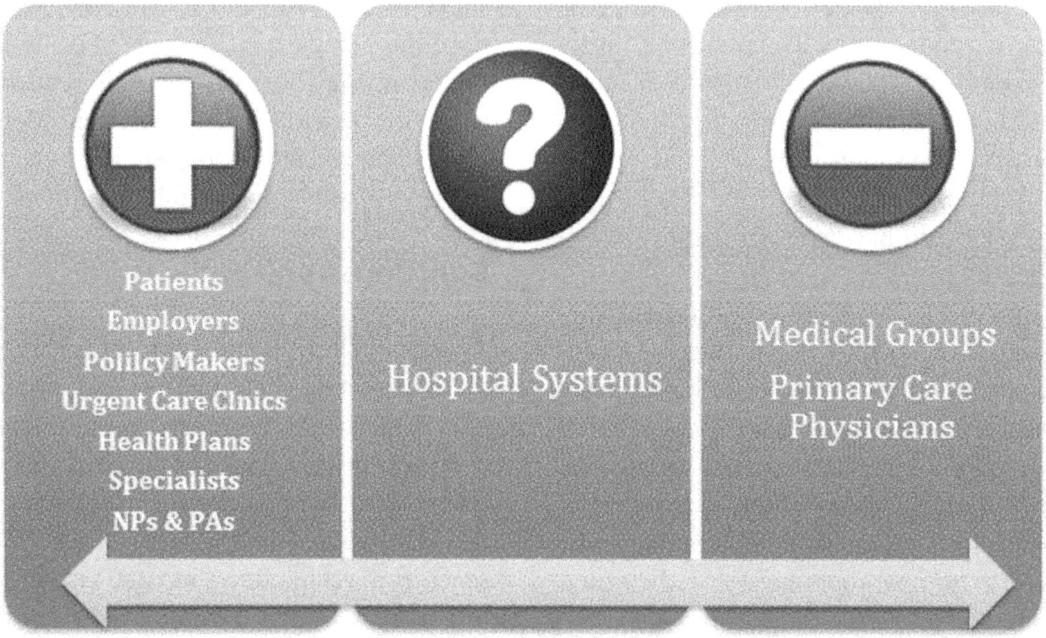

non-users) and 12% are uninsured (vs. 6% for non-users)(Market Strategies, 2007).

Subsequent academic studies found that general retail clinic consumers tend be in the 18-44 years age group. Compared to patients that visit traditional primary care physician offices, that age group has twice as many visits to retail clinics. On the other hand, patients that are younger than 18 years and older than 44 years are more likely to visit primary care physicians and hospital emergency rooms (Mehrotra et al., 2008). Similarly, younger families (those with a family respondent ages 18 to 34) are more than twice as likely as older families (those with a family respondent ages 50 to 64) to have used a retail clinic (Tu & Cohen, 2008). However, families with children were more likely to use retail clinics than single adults or couples, thus suggesting that consumers are starting to use retail clinics for their children's acute care needs (Tu & Cohen, 2008).

Among commercially insured patients, adults aged 18 to 44 years and women are more likely to visit a retail clinic than other age groups. Moreover, people living in zip codes with higher median household incomes were 2.6% more likely to use a retail clinic than those from zip codes with low median incomes (Ashwood et al., 2011). Other studies have confirmed some of these findings among all patients. Parente & Town (2009) found that retail clinic users are on average three years younger than non-users and are more likely to be female. Similarly, it was found that higher-income families (those earning at least 600% of the federal poverty level) were nearly twice as likely to have used a retail clinic as families with incomes less than 200% of poverty (Tu & Boukus, 2013).

A study focusing on baby boomers and older persons found that willingness to use retail clinics is greater among women and decreases with age. Moreover, people who are more worried about staff qualifications or misdiagnosis are less interested in using retail clinics (Leppel, 2010). It is also important to note that the demographic characteristics of retail clinic users seem to be shifting over time. A study comparing users in 2007-2009 to those in 2000-2006 found that these were more likely to be 65 years of age or older (14.7% vs. 7.5%) (Mehrotra & Lave, 2012).

An especially important characteristic among retail clinic users is that they are less likely to have a primary care physician than the general population. Mehrotra and colleagues reported that about 60% of patients that visit the clinics have no primary care physician relationship, compared to only 20% in the general population (Mehrotra et al., 2008). Tu & Cohen (2008) have also shown that families with no usual source of medical care were more likely to use retail clinics than families with a usual source of care. When retail clinic patients are asked "What would you have done today if this clinic is not an available option?" many answer "just wait and see" including self-care (30%), "visit the ER," (26%), "other care" such as trying to find a provider, or "any clinic that could see me" (26%), and "urgent care" (18%). Not surprisingly, insured patients were more likely to answer "wait to be seen by a doctor" while uninsured patients were more likely to prefer to "visit the ER"(Wang, Ryan, McGlynn, & Mehrotra, 2010).

Consumers' reasons for visiting retail clinics tend to focus on convenience, availability and wait times. In a study that interviewed 61 patients at six retail clinics, patients were asked "What is it about this clinic that made you come here today?" The reasons mentioned were short travel distance from home/work (77%); reasonable pricing (69%); fast service (62%); little or no wait time (43%); and dissatisfaction with other providers such as primary care physicians and hospital emergency rooms (36%)(Wang et al., 2010). It seemed that patients make a decision about visiting a retail clinic after taking into account the severity of their symptoms, their insurance status and ability to pay for healthcare. Some of the comments made by patients about their reason for visiting the clinics include (Wang et al., 2010, p. 10).:

I called my health provider and the closest urgent care clinic was all the way in Carmichael, which is about an hour drive from where I am. So I remember that Rite-Aid had a clinic for minor things like pinkeye and so I came to the clinic here at Rite-Aid.

Yes, they are cheap... going to the emergency room is about $3,000, $4,000, depending on what is going to be done.

... They [ER] supposedly gave me an injection and they charged me almost $2,000. .... That is to say, it's a lot of money. Yes, here it's about what $49, $50.

If I had to pay for it, I'd rather do it here. I'd bring my sister because it was $200 at urgent care. Here it'd only be $50.

... I do not know how much it [urgent care doctor] would have cost. Here the pricing is up front."

They took good care of me here and it's really quick. You don't have to do much... Wasting so much time, mainly. Because we always work double shifts, we don't have time [to see a doctor] ...

It's really convenient. I'm in and out, I get the results.

I didn't want to go search out some other kind of urgent care or something under my insurance where there's a wait. So I thought I'd stop by here and just see. And there was nobody waiting and so I was in and out, prescription turned in within ten minutes.

Even though I did wait two hours this time, I waited much longer in emergency rooms.

I thought about doing it [seeing a PCP], but quite honestly when you call them up it's like, 'are you a regular patient?' is the first question they ask you. And if you're not, I'm not sure whether they pay enough attention to you and get you kind of booted to the end of the line. And I quite honestly didn't want to sit in the doctor's office all day long when I wasn't feeling that good and I don't believe in going to the emergency room for something like a sinus infection. So there was no way I was going to do that. So I wanted to go to a... .you know, I've been to clinics before. Urgent care and stuff like that. But again you wait a long time.

More recent surveys have found that the main reason for visiting a retail clinic vs. other sites of care were "no need to make an appointment" (57%), "acceptance of insurance" (46%), convenient location (45%), "less expensive" (42%), "short wait times" (35%), "open when the physician's office is closed" (34%), "do not have a regular physicians" (18%) and "more pleasant experience than physician's office" (9%) (Richman, 2013). Preferences tend to be different among the adult and pediatric populations. When cost is an issue, the adult patient may favor retail clinics for minor conditions. However, parents of children did not make care decisions based on cost, suggesting that other factors, such as convenience, may play more of a role for this segment (Angstman, Bernard, Rohrer, Garrison, & MacLaughlin, 2012). Moreover, for parents who use retail clinics for pediatric care, 74% first considered going to the pediatrician but reported choosing the retail clinics because it had more convenient hours (36.6%), no office appointment was available (25.2%), they did not want to bother the pediatrician after hours (15.4%), or they thought the problem was not serious enough (13.0%) (Garbutt et al., 2013a). Another study of consumer preferences based on hypothetical scenarios has shown that consumers prefer to receive care from a physician at a private office vs. a retail clinic. However, if the retail clinic is cheaper, their preferences might change. All else equal, cost savings of $31.42 per visit would be enough for them to switch their care from a physician office to a retail clinic (Ahmed & Fincham, 2010).

Uninsured/Underserved

Retail clinics provide care at fixed low prices and in convenient, accessible locations. Therefore, when clinics first opened in the early 2000s, many healthcare industry analysts argued that the clinics can represent a solution for the medically uninsured. As explained in chapter 1, the medically uninsured are people who have no insurance coverage because they can't afford private health insurance plans, they work for a small employer or an employer that does not provide coverage as a benefit, are self-employed, or are not poor enough to qualify for public programs such as Medicaid. The total number of uninsured people prior to the implementation of the Patient Protection and Affordable Care Act (PPACA) was about 52 million people. It is important to note that many people are uninsured by choice- surveys show that about 40% of the uninsured can afford coverage but chose not to get it because they don't believe that they need it. The majority of this group is young and healthy people also referred to as the "young invincibles". For example, Scott (2006) maintained that "as the number of Californians without coverage (or with coverage that leaves significant out-of-pocket costs) increases, we can expect to see the emergence of options such as retail clinics to meet consumer needs.... [The clinics] are now appearing in less affluent communities where under-insured and uninsured consumers are willing to pay cash for clinic care, not only because it is convenient, but also because they have limited access to healthcare elsewhere" (p. 11). Similarly, Gallegos (2007) noted: "The goal of serving quality, affordable, and convenient healthcare to all populations of our nation is attainable. Adequate healthcare service that is blind to race, ethnicity, economic status, geographic location, and insurance coverage is not only a possibility but is also urgently needed. Retail medical clinics, in conjunction with educating patients about them and continued use of such clinics, can be one solution to reducing healthcare disparities"(p. 233). In the media, Gerencher (2010) advised in the Wall Street Journal: "If you're uninsured and seeking stop-gap care until you find coverage, you can triage your way better to better health by understanding the tradeoffs of several care options. A retail clinic or urgent care center can be a suitable fit, depending on the severity of your medical need and personal preferences" (p.1).

However, as the evidence on the location of retail clinics and the populations they serve began to accumulate, it became obvious that the clinics are not especially designed to solve the access and cost problems of the uninsured and the underserved. For example, Pollack and Armstrong (2009) examined the location of retail clinics by census tracts (county subdivisions). They found that only 13.6% of census tracts with retail clinics were located in medically underserved areas/populations. They also found that those tracts with retail clinics had a lower percentage of black and Hispanic individuals, fewer rental units, and lower rates of poverty than tracts without retail clinics. When comparing chain stores with retail clinics vs. without them, they discovered that stores with retail clinics were located in areas with more white residents, fewer black and Hispanic residents, higher rates of home ownership, higher median household incomes and lower rates of poverty, thus indicating that companies are locating clinics in more advantaged stores. The authors concluded that "...despite features such as walk-in appointments and evening and weekend hours, access by disadvantaged populations may be limited if the clinic is difficult to reach" (Pollack and Armstrong, 2009, p. 947). In an invited commentary on the article, Babara Starfield, a physician and primary care expert, asked: "Why would a retail store open a "convenience center" for nonemergency health services? It seems unlikely that the motivation is either completely or even mainly altruistic. After all, these retail establishments have to be responsive to the expectations of financial profit by their investors. It seems most likely that there are 2 main reasons: expectation of profit from customers who have insurance or who can afford the fees (generally lower than office visit fees) and as "loss leaders" by luring customers to the main offerings of the store, including (but not limited to) prescription and nonprescription medications" (Starfield, 2009, p. 950).

Several additional reasons can help explain why retail clinic operators are staying away from areas with underserved/poor populations. Medicaid reimbursement rates for fee-for-service retail clinics are very low and can undercut the clinics' viability. Also, many Medicaid enrollees are covered under Medicaid capitated plans that require the use of a primary care gatekeeper. If these enrollees want to seek care at a retail clinic, they need to obtain a referral from their primary care physician, which significantly lowers the likelihood of them seeking care (Weinick et al., 2010). However, since Medicaid is managed at the state level, the policies are different from state to state. In a survey of all 50 states concerning retail clinic policies, Takach and Wigert (2009) explain: "A few states indicated in their survey that Medicaid managed care plans include retail clinics in their networks and therefore reimburse for care provided to Medicaid beneficiaries. Some Medicaid managed care networks in Georgia, Kansas, and Tennessee include retail clinics. Arizona indicated that if services are emergent or urgent, then the plans would be obligated to pay for those services at retail clinics. But if the services provided are routine and should have been obtained from the member's primary care provider, then the health plan could deny payment for those services. Idaho and Illinois both use primary care case management programs to manage their Medicaid beneficiaries and stated that retail clinics could be used beneficiaries if prior authorization was received from the primary care provider. Retail clinic operators said prior authorization is a significant hurdle for patients and can significantly deter their use of retail clinics"(p. 4-5).

Moreover, Rudavsky and Mehrotra (2010) found that the catchment areas of retail clinics (people that live within 5-minute driving distance to a clinic) had people with higher household incomes ($52,943 vs. $46,080), better education (32.6% vs. 24.9% with college education), higher proportion of Hispanics or Latinos (17.6% vs. 15.4%) and are less likely to live below the poverty lines (10.2% vs. 12.6%) than the areas that do not have retail clinics. The authors commented that their findings "...should dispel the notion that retail clinic companies are specifically targeting the underserved. Rather, except for the differences in income and education, the urban residents that live within a retail clinic catchment area are similar to the urban population as a whole. This may not be surprising. Retail clinics are most commonly run by for-profit companies who want to reach as broad a segment of the whole population as possible" (Rudavsky & Mehrotra, 2010, p. 44).

From the perspective of the uninsured, it is important to note that while the clinic prices are lower than those of primary care physicians and urgent care centers, they are relatively expensive. Paying $80 in out-of-pocket cash for the diagnosis and treatment of an ear infection is beyond the means of many uninsured people, especially when the alternative is no care at all or free care at the county hospital emergency room.

Typical retail clinic operators are for the majority for-profit organizations and therefore are justified in their decisions to place the clinics in more profitable stores and areas. More recently, however, a number of not-for-profit and governmental health systems and community organizations have started opening retail clinics to meet the needs of the uninsured and the underserved. For example, Milwaukee Health Services, a community health center has opened a retail clinic to target underserved populations. The clinic is housed in a local supermarket with the goal of improving access to its services in an area with a shortage of providers. The clinic is integrated with the health center and therefore patients in need of follow-up care can be scheduled for visits at the center (Boulton, 2010). Similarly, the Hennepin County Medical Center, Minnesota's biggest public hospital opened its first retail clinic in 2010 to provide a vital service to the community (Yee, 2010).

Retailers

The major retailers that have been involved in the retail clinic model are CVS, Walgreens, Wal-Mart, Target, Kroger, H-E-B, Shopko and Rite Aid, among others (Kaissi & Charland, 2013a). Tables 3 and 4 show all the retailers that have opened and closed clinics between 2006 and 2012. A 2008 analyses showed that 73% of clinics were located in drug stores, 15% were located in grocery stores, 7% were located in general merchandise stores (supercenter or "Big Box" retailers such as Target or Wal-Mart), and about 4% in shopping plazas, malls, airports and government buildings (Rudavsky et al., 2009). A more recent analysis has shown slightly different numbers with 70% in drug stores, 13% in grocery stores, 15% in general merchandise stores and only 2% are standalone or in malls (Merchant Medicine, 2011b). In general, grocery stores provide more advantages in terms of foot traffic: 87% of consumers visit a grocery store every month, compared to 59% visiting a general store, 27% visiting a club store (such as Costco and Sam' Club) and only 2% visiting a drug store. Web Golinkin, CEO of RediClinic which operates clinics exclusively at H-E-B grocery stores suggests that the grocery advantage is not just about volumes: "They have more frequent shoppers, generally better shopper demographics, and greater in/out convenience than big box. And there is more for people to do in grocery stores than in drug stores if they have to wait." He added: "But drug stores have advantages, too, including greater in/out convenience and a larger percentage of health-oriented shoppers,

Table 3. Clinics still open by retailer, 2006-2012 (Kaissi & Charland, 2013a)

Retailer	Clinics still open n (%)
CVS	546 (41.5%)
Walgreens	357 (26.3%)
Wal-Mart	156 (11.5%)
Kroger	80 (5.9%)
Target	44 (3.2%)
HEB	29 (2.1%)
Shopko	19 (1.4%)
Rite-Aid	18 (1.3%)
Standalone	17 (1.3%)
Duane Reade	12 (0.9%)
Hy-Vee	12 (0.9%)
All other retailers*	70 (5.1%)
Total	1360 (100%)

*all retailers with less than 10 clinics each

Table 4. Closed clinics by retailer, 2006-2012 (Kaissi & Charland, 2013a)

Retailer	Closed clinics n (%)
CVS	160 (31.8%)
Wal-Mart	71 (14.1%)
Publix	48 (9.5%)
Kroger	37 (7.4%)
Walgreens	37 (7.4%)
Cub Foods	122 (2.4%)
All other retailers*	138 (27.4%)
Total	503 (100%)

*all retailers with less than 10 clinics each

and big box stores have the most shoppers, so each venue has its strong points"(Merchant Medicine, 2011b, p. 2-3).

For retailers, retail clinics represent an experiment into an area that they have no prior expertise in, namely delivery of healthcare services for minor, episodic conditions. Retailers are typically revenue-focused, cost-conscious and consumer-centric in any new product or service they offer, and retail clinics present a significant potential in relation to these priorities. First, as previously mentioned, retailers count on retail clinics to attract new customers to the store and increase sales of prescription drugs, over-the-counter medications and other merchandise. Second, retail clinics can help retailers better serve their existing customer base by providing an important service while they are at the store, not very different from having a money transfer company or local banking branch. Third, some retailers consider retail clinic an opportunity to reduce their employees' healthcare costs by providing them with a cheaper way to diagnose and treat low-acuity conditions. Therefore the clinics can increase productivity and decrease absenteeism by providing an in-store convenient option (Scott, 2006). In interviews with retailers, Laws and Scott (2008) confirmed that the main motivation for these companies is in "in increasing revenues through stronger consumer relationships, increased sales of prescription and over-the-counter medications, and increased sales of general merchandise" (p. 1294).

The main focus for retailers, at least initially, is not healthcare or health in general, but rather revenues, consumer satisfaction and cost saving. As Scott (2006) articulated: "In many ways, in-store health clinics are a retail experiment that has captured the attention of the healthcare industry. Their existence depends on retail leases, while their success depends on the patronage of customers who may think of their visit as an extension of a shopping trip, and not necessarily an extension of healthcare" (p. 10). When retail clinics do not deliver on their promises, retailers eliminate them from their stores. Unlike in healthcare, product life cycles in retail are very short, and retailers do not hesitate to experiment with new products and formats, and to remove lines of business that are not as profitable. In fact, 526 clinics out of 1,864 clinics have closed between 2006 and 2012, for a closure rate of 28% (Kaissi & Charland, 2013a). While this rate is unheard of in healthcare, it is very common in retail. For many retailers, the closures are not an indication of a total retreat from the retail clinic model, but rather a decision to relocate clinics to more compatible stores and more profitable markets. In many ways, this reflects the retail mentality of "fast turnaround, rapid consumer testing and constant reinvention of the model" (Scott, 2006, p. 10). It is important to note that for some retailers, especially grocery stores, the interest has lately expanded to healthcare in and of itself. Since most stores have a pharmacy on-site, a health and beauty aisle, healthy foods such as fresh produce, organic and natural foods, the retail clinic fits with this spectrum of offerings (Merchant Medicine, 2011a).

Owners/Operators

When retail clinics first started to open, the main operators were investor-owned and venture-backed companies that were independent from the retailers. For example, MinuteClinic was owned by Bain Capital, Take Care was owned by Beecken Petty O'Keefe and Company and RediClinic was owned by Revolution Health (Laws & Scott, 2008). However, as the business model proved elusive and as clinics return-on-investments (ROIs) did not live up to potential, investors' patience ran out and they began to divest their stakes in some clinics. As a result, the proportion of investor-owned clinics fell, while the proportion of drug-store owned clinics (such as CVS-owned MinuteClinic and Walgreens-owned Take Care) and hospital-owned clinics rose. Between 2007 and 2010, investor-owned retail clinics dwindled from 24% to 16%, while hospital-owned clinics soared from 9% to 18% (Laws & Scott, 2008; Tu & Boukus, 2013).

The most prominent hospital systems that own retail clinics and operate them include the Mayo Clinic in Rochester, Minnesota, Geisinger Health System in Danville, Pennsylvania, and Sutter Health in Northern California. However, for the majority of hospital systems, outright ownership and operation of retail clinics is too risky and costly, and therefore many have opted to partner/affiliate with retail pharmacy chains and other retail clinic chains. For example, CVS MinuteClinic have partnered with The Cleveland Clinic in Cleveland, the University of California-Los Angeles Health System in Los Angeles, Sharp Healthcare in San Diego and Allina Health in Minneapolis/St Paul. Similarly, RediClinic which operates retail clinics at H-E-B stores in Texas have partnered with Memorial Hermann Health System in Houston, St Davids' Health System in Austin, and Methodist Healthcare System in San Antonio. For the retail clinic operators, partnering with a local hospital systems can provide them with brand recognition and much-needed legitimacy in the eyes of the consumers. For hospital systems, retail clinics can provide relief for overcrowded emergency rooms, solution to primary care physician shortages, increase in referrals to physicians and hospitals, and possible increase in revenues (Fenn, 2008; Fottler & Malvey, 2010; Kaissi, 2010a; Lin, 2008; Newbold & O'Neil, 2008; Pollert, Dobberstein, & Wiisanen, 2008). Moreover, hospitals can "provide a complete spectrum of options for their patients, retain these patients in their networks, and raise the visibility of their "brand" in the community… [and] also promote continuity of care through their affiliated RMCs, particularly when such clinics are connected to the hospital's EMR system" (Schleiter, 2010). In Chapter 9, we discuss in depth the role of hospital systems in retail clinics in specific, and in convenient care in general.

At the time of the writing of this book, more than 30 operators owned the 1,574 clinics that are open (Merchant Medicine, 2013). Not surprisingly, MinuteClinic has the lion's share of clinics with 774, followed by Walgreens Health Clinics with 338 clinics, The Little Clinic with 109 clinics, Target Clinic with 57 clinics and RediClinic with 30 clinics. The retail clinic industry, unlike the urgent care one, is very consolidated with the five top operators in control of 86% of the market. The consolidation can be traced back to the years of 2006 and 2007 when several acquisitions were completed. In July 2006, CVS Caremark acquired MinuteClinic and established it as a wholly-owned subsidiary. In May 2007, Walgreens Co acquired Take Care Health Systems, and in May 2008 Kroger Co became a shareholder in the Little Clinic. In April 2010, Kroger bought the outstanding shares and became the sole owner of the company (Hansen-Turton & Ridgway, 2013). Table 5 shows the retail clinic operators and the number of clinics as of December 2013, while Table 6 shows the operators by the number of retail clinics closed between 2006 and 2012.

Table 5. Clinics by operator, 2013 (Merchant Medicine, 2013)

Operator	Number of Clinics
MinuteClinic	774
Walgreens Health Clinic	388
The Little Clinic	109
Target Clinic	57
RediClinic	30
FastCare	26
Baptist Express Care at Walmart	18
Aurora QuickCare	10
DR Walk-In Medical Clinics	7
Lindora Health Clinics	7
Alegent Quick Care	6
Cox Health at Walmart	5
Family Statcare	5
Access Health	4
Family Medicine Specialists at Walmart	4
Family Quick Care	4
Living Well Express Care	4
Owensboro Medical at Walmart	4
PPH Express Care	4
St Vincent Health at Walmart	4
Carson-Tahoe Health at Walmart	3
Community Express Care	3
Geisinger CareWorks	3
Heritage Valley Health	3
Mayo Express Care	3
Memorial Care Health Express	3
Mercy QuickCare	3
St Dominic Hospital at Walmart	3
Sutter Express Care	3
All Others (fewer than 3 clinics)	78
Totals	1574

Table 6. Closed clinics by operator 2006-2012 (Kaissi & Charland, 2013)

Operator	Closed clinics n (%)
Minuteclinic	177 (35.2%)
The Little Clinic	82 (16.3%)
Take Care	37 (7.4%)
Rediclinic	20 (4%)
Quick Health	15 (3%)
SmartCare	15 (3%)
NOW Express Care	11 (2.2%)
Well Spot	11 (2.2%)
All other operators*	135 (26.8%)
Total	503 (100%)

*all operators with less than 10 clinics each

Emergency Rooms and Urgent Care Centers

Retail clinics provide services for non-emergent, acute episodic illnesses and can therefore represent a solution to emergency room overcrowding and over-use for minor illnesses (discussed in Chapter 1). For example, insured patients with minor illnesses may elect to visit a retail clinic instead of an emergency room at lower co-pays and much shorter waiting and examination times. As previously mentioned, 26% of retail clinic users would have gone to the emergency room if the retail clinic was not there (Wang et al., 2010). Not surprisingly, health insurance plans are using retail clinic contracting as a strategy to reduce high emergency department utilization and overall expenses. However, many experts do not believe retail clinics can effectively channel patients away from emergency rooms. They also note that other reasons, and not non-urgent minor conditions, are responsible for long waiting times and emergency room overcrowding. In fact, many hospitals and health systems already have "fast-tracks" staffed by nurse practitioners and physician assistants to provide care for minor conditions in the emergency room (Weinick et al., 2010). Other health systems with less busy emergency rooms are not thrilled to be losing insured and paying patients to the retail clinics, with all the vanished revenue associated with these patients (Fottler & Malvey, 2010).

Urgent care centers, as described in the previous chapter, provide services that overlap with those of retail clinics, but also treat more serious illnesses and injuries, and are typically located in different settings such as strip malls. As previously mentioned, 18% of retail clinic users would have gone to the urgent care center if the retail clinic was not there (Wang et al., 2010). Therefore, retail clinics may also pose a competitive threat to the viability of urgent care centers (Weinick, 2010). An interesting recent trend has seen some companies using a hybrid model of retail clinics and urgent care centers that are sometimes located adjacent to each other. For example, Solantic (now CareSpot) has both in-store retail clinics and free-standing urgent care centers. Patients that present to retail clinics in need of services that are outside the scope of practice of these clinics are referred to the adjacent urgent care center and therefore "kept within the same company". In a previous study, a health system executive affiliating with retail clinics discussed a similar arrangement with urgent care centers as a way to alleviate the fear of primary care physicians working in the center (Kaissi, 2010a).

Physicians and Physician Groups

To date, the fiercest opposition to retail clinics has come from primary care physicians such as family physicians, internal medicine physicians and pediatricians, and their professional associations. The main concerns raised by these traditional providers have centered on quality of care, scope of practice, lack of coordination care and over-prescription of anti-biotic and other medications. The underlying fears though relate more to turf issues of competition, loss of patients and decreased revenues.

One of the first professional associations to take on retail clinics was the American Medical Association (AMA) and its state affiliates. The AMA is the largest association of physicians and medical students in the United States and it aims to improve the science and art of medicine and advance the interests of physicians and their patients (AMA, 2013). In June of 2006, the AMA passed a resolution that called for the retail clinic industry to adopt specific principles:

1. "Store-based health clinics must have a well-defined and limited scope of clinical services, consistent with state scope of practice laws.
2. Store-based health clinics must use standardized medical protocols derived from evidence based practice guidelines to ensure patient safety and quality of care.
3. Store-based health clinics must establish arrangements by which their healthcare practitioners have direct access to and supervision by MD/DOs, as consistent with state laws.
4. Store-based health clinics must establish protocols for insuring continuity of care with practicing physicians within the local community.
5. Store-based health clinics must establish a referral system with physician practices or other facilities for appropriate treatment if the patient's conditions or symptoms are beyond the scope of services provided by the clinic.
6. Store-based health clinics must clearly inform patients in advance of the qualifications of the healthcare practitioners who are providing care, as well as the limitation in the types of illnesses that can be diagnosed and treated.

7. Store-based health clinics must establish appropriate sanitation and hygienic guidelines and facilities to insure the safety of patients.
8. Store-based health clinics should be encouraged to use electronic health records as a means of communicating patient information and facilitating continuity of care.
9. Store-based health clinics should encourage patients to establish care with a primary care physician to ensure continuity of care" (Weinick et al., 2010).

However, the AMA did not stop at the principles. At the annual AMA House of Delegates meeting in June of 2007, many physicians and physicians groups called on the association to ban retail clinics all together. For example, one of the physicians attending the meeting at the time declared: "There is no more urgent issue than this for the AMA....This issue speaks to what all of us do every day in practice. If the AMA does nothing, in five years, the chairs [at the AMA] meeting will be filled with representatives from Walgreens, Wal-Mart and other retail outlets" (Jaspen, 2007, p. 1). Instead, the AMA called for the retail clinics to be investigated for potential conflicts of interest arising from inducing patients to fill their prescriptions at the same in-store pharmacies, and to prohibit health insurance companies from waiving or lowering co-payments only for patients that receive services at the clinics. The AMA feared that this financial incentive might influence patients to seek treatment at the clinics on the basis of cost rather than quality of care (Paddock, 2007).

Before too long, other professional associations representing physicians of different specializations joined the opposition movement. Given that retail clinics provide primary care services for conditions traditionally treated by family physicians, it is no surprise that the America Academy of Family Physicians (AAFP) was in the lead. The AAFP represents more than 110,000 family physicians, family medicine residents, and medical students (AAFP, 2013). In October of 2007, the AAFP Congress of Delegates passed a policy that clearly stated its opposition to retail clinics. Similar to the AMA's, the policy specified some principles for retail clinics to abide by:

"AAFP does not endorse Retail Health Clinics (RHC), believes that they could interfere with the medical home and opposes expansion of their scope of service, in particular, to include the diagnosis, treatment and management of chronic medical conditions in this setting. The AAFP is committed to the development of a healthcare system based on high quality, cost effective, team-based and patient-centered primary care and on the tenants of first contact, comprehensive, coordinated and continuing care for all persons (i.e., a medical home). The AAFP believes that the RHC model of care is not a medical home and has the potential to further fragment patient care. In those markets where RHC's exist, the AAFP has defined a set of attributes related to their design and operation that are important to the patient care offered in this setting. It is the individual physician's choice whether or not to sponsor or work cooperatively with a retail clinic, however the AAFP urges all retail clinics to abide by the following attributes:

1. **Scope of Service:** Retail clinics must have a well-defined and limited scope of clinical services.
2. **Evidence-based Medicine:** Clinical services and treatment must be evidence based and quality improvement–oriented.

3. **Team-based Approach:** The clinic should have a formal connection with physician practices in the local community, preferably with family physicians, to provide continuity of care. Non-physician health professionals practicing in this setting, such as nurse practitioners and physician assistants, should operate in accordance with state and local regulations, as part of a "team-based" approach to healthcare and under responsible supervision of a practicing, licensed physician.
4. **Referrals:** The clinic must have a referral system to physician practices or to other entities appropriate to the patient's symptoms beyond the clinic's scope of services. The clinic should encourage all patients to have a "medical home."
5. **Electronic Health Records (EHR):** The clinic should include an EHR system sufficient to gather and communicate the patient's information with the family physician's office, preferably one that is compatible with the Continuity of Care Record supported by AAFP and others" (Weinick et al., 2010, p.60).

After the policy was drafted, the three largest retail clinic operators (MinuteClinic, Take Care and RediClinic) agreed to the AAFPs desired attributes. Hal Rosenbluth, Take Care Health co-founder and board chair, announced: "The key from our perspective is that everybody try and find a way to do what's in the best interest of a patient. [...] We believe very strongly in the medical home and we believe very strongly in the role of physicians" (O'Reilly, 2007, p. 1). The AMA blessed the agreement, with one AMA trustee stating "While store-based health clinics can never replace the patient-physician relationship, with guidance from the AMA and AAFP, they can offer patients a viable option for routine healthcare services" (O'Reilly, 2007, p. 2). Around the same time, the AAFP started working with the Convenient Care Association (CCC) to develop common quality-of-care standards and build a CCC clinical advisory group that will include physician representatives. Callahan (2007) described the AAFPs' view of retail clinics as "realistic." Rick Kellerman, MD, then-president of AAFP noted: "The major lesson is that patients want convenience. Mothers who work and have a sick child do not want to take off work and wait a day or two for the child to be seen. We have also told our members they can compete with retail clinics by expanding office hours and decreasing waiting times through innovations in scheduling. We have witnessed a number of physician office innovations: sick clinics at noon and after hours, no-wait visits during the day, [etc.]" (Callahan, 2007). However, the agreement between the clinic operators (joined later by Bellin Health) and the academy was abruptly terminated by the physician group in 2010 (AAFP, 2010). The main reason that triggered the change was the expansion of some retail clinic operators' services to the diagnosis, treatment and management of chronic medical conditions (discussed later in this chapter). Since then, no agreements between the AAFP and operators have been signed.

It is important to note that many of the concerns raised by the physician groups have proved to be unfounded, especially those related to quality of care, adherence to protocols, and coordination of care. Rigorous research studies (which we cover in depth later in this chapter) have shown that quality of care in retail clinics is similar to, if not better than, care provided in physician offices and other settings. Research also shows that providers strongly adhere to protocols, and that retail clinics, for the most part, do not disrupt the patient-physician relationship.

While the AMA and AAFP have had a firm stand on retail clinics with some occasional flexibility, the position of the American Academy of Pediatrics (AAP) can be described as vehement opposition. The AAP is the professional association of pediatricians, has about 60,000 members and is "dedicated to the health and well-being of infants, children, adolescents and young adults" (AAP, 2013). In its 2006 "Work Policy Statement", the AAP specified:

"The American Academy of Pediatrics (AAP) opposes retail-based clinics (RBCs) as an appropriate source of medical care for infants, children, and adolescents and strongly discourages their use, as the AAP is committed to the medical home model. The medical home model provides accessible, family-centered, comprehensive, continuous, coordinated, compassionate, and culturally effective care for which the pediatrician and the family share responsibility. Given that the RBC is not a medical home model, the AAP is particularly concerned with the effects of the following attributes of an RBC on healthcare for children and adolescents:

- Fragmentation of care.
- The possible effects on quality of care.
- Provision of episodic care to children with special healthcare needs and chronic diseases, who may not be readily identifiable.
- Lack of access to and maintenance of a complete, accessible, central health record that contains all pertinent patient information.
- The use of tests for the purposes of diagnosis without proper follow-up.
- The possible public health issues that could occur when patients with contagious diseases are in a commercial, retail environment with little or no isolation (e.g., fevers, rashes, mumps, measles, strep throat, etc.).
- Seeing children with "minor" conditions, as will often be the case in an RBC, is misleading and problematic. Many pediatricians use the opportunity of seeing the child for something minor to address issues in the family, discuss any problems with obesity or mental health issues, catch up on immunizations, identify undetected illness, and continue strengthening the relationship with the child and family. These visits are important and provide an opportunity to work with patients and families to deal with a variety of other issues.

The AAP acknowledges that the shifting economic and organizational dynamics of the current healthcare system will likely support the continued existence and expansion of RBCs. However, the aforementioned concerns and the overall effects these clinics will have on pediatric practice have led the AAP to respond with the following principles:

1. **Supporting the Medical Home Model:** RBCs should support the medical home model by referring the patient back to the pediatrician or other primary care physician for all future care. In the event that the patient does not have a relationship with a pediatrician or primary care physician, RBCs should have the means to assist the family in establishing contact with one within a medical home. Third

party payers are encouraged to provide appropriate incentives to plan members to access the medical home as the best practice model for pediatric primary care.

2. **Communication:** The AAP recommends that RBCs promptly communicate with the patient's pediatrician or other primary care physician within 24 hours of the visit. At a minimum, the following information should be included: patient's name, date of birth, at least 2 additional pieces of identifying information (e.g., parents' name and/or address), reason for visit, diagnosis and disposition, findings, laboratory results (if any), and an indication as to whether any follow up is needed.
3. **Using Evidence-Based Medicine:** The AAP recommends that all those providing care to children follow all AAP clinical guidelines as well as those guidelines developed by other medical organizations that have the support and endorsement of the AAP. RBCs should be required to participate in ongoing quality-improvement and quality-assurance processes, as required of pediatric and other primary care practices. RBCs must meet all requirements related to quality assurance and ensure full compliance with state licensure requirements for oversight or collaborative protocols relative to scope of practice.
4. **Contagious Diseases:** By providing medical care to individuals in a retail-based setting, RBCs must take the necessary precautions to prevent the spread of contagious diseases. Although the RBC may have policies that limit the scope of services, this may not prevent individuals with contagious diseases from seeking care at RBCs. This presents a potential public health hazard to retail staff and customers who may come in contact with a contagious individual. RBCs should be subject to and comply with all healthcare facility standards (e.g., hygiene, safety, regulations of the Occupational Safety and Health Administration, policies and procedures for children with communicable diseases, etc.).
5. **Financial Incentives:** The AAP is opposed to waiving or lowering copays or offering financial incentives for visits to RBCs in lieu of visits to pediatricians' or other primary care physicians' offices. The AAP believes the medical home model is the optimal standard of care, and RBCs are not medical homes. Payer incentives should not promote fragmentation of care but should instead recognize and reward systems of care that promote continuous, coordinated, and comprehensive care" (AAP, 2006).

A recent survey of pediatricians and pediatric nurse practitioners showed that these providers agree with the positions taken by the AAP (Garbutt et al., 2013b). About 90% of the providers were aware that their patients had used a retail clinics, and 81% considered the clinics as competition that has taken away some of their business. In addition, 91% of the providers suggested that patients needed to seek additional care from them after visiting a retail clinic, with suboptimal care being the reason for the additional office visits. The pediatricians indicated that with patients visiting retail clinics, they have experienced incorrect diagnoses (81%); overuse and misuse of antibiotics (77% and 68%, respectively); failure to conduct diagnostic tests (68%); or ignoring the test results when making a treatment decision (69%). Only 15% of the physicians reported that the retail clinic notified them within 24 hours that their patient was seen at the clinic. When that happened, providers were more likely to report that the clinics followed recommended care guidelines and were less likely to report that the clinics provided suboptimal care. Moreover, pediatricians have responded to the business threat of retail clinics by adjusting their office hours, providing walk-in appointment options and discussing retail clinics with the parents.

The main rationale behind the pediatricians' opposition seems to be that providers at retail clinics treat children without having any specialized training in pediatrics. It is important to note that Massachusetts is the only state that has prohibited retail clinics from providing services to children less than 24 months of age and from providing childhood immunizations (Takach & Witgert, 2009). AAP's strong opposition to retail clinics has trickled down to the local pediatrician level. A recent e-mail correspondence with a pediatrician in San Antonio raises many quality concerns about retail clinics' treatment of patients (Appendix B). That same pediatrician shared a letter sent on behalf of the San Antonio Pediatric Society to the Methodist Healthcare System, when the health system announced its affiliation with RediClinics to operate retail clinics at H-E-B stores in various San Antonio locations (Appendix C).

Convenient Care Association

When the retail clinic industry started its growth, it did not have a trade association to represent the interests of retail clinic operators and lobby on their behalf. A summit was held in 2006 by Hal Rosenbluth, the founder of Take Care Health Systems, with the purpose of shaping the future of the industry. At the summit, attended by clinic operators, providers, and other stakeholders, two main priorities emerged: quality of care and adherence to standards (Hansen-Turton & Ridgway, 2013). Donna Shalala, former secretary of the U.S. Department of Health and Human Services was attending the summit. She advised the stakeholders that unless they formed a trade association, the industry will not succeed or be taken seriously (Hansen-Turton, personal interview, 2013). Per her advice, the operators formed the Convenient Care Association (CCA).

The CCA, incorporated in October of 2006, "works primarily to enhance and sustain the growth of the Convenient Care industry through sharing of best practices and common standards of operation" (CCA, 2013). In November, the first board meeting of the CCA was held to establish quality and safety standards for the industry and to have a certification program (described elsewhere in this chapter). The standards, the certification program and many advocacy efforts against anti-retail clinic legislation count among the association's achievement to date (Hansen-Turton & Ridgway, 2013). The goals of the CCA are:

- "Sharing best practices, common standards of operation, experiences and ideas
- Developing common standards of operation to ensure the highest quality of care throughout all CCCs
- A united voice to advance the needs of CCCs and their customers
- A unified effort to promote the concept of CCCs, and to respond to questions about this evolving industry

- Reaching out to the existing medical community and creating new partnerships
- Building synergies with traditional medical service providers" (CCA, 2013).

Today, the CCA represent 95% of retail clinics operating in the United States and holds an annual "Retail Clinician Education Congress"(CCA, 2013).

In summary, insured patients living in suburban areas with high incomes seem to appreciate having a close-by retail clinic as a convenient alternative for care for minor conditions. Uninsured and underserved patients living in less affluent areas are less likely to have a retail clinic within short driving distance, and may find the prices of the retail clinics unaffordable. Retailers hope that clinics increase revenue, decrease employee healthcare costs, and boost purchases of drugs and other goods sold in their stores. However, their patience for clinics not performing is limited and they pull the plug on some of them in favor of better-performing ones in other stores and locations. Retail clinic operators, whether investor-owned companies or hospital systems are still trying to refine the business model in order to grow revenues and maintain patient satisfaction and quality of care. Hospital emergency rooms can see retail clinics as release valves, but are concerned about lost patients and revenues, and so are urgent care centers. Physicians groups, especially family physicians and pediatricians continue to feel the threat of retail clinics and to raise concerns about their quality, although their resistance has somehow waned in the last few years. The Convenient Care Association has positioned itself as nationally recognized organization that advocates on behalf of retail clinics and ensures quality and safety standards are regularly followed.

4. OUTCOMES AT RETAIL CLINICS

Retail clinics have been drummed up as a low-cost, high-quality and convenient alternative to traditional primary care physician offices and hospital emergency rooms. In this section, we examine the evidence surrounding quality of care, patient satisfaction, savings and costs of care at retail clinic and assess their effects on care coordination and patient relationships with primary care physicians.

Quality of Care

As mentioned in the previous section, the retail clinic industry came under severe fire from physicians and the associations representing them for their potential to jeopardize quality care of care and lead to medical mistakes and injuries. While the CCA worked to address the concerns by establishing standards and certification protocols, the general public was still hesitant about the quality of care provided at retail clinics. In the early years, many patients perceived retail clinics as a lower-quality alternative to care provided in private physician offices. It wasn't until rigorous third-party research on quality of care was published in peer-reviewed journals that the evidence on quality of care was established. Retail clinic operators (who we interviewed in summer of 2009) breathed a sigh of relief as the first studies showed favorable quality outcomes in their clinics.

Evidence on quality of care in retail clinics first appeared in 2007. Woodburn, Smith and Nelson (2007) examined rates of adherence to an acute pharyngitis practice guideline in a population of 57,331 patient visits in retail clinics. For patients with a negative rapid strep test result, clinic providers adhered to guidelines by withholding unnecessary antibiotics in 99.05% of the cases. For patients with a positive rapid strep test result, adherence to guidelines by prescribing an appropriate antibiotic was observed in 99.75% of the cases. Therefore, the combined guideline adherence rate for both groups of patients was 99.15%. Another guideline required providers to conduct a strep culture for patient with a negative rapid strep test. The rate of adherence to that standard was 99.1% of patients. Of those, 96.2% were appropriately treated with an antibiotic. Only 0.95% of patients with a negative rapid strep test result were provided an antibiotic, which is considered against the clinical guidelines. However, for half of these prescriptions the providers submitted documentation of clinical concerns for which an antibiotic was a reasonable choice. These rates compare extremely favorably with documented rates of adherence to guidelines in the care of acute pharyngitis in primary care physician offices (Gonzales, Malone, Maselli, & Sande, 2001), a testament to the quality of care provided in retail clinics. These results helped alleviate fears that retail clinics over-prescribe antibiotics to boost sales in the in-store pharmacies (Woodburn et al., 2007).

In 2008, Rohrer, Yapuncich, Adamson, and Angstman published results from a retrospective cohort study of medical records of patients in a retail clinic and physician office. The observation group consisted of the first 200 consecutive pediatric patients (younger than 18 years of age) seen in a new retail clinic during its first 3 weeks of operation. The comparison group consisted of 200 consecutive pediatric patients seeking care at a physician office. The two groups were measured on repeat visits. Repeat visits are considered a measure of low quality (as well as cost of care), because "high rates of repeat visits may indicate that the care provided at the initial visit was incomplete"(Weinick et al., 2010, p. 29). The study found no differences in risk of early return visit (within two weeks) between retail clinic patients and physician office patients (Rohrer, Yapuncich, Adamson & Angstman, 2008). One year later, Rohrer and his colleagues at the Mayo Clinic conducted a similar study measuring repeat visits, but for adult patients (Rohrer, Angstam, & Furst, 2009a). They compared three groups of patients in Minnesota: those using a retail clinic, those using a regular physician office care, and those using a same-day acute care clinic in a medical office. For retail clinic patients, 14% of visits lead to a return office visit, compared to 24.4% for physician office patients and 20.6% for same-day acute care clinic patients. After adjusting for other variables such as age, sex, marital status, acuity, and number of office visits in the previous six months, no significant differences in risk of early return visits were found among the groups, and the authors concluded that "... retail walk-in clinics appeared to increase access without increasing early return visits" (Rohrer et al., 2009a, p. 18).

Also in 2008, Thygeson, Van Vorst, Maciosek, and Solberg reported on clinical quality data for MinuteClinics from the Minnesota public performance measures. They concluded that "MinuteClinics' performance on the Health Plan Employer Data and Information Set (HEDIS) pharyngitis measure is excellent (100 percent), while performance on the HEDIS upper respiratory tract infection measure for children is only average (86 percent) compared to other Minnesota provider groups" (Thygeson, Van Vorst, Maciosek, & Solberg, 2008, p. 1291).

Arguably, the most influential study on retail clinic quality is the one conducted by the Rand Corporation and published in 2009 (Mehrotra et al., 2009). The researchers examined episodes of care (initial and follow-up visits, pharmaceutical and ancillary tests) for three conditions: otitis media (ear infection); pharyngitis and urinary tract infections. They constructed 14 quality indicators based on guidelines published by the American Academy of Pediatrics, the American Academy of Family Physicians, and the Infectious Diseases Society of America, and created an aggregate quality score for all conditions. They also measured whether patients received specific preventative services in the three months following their visits. They compared care provided for the three conditions in retail clinics, physician offices, urgent care centers and hospital emergency rooms. Overall, aggregate quality scores were similar at retail clinics (63.6%), physician offices (61.0%) and urgent care centers (62.6%), but were lower for emergency rooms (55.1%). Individual quality scores on the specific measures showed that retail clinics performed better than or as good as other settings. For example, for otitis media, the pass rate for "duration of therapy for at least 10 days" was 91.7% at retail clinics, 89.0% at physician offices, 93.4% at urgent care centers and 89.1% at emergency rooms. For pharyngitis, the pass rate for "culture or rapid strep test was obtained in diagnosis of GABHS (Group A ß-hemolytic streptococcal) for children" was 86.6% at retail clinics, 77.9% at physician offices, 72.7% at urgent care centers and 52.4% at emergency rooms. For urinary tract infections, the pass rate for "antibiotics prescribed for seven days or less for uncomplicated lower tract infections" was 60.1% for retail clinics, 57.1% for physician offices, 58.5% for urgent care centers and 55.4% for emergency rooms. The only measure in which retail clinics scored lower than other settings was for "urine culture obtained for all high-risk patients" for urinary tract infections. On this measure, the pass rates for retail clinics was 29.6%, compared to 56.8%, 58.1%, and 54.8% at physician office, urgent care centers and emergency rooms, respectively. On preventative care, the results were similar to quality scores as retail clinics had similar rates of preventative services (14.5%), when compared to physician offices (14.2%) and urgent care centers (13.7%), while emergency rooms had significantly lower rates (10.7%).

In 2011, Jacoby and his colleagues examined rates of adherence to two quality measures in a pediatric retail clinic. The measures were modeled after Heathcare Effectiveness Data and Information Set (HEDIS) measures and included appropriate testing for children with pharyngitis and appropriate treatment for children with upper-respiratory infection. Retail clinics achieved a 90th percentile ranking for the pharyngitis measure and a 70th percentile ranking for the upper respiratory infection (Jacoby, Crawford, Chaudhari, & Goldfarb, 2011)

In the last couple of years, Rohrer and co-authors continued their work on repeat clinic visits and found similar results. They examined the electronic medical records of adult primary care patients seen in a large group practice in Minnesota for the treatment of sinusitis. Comparing retail clinic patients to regular physician office patients revealed no difference in return visits made within two weeks (Rohrer, Garrison, & Angstam, 2012). They also examined the records of pediatric patients treated for otitis media in the same group practice and found the percentage of patients returning for later visits was much lower for retail clinics (11.2%) than for physician offices (21.0%) (Rohrer et al., 2012). In a recent examination of cases of acute bronchitis treated in primary care physician offices, the adherence to clinic guidelines (in terms of not prescribing an antibiotic) was only 31%.

The adherence rate in a comparable group of retail clinic cases was 86% (Grossman, 2013).

The evidence is overwhelming that, for the minor conditions that they treat, retail clinic providers adhere strongly to clinical guidelines and strict standards, and provide adequate care that patients do not need to have another visit soon. Despite fierce criticisms from physicians, retail clinics seem to provide high quality of care when compared to other alternatives.

Continuity of Care and Effect on Primary Care Physicians

One of the main arguments raised by physicians against retail clinics is that they lead to fragmentation of care and have a negative effect on the patient-primary care provider relationship. Reviewing the evidence from the literature reveals whether these concerns are warranted or not. In a 2007 study conducted by Market Strategies Inc., among retail clinic users with a primary care physician, only 12% agreed with the statement "retail clinics have mostly or completely replaced my primary care physician for the type of treatments offered at retail clinics" (Market Strategies, 2007). In their 2008 study, Mehrotra and his colleagues found that 61.3% of patients visiting a retail clinic did not have a primary care physician. The authors commented on this finding: "Some have raised the concern that retail clinics may disrupt primary care relationships. We found that three-fifths of patients did not report having a PCP, so for these patients there is no relationship to disrupt" (Mehrotra et al., 2008, p. 1279). Clayton Christensen and coauthors made a similar point in "The Innovator's Prescription". They argued that since most retail clinic patients do not have a physician, retail clinics represent more a 'new market,' rather than a 'low-end' disruption, in that they mostly compete against non-consumption and not against physicians (Christensen, Grosmman, & Hwang, 2008). In a previously mentioned study, Wang and her co-authors found that only 38% of retail clinic users would have waited to be seen by a physician if the retail clinic was not an available option. The authors explained the findings: "Our analyses of patient interviews revealed that patients did not wish to replace their PCPs. Rather they used retail clinics as a back-up or alternative for minor healthcare needs. For more serious issues or chronic illnesses they would continue to see their PCPs. Although retail clinic visits could potentially undermine provider-patient relationship, patients with PCPs mentioned that retail clinics helped them avoid unnecessary visits to the ED when their PCPs were not available" (Wang et al., 2010, p. 4).

More recent studies have raised some red flags. Reid et al. (2012) examined the association between retail clinic use and receipt of key primary care functions. They found that patients that visited a retail clinic instead of a primary care physician had a reduction of 27.7 visits per 100 patients in terms of subsequent visits to primary care physicians for new simple conditions. Those patients also had an increase of 33.8 subsequent visits per 100 patients to retail clinics for new conditions. Moreover, visiting a retail clinic instead of a primary care physician was associated with a decrease in subsequent continuity of care (a 10.9% decrease on the continuity of care score as measured by the Bice-Boxerman index). However, there was no difference among patients who visited a retail clinic vs. a primary care physician in terms of receipt of preventative health examinations such as screening for breast cancer, cervical cancer, colorectal cancer, or Chlamydia, or receipt of diabetes management such as hemoglobin A1c testing, eye examinations, LDL testing and nephropathy care. The authors suggested that these findings send some mixed messages about retail clinics: "Taken together, the interpretation of our findings depends on one's view on the relative importance of different aspects of primary care. Some might contend that continuity is the cornerstone of primary care and, therefore, retail clinics' negative impact on continuity is critical. Others might argue that continuity and first-contact care are less important than preventive care, especially for a healthy patient population. In this light, retail clinics' impact on primary care may not be as great as feared" (Reid et al., 2012, p. 509). Rohrer and his colleagues also examined continuity of care in a sample of patients using retail clinics vs. those using standard physician office care. They defined continuity as percentage of subsequent visits made to the patient's primary care physician (all patients are part of the same large multispecialty group practice and therefore all have a primary care physician). The mean continuity of care score for patients who visited a retail clinic was 0.17, compared to 0.44 for patients who used a standard physician office. More than half of patients (54.5%) who visited a retail clinic did not make any visits to their primary care physician, compared to only 31% for those who did not use a retail clinic. The authors contended that "continuity of care is associated with many positive outcomes, including improved delivery of preventive services, decreased hospitalization, lower healthcare costs and improved chronic disease management. Having a greater number of visits and a recent health maintenance visits with a primary care physician is associated with successful delivery of preventative services. The decreased continuity of care and the large number of zero visit outliers seen among retail clinic users may undermine these goals" (Rohrer, Angstram, Garrison, Maxson, & Furst, 2013, p. 152).

Another measure of continuity of care, especially among pediatric patients, is whether the retail clinic and/or parents notified the pediatrician that a visit to a retail clinic has taken place. A recent study has shown that only 41.8% of parents who had sought care at a retail clinic have informed their pediatrician about the visit. The reasons cited for not informing the pediatrician were not thinking that the visit was important (37.5%), not having seen the pediatrician since the retail clinic visit (34.0%), forgetting to tell the pediatrician (18.8%), or assuming the clinic would do so (3.5%) (Garbutt et al., 2013a). The authors put these findings into context: "Virtually no parents reported that their pediatrician had raised the topic of RC [retail clinic] care with them, and fewer than half volunteered information about their RC visit to the PCP. Effective communication about care is essential to avoid duplication of services and ensure safety and effective care coordination. This will become even more important if RCs assume a more active role in management of chronic diseases. In settings where RCs are affiliated with a hospital system, an integrated electronic medical record can facilitate communication between the RC and the child's medical home within 24 hours of a clinic visit, as recommended by the American Academy of Pediatrics. However, most RCs are independently owned, and in this setting, PCPs rely more on parents to inform them about RC visits" (p. 849).

The evidence around the effect of retail clinics on coordination and continuity of care is mixed at best. For patients who do not have a primary care physician relationship, there is no argument to be made about fragmentation of a care that does not exist in the first place. However, for patients who already have such relationship, retail clinics may reduce subsequent visits to the patient's physician. It could be argued that once patients experience the convenience and easy access of retail clinics, they become less likely to accept the frustrations and irritations associated with physician offices. Moreover, continuity of care cannot always be defined by physical visits to the physician, as patients are seeking to communicate more with physicians over the phone and by e-mail and chat sessions.

Patient Satisfaction

Patients in the United States are not satisfied with the traditional primary care system. About 25% of patients complain that they wait 30 minutes or longer in the exam room before being seen by the physician. Other patients' complaints include not being able to schedule an appointment within one week, the physician spending too little time with them, test results not provided in a timely manner, and physicians not responding to phone calls promptly (Hitti, 2007). At the same time, primary care physicians are not satisfied with their patients. About 2/3 of physicians complain that patients do not follow proper procedures. Moreover, physicians are frustrated that patients wait too long before making an appointment and that they request unnecessary tests and prescriptions (Hitti, 2007). Kissinger describes the situation as "a growing disconnect between patients and physicians and signals ongoing frustration but is indicative of primary care delivery trends…" (Kissinger, 2008, p.315). More recent surveys assessing patient perceptions of primary care show that only 76% of patients are satisfied with their primary care physician. However that percentage dwindles down to 65% for the 18-24 years age group, and to 69% in the 25-44 years age group (Deloitte Center for Health Solutions, 2012).

In this context, it is not surprising that patients would embrace a new delivery approach of primary care services such as retail clinics where appointments are not needed and wait times are minimal. In 2005, the Wall Street Journal Online Interactive Health-Care Poll showed that 78% of consumers believe that retail clinics provide a convenient way for people to receive basic medical services (Gullo, 2005). A 2007 Harris Interactive poll indicated high overall patient satisfaction with retail clinics in four areas: cost (80% satisfaction), convenience (83% satisfaction), having qualified staff to provide care (85%) and quality of care (90%) (Harris Interactive, 2007). A 2008 survey showed that 2 out of 3 parents who have used a retail clinic for their children were "likely or very likely to return" to the clinic (Colihan, 2008). Subsequent polls have shown increasing satisfaction with 93% of consumers somewhat satisfied or very satisfied with convenience, 88% with having qualified staff to provide care, 86% with cost of care, and 90% with quality of care. Some of the positive comments posted online by patients included (Harris Interactive Online Onsite Health Clinic Bulletin Board, 2007):

- "I was satisfied, because I only needed to drive 1 mile, wait 5 minutes, see the doctor for 10 minutes, walk over to the pharmacy counter, get my prescription, and back home in under 30 minutes."
- "I like that it's convenient and I didn't have to wait too long."

- "What I like most about the rhc [retail health clinic] is: easy to find, usually open, takes insurance if you have it, affordable if you don't."
- "I liked how friendly and efficient the clinic was."

However, some patients expressed dissatisfaction with some aspects of the clinics:

- "Sometimes I feel they are rushing me through… I am sometimes not completely satisfied with the attention they give."
- "There is no doctor there if the situation is more serious than thought to be."
- "No bonding and not private enough for me."
- "My doctor not being there, dealing with a new person, having to give all of my information to another company."

Similarly, other innovative research used social media posts made by patients about their experience at CVS and Walmart retail clinics (Aversa, 2013). The results showed that 67% of users made positive comments about Walmart's clinic and 59% about CVS's MinuteClinic. More specifically, "lifecasting" (general discussion about *experience* in the context of day-to-day life) and general praise accounted for the largest portion of the conversations. Walmart clinic's convenience was praised especially its accessibility, ease, and speed, while CVS patients were mostly satisfied with affordability. But not all comments were positive, as some patients complained about the unexpected long wait times: "Wait if it's called a "minute clinic" then WHY IS MY WAIT TIME AN HOUR, CVS literally sits on a throne of lies". Interestingly, 17% of Walmart clinic users stated that they were embarrassed to admit they used the clinic and that they saw it as a desperate last resort (Aversa, 2013). More recent polls have shown some concerning results for retail clinics. Less than half of users said they were "extremely" or "very" satisfied with the care they received, while about 18% were "somewhat" satisfied" or "not at all" satisfied (Gardner, 2013). In peer-reviewed research, Hunter, Weber, Morreale and Wall (2009) found with varied incomes and different ethnicities were very satisfied with clinics' location, no appointment necessary, short wait time, and low cost. Wang, and colleagues found that 67% of patients expressed satisfaction with the care that they received at retail clinics, with the main reasons for satisfaction being that the provider was caring, the provider spoke Spanish, the care was thorough, the provider was knowledgeable and the provider was trustworthy (Wang et al., 2010).

In general, patients seem to be satisfied with various aspects of retail clinics' care. However, some concerns relating to wait times, feeling rushed, and not feeling a connection with the provider should be taken seriously by the clinic operators.

Costs of Care and Savings

The costs of delivering care in the American healthcare system are exponentially higher than in any other country. Therefore, for any innovation to prove its worth, it should have markedly lower costs than the traditional alternatives. Retail clinics can provide care at lower costs because they use less expensive providers, provide care in smaller settings, and specialize in low-acuity conditions. Research that has examined costs in retail clinics became abundant in the last few years.

The previously mentioned 2009 study by Mehrotra and colleagues that assessed quality of care at various settings of care also compared costs of care. Episodes of care initiated at retail clinics cost $110, compared with $166 for those originating at physician offices, $156 at urgent care clinics and $570 at hospital emergency rooms. The main difference was for "evaluation & management" visits, where retail clinic costs were significantly lower ($66) than other settings ($106 for physician offices, $103 in urgent care centers, and $358 in emergency departments). Costs for laboratory and imaging services were $15 at retail clinics compared to $33, $27, and $113 for physician offices, urgent care centers and hospital emergency rooms, respectively. Prescription costs were similar in retail clinics, physician offices and urgent care centers (ranging between $21-$22), but higher in emergency rooms ($26). Despite the evidence provided in these findings that retail clinics have overall lower costs, the authors cautioned that "because retail clinics are very convenient to use, patients who would not have sought any care previously may now go to a retail clinic. This would increase overall healthcare utilization and in turn increase costs" (Mehrotra, et al., 2008). This suggests that while retail clinics may be cheaper when comparing individual episodes of care, they might lead to overall increase in healthcare costs due to new utilization.

Similar results were found in a study comparing patients using retail clinics with those using standard physician office care for five common conditions (pink eye, sore throat, viral illness, bronchitis, and cough)(Rohrer, Angstram & Bartel, 2009b). The cost of the retail clinic visit was $88.10, whereas cost for a physician office visits was $126.30. However, given the unique setting where the study was conducted, the authors were wary of generalizing the results "The retail clinic utilized in this study is integrated into our electronic medical record and ordering system. This may limit how broadly results might be generalized. The impact on utilization of healthcare resources may be different in a different clinical environment"(p.335). Also, in an unpublished study examining the ten most common conditions treated, care at retail clinics were, on average, 64% less expensive than care in other settings, which translates to a difference of approximately $153 between care delivered in the retail setting and the physician's office (Parente & Town, 2009). The authors also estimated that the total welfare from the introduction and diffusion of retail clinics is $449.1 million or approximately $2.05 across every insured U.S. resident under-65 years of age.

An in-depth analysis of costs of care for visits at MinuteClinic vs. other care setting examined sore throat, otitis media (inflammation of the middle ear), acute sinusitis, conjunctivitis, and urinary tract infection. For a MinuteClinic episode, the average cost was $51 less than in an urgent care center, $55 less than in a physician office, and $279 less than in a hospital emergency room. The average cost per episode increased only by 12.2% in the retail clinic setting, compared to 20.3% in emergency room, 12.7% in the physician office, and 11.9% in the urgent care center (Thygeson et al., 2008).

Weinick, Burns and Mehrotra (2010) examined visits to hospital emergency rooms and estimated that 13.7% to 27.1% of them could take place at retail clinics and urgent care centers, with potential annual savings of $4.4 billion annually. Similarly, a study by Take Care Health has estimated that if visits to hospital emergency rooms, urgent care centers or primary care physician offices that happen when retail clinics are open took place in these clinics instead, there would be costs savings of $135.53 million per year (Patwardhan, Davis, Murphy & Ryan, 2012). A recent analysis of cost of care for simple conditions such as sinusitis or colds shows that retail clinic visits cost almost seven times less than visits to hospital emergency rooms (PwC, 2013). Calculations by Athena Health examined the cost of flu shots. Currently 50% of these shots are administered in physician offices at a cost of $3 Billion per year. If retail clinics administered these shots instead, the cost could be reduced to $2.4 Billion, a 21% decrease (Grossman, 2013).

The evidence is very clear that retail clinics provide services at a lower cost than other sites of care, with substantial savings for the healthcare system at large. Some experts have argued that if retail clinics lead to new utilization, the cost savings may be lower. It remains to be seen whether this argument is valid or not. We contend, however, that even if retail clinics are inducing demand by bringing in non-users to the healthcare system, there are long-term savings as these patients tend not to delay their care, get preventative services and deal with minor problems before they become larger and costlier.

5. FUTURE OF RETAIL CLINICS

Despite the remarkable growth in retail clinics in the last seven years, many questions remain about their potential and future viability in the healthcare system at large. In a study of executives of hospital systems that own/affiliate with retail clinics, we examined whether retail clinics were a fad or were here to stay. We reported on the results: "I don't see great growth for retail clinics. It is just a relieve valve for the health system, not a primary revenue stream. [Retail chains] are cutting back. The model does not make sense, the retail clinics will not make money or be self-sustaining. At best they will break even." Another commented that "there is not the financial gain that we thought originally would happen" and yet another one cautioned that "this is not going to be a significant part of the healthcare system." Others were less critical but still very pragmatic in their assessment: "They will continue to serve a need, which is access for patients. This is just another access point, with convenient times and locations, not a whole new way of treating patients," and "from a convenience point of view it is fine, but patients still need a medical home so care would not be fractured for people with chronic conditions." Only one of the respondents was very optimistic about the future of retail clinics and described the trend as "a transformational development in healthcare that is taking hold" (Kaissi, 2010b, p. 225-226). The respondents suggested that the keys to success were a good location, vertical integration with a healthcare system, better marketing of services and focus on a specific niche.

Tom Charland, industry expert and CEO of Merchant Medicine, was equally cautious in his most recent assessment of the industry. He noted that "it is still unclear whether all four of the large retailer-owned clinic operators – CVS/MinuteClinic, Walgreens/Take Care, Kroger/The Little Clinic and Target Clinic – will continue to grow. It would not surprise us if one or two of these players begins to scale back.... Apart from CVS, the modest growth by the other major retailers can be explained by a lack of clarity around the changing economic forces in healthcare. It's still too early to say whether shared savings and narrow networks will cause traditional healthcare providers to start referring simple cases into retail clinics. If they do, expansion should be a no-brainer for Walgreens, Kroger and Target. But that clarity won't come until 2014 at the earliest. CVS has always been more willing to roll the dice in this space than other retailers, which explains why they have nearly twice as many clinics as their nearest competitor" (Merchant Medicine, 2013, p. 3).

Surprisingly, Christine Cassel, a physician, recently observed in JAMA, the official Journal of the American Medical Association: "Retail clinics hold potential for a uniquely US solution to the problem of access to primary care. Although questions remain about their future, evidence suggests that retail clinics may have an important role in US healthcare. There are challenges, but this is happening already. The question is whether this phenomenon will grow and flourish [...] or whether 20th-century attitudes about physician and hospital dominance in healthcare will prevent market-based solutions to the healthcare access and cost crisis. This model is a challenge to medical and hospital leadership, as well as to leaders in the retail health clinic industry, as they pursue the potential opportunities and benefits for the American people" (Cassel, 2012, p. 2151-2152). Some industry observers agree that retail clinics are here to stay and thrive. Tine Hansen-Turton, a retail clinic expert and CEO of the CCA suggests that "retail clinics are becoming more main stream and will only continue to grow. The incentives are now aligned between providers and insurers and consumers. It is no more seen as a stretch, but as an opportunity to provide the right care in the right place at the right time..... [we] have created a consumer group in their 30-40's and they will continue to use retail clinics as their main source of care for the rest of their lives" (Hansen-Turton, personal interview, 2013). Web Golinkin, CEO of RediClinic, suggests that the most important recent growth has been in utilization rather than the number of new clinics. He posited that "the industry will continue to grow in both respects, but some operators won't be successful, not due to lack of demand, but because they don't understand the operational challenges or lack sufficient capital to wait for consumer- and market-driven rationality to prevail. So there will be growth, and very significant growth in the long term, but there may be failures along the way" (Golinkin, personal interview, 2013).

A recent estimate by GBI Research sheds some light on future clinic growth. It forecasts that the CAGR (Compound Annual Growth Rate- which is the year-over-year growth rate of an investment over a specified period of time) for retail clinics for the period 2011-2018 will be 11.2% and that the number of clinics is expected to reach 2,854 by 2018 (GBI Research, 2012). Consulting firm Accenture was more optimistic as it expected the number to reach 2,400 by only 2015, covering about 10.8 million visits per year (Accenture, 2013). It remains to be seen whether these numbers come true or whether they fall short, like overly optimistic estimates in the past have.

Expansion of Scope

The original formula of retail clinics consisted of a nurse practitioner or physician assistant that handles a basic menu of preventative and easy-to-diagnose routine conditions. In the last few years, there have been many signs that clinic operators are seeking to change that formula by expanding the scope of services offered. As previously mentioned, some of these strategies to expand into chronic disease management, have severely angered physician groups and have led to the severance of the agreement between the AAFP and major retail clinic operators.

For visits to retail clinics between 2007-2009, only 1% were for chronic disease care (Mehrotra & Lave, 2012). Similarly, a study of visits in 2007 showed that chronically ill patients used the clinics only for minor conditions. For their chronic conditions, these patients saw a physician at rates similar to or higher than those of patients who did not use the retail clinic (Wilson et al., 2010). However, there are many reasons to believe that these numbers will soon rise. A 2009 report by Deloitte Center for Health Solutions claimed that "the retail clinic business model is capable of supporting additional revenue streams unrelated to its core operations (i.e., services around a non-urgent primary care visit and prescription dispensing)" (p. 9). It maintained that current retail clinic services fall under "Zone One" services such as primary care services, contracted diagnostic testing (lab, biometrics, imaging), prescription/over-the-counter (OTC) remedies and basic preventive screenings. However, retail clinics could expand into "Zone Two" including pharmacy dispensing and delivery (infusion/injection), optometry, hearing, home health aides, and additional prevention programs around wellness and healthy living, and even "Zone Three" services such as advanced care/disease management, referral management and health insurance programs (in partnership with a health plan/employer). Weinick and her colleagues interviewed major retail clinics stakeholders and reported the following views: "A representative from one retail clinic operator noted that this is a logical extension of current services, since midlevel providers, such as nurse practitioners, are trained to offer this type of care, and it can be cost-effective for them to do so. At the same time, this individual stated that retail clinics could not address all aspects of chronic disease management: Some types of care would require referrals to physicians, more-extensive testing than is available in retail clinic settings, or be better addressed in the context of an ongoing provider-patient relationship. Another retail clinic representative described the operator's organizational approach to expanding into screening for and treatment of hypertension and potentially managing asthma care. A representative of a health system that owns retail clinics described its hope of providing care for mild hypertension and hyperlipidemia. Another representative of a health system with formal ties to a retail clinic operator reported discussing the possibility of retail clinics monitoring patients who are taking blood thinners" (Weinick et al., 2010, p. 39).

In a 2010 study, we asked the health system executives about this trend. One of them responded: "I think this is a very positive trend. If we could turn them into chronic disease management centers for example to provide diabetes care, education and counseling sessions, that will be a strength, a real potential, if insurance companies are willing to pay for long term disease management" and predicted that this will be "the natural evolution of the clinics: they will focus more and more on chronic management and life-style behavior changes." Others linked the expansion with the financial difficulties that retail clinics face: "It is not surprising that they are going in that direction to increase profits," and "tinkering with the scope is important for their long-term success. There is a financial incentive to increase revenue." However, the large majority of the respondents were critical of this trend for various reasons. The first objection related to continuity and quality of care: "it cannot work if is not integrated with a care model, so the patient can go somewhere in case things escalate. You cannot do chronic management in a retail setting. Retail clinics are trying to make themselves valuable this way, but people with chronic conditions need more," and "I don't agree with it, they are not a primary care home, they do not have a 24/7 on-call." One respondent was specifically concerned about physician reactions: "Physicians don't agree with that, they think chronic care will not be handled well. Especially that retail clinics have lots of turnover and lack of continuity." The other objection raised was more of a practical nature: "If they start doing chronic care, the downside is patients will have to wait 45 minutes, and that will impact satisfaction" (Kaissi, 2010b, p. 226-227.)

The argument for expansion is that many patients do not normally adhere to their physician recommendations and do not visit their offices regularly because of lack of convenience. Therefore, allowing patient monitoring on a convenient walk-in basis can lead to improved access and better outcomes. Moreover, nurse practitioners are well equipped to provide these services as many of them already manage patient chronic diseases in physician offices. However, the potential for care fragmentation is very significant. Weinick et al. (2010) described these concerns as raised by their panel of experts: "monitoring of blood pressure, cholesterol, or blood sugar may be done at a retail clinic, but patients may need medication adjustments or further counseling from their physician. The results of the retail clinic testing might not be available at the primary care office unless the communication challenges discussed in previous chapters are addressed. In addition, as one health system representative suggested, this trend could lead to duplication of care and increased costs. If retail clinics focus on just a subset of chronic conditions, such as mild hypertension, patients must self-triage to the most appropriate site of care- a decision that may require clinical knowledge that they do not possess, such as understanding the distinction between mild and moderate hypertension. Finally, if the routine monitoring done at the retail clinic indicates normal results or no unexpected changes, there could be missed opportunities to identify related problems that would normally be addressed in a broader-scope primary care visit" (Weinick, 2010, p. 40).

Several examples of expansion of scope in the last couple of years are worth illustrating. In May of 2011, RediClinic launched Weigh Forward, a comprehensive, medically-supervised weight management program. The rationale for this service had many dimensions: "First, weight management was a large growing market that appealed to RediClinic's core 'Soccer Mom' customer, as well as to third-party payers who understood that obesity is a core healthcare cost driver. Second, it could be delivered by RediClinic's existing clinical staff. Third, it could be differentiated from other commercial weight loss programs by taking advantage of RediClinic's clinical infrastructure and grocery store venue. And fourth, a multi-visit program with a product sales component could be profitable" (Merchant Medicine, 2012b, p. 4). Web Golinkin describes it as "really a lifestyle management program being marketed as a weight management program, since it addresses all of the key elements of a healthy lifestyle and many of the risk factors that need to be controlled in chronic disease management" (Golinkin, personal interview, 2013). The program lasts 10 weeks, with in-clinic and online components. It starts and ends with a thorough medical evaluation and a complete panel of lab tests, and it focuses on behavior modification, diet/nutrition, and physical activity. Patients are provided with weekly meal plans with recipes and a shopping list. Patients typically get out of the clinic straight to the grocery store and purchase the items they need from the list (Merchant Medicine, 2012b).

More controversially, Walgreens announced in April of 2013 that its clinics, renamed Healthcare Clinics, will start diagnosing and treating chronic conditions such as diabetes and hypertension. The decision has been seen by many traditional providers such as hospitals and health systems as a declaration of war. Walgreens has responded that it is not acquiring physician practices, offering imaging or treating inpatients. Rather, it wants to be the front door to primary care in the U.S., and part of population health under healthcare reform. Alan London, M.D., the Chief Medical Officer of Healthcare Clinics explained. "I like to tell hospital executives that our Walgreens stores are already built. They're located on some of the most popular and well-traveled intersections in the country. The lights are on; the air conditioning is on. It's very simple for us to expand our model to locations that help expand the hospital's reach, and not cost them a lot of capital to expand it on their own"(Stempniak, 2013, p. 1). Naturally, hospital executives and physicians are not assured, and many worry about the possible disruptions in the continuum of care.

6. CONCLUSION

The retail clinic industry seems to be at a crucial point in its growth. As Yee (2010) described, "the industry is going through an awkward adolescence. It's no longer the brash young upstart, but neither is it quite sure what it wants to be when it grows up" (p. 1). Many of the external challenges that were originally faced by the industry seem to have eased: contract with insurance companies, opposition from the medical community, and consumer attitudes. The basic value proposition of convenience, affordability and quality is starting to become accepted by the healthcare industry and the consumers. However, serious internal challenges remain, such as increasing utilization, having a sustainable business model and offering a new menu of non-routine services.

REFERENCES

Accenture. (2013). *Retail medical clinics: From foe to friend?* Retrieved from http://www.accenture.com/SiteCollectionDocuments/PDF/Accenture-Retail-Medical-Clinics-From-Foe-to-Friend.pdf

Advance Healthcare Network for NPs and PAs. (2012). *What do NPs and PAs think about convenient care?* Retrieved from http://nurse-practitioners-and-physician-assistants.advanceweb.com/Columns/Retail-Health-Report/What-do-NPs-and-PAs-think-about-convenient-care.aspx

Ahmed, A., & Fincham, J. E. (2010). Physician office vs. retail clinic: Patient preferences in care seeking for minor illnesses. *Annals of Family Medicine*, *8*(2), 117–123. doi:10.1370/afm.1052 PMID:20212298

American Academy of Family Physicians. (2010). *AAFP board revises retail health clinic policy academy opposes ongoing expansions in scope of service*. Retrieved from http://www.aafp.org/news-now/inside-aafp/20100224retail-policy.html

American Academy of Family Physicians. (2013). Retrieved from http://www.aafp.org/home.html

American Academy of Pediatrics. (2006). AAP principles concerning retail-based clinics. Retail-Based Clinic Policy Work Group. *Pediatrics*, *118*(6), 2561–2562. doi:10.1542/peds.2006-2681 PMID:17142546

American Academy of Pediatrics. (2013). Retrieved from http://www.aap.org/en-us/Pages/Default.aspx

American Medical Association. (2013). Retrieved from http://www.ama-assn.org/ama

Angstman, K. B., Bernard, M. E., Rohrer, J. E., Garrison, G. M., & MacLaughlin, K. L. (2012). Repeat retail clinic visits: Impact of insurance coverage and age of patient. *Population Health Management*, *15*(358), 358–361. doi:10.1089/pop.2011.0088 PMID:22788953

Ashwood, J. S., Reid, R. O., Setodji, C. M., Weber, E., Gaynor, M., & Mehtrotra, A. (2011). Trends in retail clinic use among the commercially insured. *The American Journal of Managed Care*, *17*(11), e443–e448. PMID:22200061

Aversa, S. (2013). *Comparing social sentiment on convenient care clinics*. Business-2Community. Retrieved from http://www.business2community.com/social-media/comparing-social-sentiment-on-convenient-care-clinics-0591279#t7OZE2fH8e2wkolg.99

Banjo, S. (2012). Wal-Mart lags in clinic race. *Wall Street Journal*. Retrieved from http://online.wsj.com/news/articles/SB10001424052702304458604577490680107844876

Boehringer Ingelheim Pharmaceuticals, Inc. (2010). *Boehringer Ingelheim Pharmacy Satisfaction™: Retail Clinic Outlook*. Retrieved from http://www.pharmacysatisfaction.com/resources/pdf/MI73586TRF_RCO_Appendix.pdf

Bohmer, R. (2007). The rise of in-store clinics: Threat or opportunity? *The New England Journal of Medicine*, *356*(8), 765–768. doi:10.1056/NEJMp068289 PMID:17314334

Bohmer, R. M. J., & Groberg, J. P. (2002, July). *QuickMedx Inc*. (Case 603-049). Harvard Business School.

Boulton, G. (2010, January 5). New clinic boosts access: Health center in Lena's market helps low-income residents. *Milwaukee Journal Sentinel*.

Callahan, E. (2007, August 20). Retail clinics can be a valuable source partner. *Medical Staff Briefing*.

Cassel, C. K. (2012). Retail clinics and drugstore medicine. *Journal of the American Medical Association*, *307*(20), 2151–2152. doi:10.1001/jama.2012.3966 PMID:22618918

Champy, J. (2011). *What's really working in business. What it takes to win, big, now! Jim Champy brings together breakthrough approaches to strategy, marketing, and execution!* FT Press.

Christensen, C., Grossman, J. H., & Hwang, J. (2008). *The innovator's prescription: A disruptive solution for healthcare*. New York: McGraw-Hills.

Colihan, K. (2008, August 12). Parents like retail clinics for kids: Survey shows popularity of health clinics located in stores. *WebMD Health News*.

Convenient Care Association. (2013). Retrieved from http://www.ccaclinics.org/index.php?option=com_content&view=article&id=4&Itemid=116

Costello, D. (2008). A checkup for retail medicine. *Health Affairs*, *27*(5), 1299–1303. doi:10.1377/hlthaff.27.5.1299 PMID:18780914

C.S. Mott's Children Hospital. (2007). Retail Clinics: An Emerging Source of Healthcare for Children. C.S. *Mott Children's Hospital National Poll on Children's Health.*, *4*(3), 1–2.

Deloitte Center for Health Solutions. (2008). *Growth of retail clinics: 2008 survey of healthcare consumers*. Author.

Deloitte Center for Health Solutions. (2009). *Retail clinics: Update and implications*. Author.

Deloitte Center for Health Solutions. (2012). *Survey of US Health Consumers*. Retrieved from http://www.deloitte.com/assets/dcom-unitedstates/local%20assets/documents/health%20reform%20issues%20briefs/us_chs_issuebrief_2012consumersurvey_061212.pdf

Dolan, P. L. (2009, March 30). Seasonal slump shutters 89 MinuteClinic Locations. *American Medical News*. Retrieved from http://www.ama-assn.org/amednews/2009/03/30/bisa0330.htm

Eder, R. (2005). A crowded market emerges to fill growth prescription. *Drug Store News*. Retrieved from http://business.highbeam.com/413375/article-1G1-135665176/crowded-market-emerges-fill-growth-prescription

Fenn, S. (2008). Integrating retail clinics into the hospital system. *Frontiers of Health Services Management*, *24*(3), 33–36. PMID:18435359

Fottler, M., & Malvey, D. (2010). *The retail revolution in healthcare*. Santa Barbara: Praeger.

Gallegos, A. (2007). Retail medicine: The cure for healthcare disparities? *Journal of Healthcare Management*, *52*(4), 227–234. PMID:17695958

Garbutt, J. M., Mandrell, K. M., Allen, M., Sterkel, R., Esptein, J., & Kreusser, K. et al. (2013). Parents' experiences with pediatric care at retail clinics. *Journal of the American Medical Association Pediatrics.*, *167*(9), 845–850. PMID:23877236

Garbutt, J. M., Mandrell, K. M., Sterkel, R., Epstein, J., Stahl, K., & Kreusser, K. et al. (2013). Pediatric providers' attitudes toward retail clinics. *The Journal of Pediatrics, 163*(5), 1384–1388, 1388.e6. doi:10.1016/j.jpeds.2013.05.008 PMID:23810720

Gardner, A. (2013). *Popularity of 'walk-in" retail health clinics growing: Poll trend driven by convenience, low cost and shortage of primary care doctors, Harris Interactive/HealthDay survey finds.* HealthDay. Retrieved from http://consumer.healthday.com/general-health-information-16/doctor-news-206/popularity-of-walk-in-retail-health-clinics-growing-poll-672127.html

Gerencher, K. (2010, February 14). Yes, the uninsured can get care. *Wall Street Journal.*

Gonzales, R., Malone, D. C., Maselli, J. H., & Sande, M. A. (2001). Excessive antibiotic use for acute respiratory infections in the U.S. *Clinical Infectious Diseases, 33*(6), 757–762. doi:10.1086/322627 PMID:11512079

Grossman, E. (2013). *Retail clinics: what the data shows.* Paper presented at Retail Clinician Education Congress. New York, NY.

Gullo, K. (2005). Many agree on potential benefits of onsite clinics in major retail stores that can provide basic medical services, yet large numbers are also skeptical. *The Wall Street Journal, 14*(21).

Hansen-Turton, T., & Ridgway, C. (2013). The future of accessible, affordable, quality healthcare. In J. Riff, S. F. Ryan, & T. Hansen-Turton (Eds.), *Convenient Care Clinics.* New York: Springer Publishing Company.

Hansen-Turton, T., Ridgway, C., Ryan, S. F., & Nash, D. B. (2009). Convenient care clinics: The future of accessible healthcare- The formation years 2006-2008. *Population Health Management, 12*(5), 231–240. doi:10.1089/pop.2009.0041 PMID:19848565

Hansen-Turton, T., Ryan, S., Miller, K., Counts, M., & Nash, D. (2007). Convenient care clinics: The future of accessible healthcare. *Disease Management, 10*(2), 61–73. doi:10.1089/dis.2006.636 PMID:17444791

Health Research Institute, Price Waterhouse Coopers. (2013). Top Industry. *Issues (National Council of State Boards of Nursing (U.S.)),* 2014.

Hitti, M. (2007). Waiting room tops patient complaints: Patients generally satisfied with doctor-patient relationship, but both sides have gripes. *WebMD Health News.* Retrieved from http://www.webmd.com/health-insurance/20070108/waiting-room-tops-patient-complaints

Horwitz-Bennett, B. (2013, February 4). Burgeoning retail clinics require unique designs. *Healthcare Design.* Retrieved from http://www.healthcaredesignmagazine.com/article/burgeoning-retail-clinics-require-unique-designs?page=3

Hunter, L. P., Weber, C. E., Morreale, A. P., & Wall, J. H. (2009). Patient satisfaction with retail health clinic care. *Journal of the American Academy of Nurse Practitioners, 21*(10), 565–570. doi:10.1111/j.1745-7599.2009.00447.x PMID:19796291

Harris Interactive. (2007) Most Adults Satisfied with Care at Retail-Based Health Clinics. *Health-Care Poll, 6*(6).

Jacoby, R., Crawford, A. G., Chaudhari, P., & Goldfarb, N. I. (2011). Quality of care for 2 common pediatric conditions treated by convenient care providers. *American Journal of Medical Quality*, *26*(1), 53–58. doi:10.1177/1062860610375106 PMID:20861514

Jaspen, B. (2007, June 25). AMA takes on retail clinics: Doctors groups say patients in danger. *Chicago Tribune*.

Joint Commission. (2013). *Comprehensive Accreditation Manual for Ambulatory Care*. CAMAC.

Kaissi, A. (2010a). Hospital- affiliated and hospital-owned retail clinics: Strategic considerations and operational challenges. *Journal of Healthcare Management*, *55*(5), 324–337. PMID:21077582

Kaissi, A. (2010b). The future of retail clinics in a volatile healthcare environment. *The Health Care Manager*, *29*(3), 223–229. doi:10.1097/HCM.0b013e3181e93149 PMID:20686393

Kaissi, A., & Charland, T. (2013a). The evolution of retail clinics in the United States, 2006-2012. *The Health Care Manager*, *32*(4), 336–342. doi:10.1097/HCM.0b013e3182a9d73f PMID:24168869

Kaissi A. & Charland, T. (2013b). Hospital-owned retail clinics in the United States: Operations, patients and marketing. *Primary Healthcare, 3*(1).

Kaissi, A., & Charland, T. (2013c). How satisfied are hospital systems with their ownership of retail clinics? *Journal of Healthcare Management*, *58*(2), 143–153. PMID:23650698

Kalorama Information. (2012*). Retail clinics 2012: Growth of stores, consumer opinion surveys, winning competitors, supplier sales of products to clinics, clinic sales forecasts and trends*. Author.

Kamerow, D. (2007). Retail health clinics-threat or promise? *British Medical Journal*, *335*(21).

Kissinger, M. (2008). Retail health clinics drive innovation into primary care practices. *The Journal of Medical Practice Management*, *23*(5), 314–319. PMID:18472612

Landro, L. (2006). The new force in walk-in clinics: Hospitals and doctors seek slice of burgeoning business; getting referrals at ShopRite. *Wall Street Journal*, 1-4.

Laws, M., & Scott, M. K. (2008). The emergence of retail-based clinics in the United States: Early observations. *Health Affairs*, *27*(5), 1293–1298. doi:10.1377/hlthaff.27.5.1293 PMID:18780913

Leppel, K. (2010). Factors influencing willingness to use convenient care clinics among baby boomers and older persons. *Healthcare Manage Review, 35*(1), 13-22.

Lin, D. Q. (2008). Convenient care Ccinics: Opposition, opportunity, and the path to system integration. *Frontiers of Health Services Management*, *24*(3), 3–11. PMID:18435355

Malvey, D., & Fottler, M. D. (2006). The retail revolution in healthcare: Who will win and who will lose? *Health Care Management Review*, *31*(3), 168–178. doi:10.1097/00004010-200607000-00002 PMID:16877884

Market Strategies. (2007). *MinuteClinic – The evolving face of consumerism in healthcare*. Author.

Market Strategies Inc. (2007). *One in ten retail clinic users replacing their primary care physician with retail clinic for treatment of common ailments*. Retrieved from http://www.marketstrategies.com/news/2014/1/One-in-Ten-Retail-Clinic-Users-Replacing-Their-Primary-Care-Physician-With-Retail-Clinic-for-Treatment-of-Common-Ailments.aspx

Martin, E. (2003, March). QuickMedx preps to take clinic concept national. *Upsizemag.com*.

Massachusetts Department of Public Health. (2008). Retrieved from www.massleague.org/CHCManual/105CMR140.pdf

Medicine, M. (2010). *MinuteClinic ends 2009 with more closures*. Retrieved from http://www.merchantmedicine.com/News.cfm?view=77

Medicine, M. (2011a). *The ConvUrgent Care Report*, *4*(1), 1–6.

Medicine, M. (2011b). *The ConvUrgent Care Report*, *4*(8), 1–6.

Medicine, M. (2012a). *The ConvUrgent Care Report*, *6*(2), 1–6.

Medicine, M. (2012b). *The ConvUrgent Care Report*, *5*(3), 1–6.

Medicine, M. (2012c). *The ConvUrgent Care Report*, *5*(10), 1–7.

Medicine, M. (2012d). *The ConvUrgent Care Report*, *5*(5), 1–6.

Medicine, M. (2013). *The ConvUrgent Care Report*, *6*(2), 1–4.

Medicine, M. (2014). Retrieved from http://www.merchantmedicine.com

Mehrotra, A., & Lave, J. R. (2012). Visits to retail clinics grew fourfold from 2007 to 2009, although their share of overall outpatient visits remains low. *Health Affairs*, *31*(9), 2123–2129. doi:10.1377/hlthaff.2011.1128 PMID:22895454

Mehrotra, A., Liu, H., Adams, J. L., Wang, M. C., Lave, J. R., & Thygeson, M. et al. (2009). Comparing costs & quality of care at retail clinics with that of other medical settings for 3 common illnesses. *Annals of Internal Medicine*, *151*(5), 321–328. doi:10.7326/0003-4819-151-5-200909010-00006 PMID:19721020

Mehrotra, A., Wang, M. C., Lave, J. R., Adams, J. L., & McGlynn, E. A. (2008). Retail clinics, primary care physicians, and emergency departments: A comparison of patients' visits. *Health Affairs*, *27*(5), 1272–1282. doi:10.1377/hlthaff.27.5.1272 PMID:18780911

Miller, J. (2007). Right size engineering: MinuteClinic CEO Michael Howe puts retail service suite in context. *Managed HealthCare Executive*. Retrieved from http://managedhealthcareexecutive.modernmedicine.com

Miller, J. M., & Nash, D. B. (2013). Quality metrics and initiatives in the clinic setting. In Convenient Care Clinics. New York: Springer Publishing Company.

MinuteClinic. 2013. Retrieved from http://www.minuteclinic.com/

National Conference of State Legislatures. (2012). *Retail health clinics: State legislatures and laws*. Retrieved from http://www.ncsl.org/research/health/retail-health-clinics-state-legislation-and-laws.aspx

Newbold, P., & O'Neil, M. J. (2008). Small changes lead to large effects. *Frontiers of Health Services Management, 24*(3), 23–27. PMID:18435357

O'Reilly, K. B. (2007, March 5). Big retail health clinics agree to AAFP operating guidelines-2007: A newly formed quick-care trade group also aims to collaborate with physician organizations. *American Medical News.*

Paddock, C. (2007, June 26). AMA calls for investigation of retail health clinics. *Medical News Today.*

Parente, S. T., & Town, R. (2009). *The impact of retail clinics on cost, utilization and welfare.* University of Minnesota, unpublished paper.

Patwardhan, A., Davis, J., Murphy, P., & Ryan, S. F. (2012). After-hours access of convenient care clinics and cost savings associated with avoidance of higher-cost sites of care. *Journal of Primary Care & Community Health, 3*(4), 243–245. doi:10.1177/2150131911436251 PMID:23804168

Pollack, C. E., & Armstrong, K. (2009). The geographic accessibility of retail clinics for underserved populations. *Archives of Internal Medicine, 169*(10), 945–949. doi:10.1001/archinternmed.2009.69 PMID:19468086

Pollert, P., Dobberstein, D., & Wiisanen, R. (2008). Jumping into the healthcare market: Our experience. *Frontiers of Health Services Management, 24*(3), 13–21. PMID:18435356

PwC. (2013). *Medical cost trend: Behind the numbers 2014.* Health Research Institute.

RediClinic. (2013). Retrieved from http://www.rediclinic.com/about/faqs/

Reid, R. O., Ashwood, J. S., Friedberg, M. W., Weber, E. S., Setodji, C. M., & Mehrotra, A. (2013). Retail clinic visits and receipt of primary care. *Journal of General Internal Medicine, 28*(4), 504–512. doi:10.1007/s11606-012-2243-x PMID:23070656

GBI Research. (2012). *Retail Clinics – 2012 Yearbook.* Author.

Richman, D. (2013). *Harris interactive: Consumer trends in retail medicine.* Paper presented at Retail Clinician Education Congress.

Rohrer, J. E., Angstam, K. B., & Furst, J. W. (2009a). Impact of retail walk-in care on early return visits by adult primary care patients. *Quality Management in Health Care, 18*(1), 19–24. doi:10.1097/01.QMH.0000344590.61971.97 PMID:19148026

Rohrer, J. E., Angstram, K. B., & Bartel, G. A. (2009b). Impact of retail medicine on standard costs in primary care: A semiparametric analysis. *Population Health Management, 12*(6), 333–335. doi:10.1089/pop.2009.0007 PMID:20038259

Rohrer, J. E., Angstram, K. B., Garrison, G. M., Maxson, J. A., & Furst, J. W. (2013). Family medicine patients who use retail clinics have lower continuity of care. *Journal of Primary Care and Community Health, 4*(2), 150–153. doi:10.1177/2150131912471683 PMID:23799725

Rohrer, J. E., Garrison, G. M., & Angstman, K. B. (2012). Early Return Visits by Pediatric Primary Care Patients With Otitis Media. *Quality Management in Health Care, 21*(1), 44–47. doi:10.1097/QMH.0b013e3182418157 PMID:22207018

Rohrer, J. E., Yapuncich, K. M., Adamson, S. C., & Angstam, K. B. (2008). Do retail clinics increase early return visits for pediatric clinics? *Journal of the American Board of Family Medicine*, *21*(5), 475–476. doi:10.3122/jabfm.2008.05.080072 PMID:18772304

Rubenstein, S. (2009). CVS shutters 90 retail clinics for the season. *Wall Street Journal.*

Rudavsky, R., & Mehrotra, A. (2010). Sociodemographic characteristics of communities served by retail clinics. *Journal of the American Board of Family Medicine*, *23*(1), 42–48. doi:10.3122/jabfm.2010.01.090033 PMID:20051541

Rudavsky, R., Pollack, C. E., & Mehrotra, A. (2009). The geographic distribution, ownership, prices, and scope of practice at retail clinics. *Annals of Internal Medicine*, *151*(5), 315–320. doi:10.7326/0003-4819-151-5-200909010-00005 PMID:19721019

Salganik, M. W. (2004, August 8). Selling quick fix for minor ailments- health: Clinics promising inexpensive, convenient care are to open in local Target stores. *The Baltimore Sun.* Retrieved from http://articles.baltimoresun.com/2004-08-08/news/0408080212_1_target-health-clinics-pizza-hut

Schleiter, K.E. (2010). Retail medical clinics: Increasing access to low cost medical care amongst a developing legal environment. *Annals of Health Law*, *19*(3), 527–575. PMID:21456398

Scott, M. K. (2006). *Healthcare in the express lane: The emergence of retail clinics.* California HealthCare Foundation.

Scott, M. K. (2013). Building and marketing a retail clinic. In J. Riff, S. F. Ryan, & T. Hansen-Turton (Eds.), *Convenient Care Clinics*. New York: Springer Publishing Company.

Spetz, J., Parente, S. T., Town, R. J., & Bazarko, D. (2013). Scope-of-practice laws for nurse practitioners limit cost savings that can be achieved in retail clinics. *Health Affairs*, *32*(11), 1977–1984. doi:10.1377/hlthaff.2013.0544 PMID:24191089

Starfield, B. (2009). The geographic accessibility of retail clinics for underserved populations – Invited Commentary. *Archives of Internal Medicine*, *169*(10), 950–951. doi:10.1001/archinternmed.2009.110

Stempniak, M. (2013, October). Retail clinics: Threat or opportunity? *Hospitals & Health Networks*. PMID:24303633

Takach, M., & Witger, K. (2009). *Analysis of state regulations and policies governing the operation and licensure of retail clinics.* Washington, DC: National Academy for State Health Policy.

Taylor, H. (2008). *Innovations in care delivery: Retail clinics. Retail clinics: A new trend in healthcare*. Paper presented at a National Consumers League Stakeholders Forum. New York, NY.

Thygeson, M., Van Vorst, K. A., Maciosek, M. V., & Solberg, L. (2008). Use and costs of care in retail clinics versus traditional care sites. *Health Affairs*, *27*(5), 1283–1292. doi:10.1377/hlthaff.27.5.1283 PMID:18780912

Truven Health Analytics. (2012). *Data-driven marketing strategy brings new clients to innovative retail clinic.* Retrieved from http://truvenhealth.com/assets/HOSP_11467_0712_HeartlandHealth_CS_Web.pdf

Tu, H. T., & Boukus, E. R. (2013). *Despite rapid growth, retail clinic use remains modest (Research Brief 29).* Center for Studying Health System Change.

Tu, H. T., & Cohen, G. R. (2008). Checking up on retail-based health clinics: Is the boom ending? *Commonwealth Fund, 1199* (48), 1-11.

Uscher-Pines, L., Harris, K. M., Burns, R., & Mehrotra, A. (2012). The growth of retail clinics in vaccination delivery in the U.S. *American Journal of Preventive Medicine*, *43*(1), 63–66. doi:10.1016/j.amepre.2012.02.024 PMID:22704748

Walgreens. (2013). Retrieved from http://www.walgreens.com/topic/pharmacy/healthcare-clinic/price-menu.jsp#treatment

D. R. *Walk-in Medical Clinics*. (2013). Retrieved from http://www.drwalkin.com/

Wang, M. C., Ryan, G., McGlynn, E. A., & Mehrotra, A. (2010). Why do patients seek care at retail clinics and what alternatives did they consider. *American Journal of Medical Quality*, *25*(2), 128–134. doi:10.1177/1062860609353201 PMID:20142442

Weinick, R. M., Pollack, C. E., Fisher, M. P., Gillen, E. M., & Mehrotra, A. (2010). *Policy implications of the use of retail clinics.* Rand Health Technical Report.

Wilson, A. R., Zhou, X. T., Shi, W., Rodin, J., Bargman, E. P., Garrett, N. A., & Sandberg, T. J. (2010). Retail clinics versus office setting: Do patients choose appropriate providers? *The American Journal of Managed Care*, *16*(10), 753–759. PMID:20964471

Woodburn, J. D., Smith, K. L., & Nelson, G. D. (2007). Quality of care in the retail healthcare setting using national clinical guidelines for acute pharyngitis. *American Journal of Medical Quality*, *22*(6), 457–462. doi:10.1177/1062860607309626 PMID:18006426

Yee, C. M. (2010, April 13). HCMC is late entry in retail clinic race. *Minnesota Star Tribune*.

KEY TERMS AND DEFINITIONS

Cost of Care: The amount in dollars spent on healthcare services within a certain healthcare system.

Nurse Practitioner: A nurse who is qualified to treat certain medical conditions without the direct supervision of a doctor.

Patient Satisfaction: Patient expectation and attitudes regarding the quality of healthcare services received.

Physician Assistant: healthcare professional licensed to practice medicine with supervision by a licensed physician.

Quality of Care: The extent to which healthcare services provided to individuals and patient populations improve desired health outcomes.

Retail Clinics: Small clinics located in general merchandise or drug stores and offering a limited scope of diagnostic and treatment services for common medical conditions.

APPENDIX 1: QUICKMEDX/MINUTECLINIC

Rick Krieger is the founder of QuickMedx (which became Minute Clinic later) and so is credited for being the father of retail clinics. In 1999, Krieger's son had a sore throat. Realizing that he needed to test him for strep, he drove him to an urgent care center in Minneapolis. After waiting for two hours, the physician performed a strep test that turned out to be negative. Krieger recalls: "We started talking about why there was not a way to just get a simple question answered or a simple test, like strep throat, done. Why was there not a way to just slip in and be seen quickly? Wasn't there some way to get care in a timely manner for a relatively simple illness? A quick, convenient way to diagnose without waiting in the ER or clinic for two hours? We are not talking about diabetes, cancer, or heart disease! We are talking about colds and throat and ear infections" (Bohmer & Groberg, 2002). Along with two business partners, Krieger set up pilot clinics in the Cub Foods grocery store chain. The company was backed by 14 local investors.

In the early days, business was very slow and the clinics treated only 8-12 patients per day. And then Krieger formed an agreement with a local union. The union was dissatisfied with the high healthcare costs it was paying when its members used the physician's office. The union was paying 80% for physician visits that cost a $100 on average. Instead, they decided to pay 100% of the $35 flat fee at the retail clinics, a $45 saving per visit. After that, QuickMedx recruited unions of bakery drivers, meat packers, auto dealers and electricians (Champy, 2011).

Despite the agreements with the unions, QuickMedx clinics saw only 49,000 patients and lost $2.8 million in its first two years. The company attracted little interest from venture capitalists until Bain Capital Ventures bought a 28% stake in the company. Soon after, the original founders left the company and a new management team was brought in.

Linda Hall Whitman was hired as Chief Executive Officer and Dr. Glenn Johnson became Chairman of the Board. The company raised $4 million in capital, increased its prices, expanded its menu of services, and updated its software to reflect practice guidelines. The company tried to expand outside of Minnesota, but then learned that the "QuickMedx" name was already trademarked in another state. Therefore, they decided to change the name to Minute Clinic. But growth in Minnesota was first priority as additional clinics were set up at Target stores, Best Buy and Guidant. In 2005, Whitman was replaced by Michael C. Howe. He grew the company from 19 clinics in two states to 83 clinics in 10 states in two years. Minute Clinic was then acquired by CVS Caremark. In 2006, it became the first retail clinic operator to earn accreditation from the Joint Commission. In 2007, Howe stated: "Consumers have already voted. In 2004, MinuteClinic recorded 60,000 patient visits. In 2005, we recorded about 175,000 visits. In 2006, we recorded 350,000 patient visits, and we'll record close to 1 million in 2007. That's a confirmation from the consumer" (Miller, 2007). CVS Minute Clinic is today the largest retail clinic operator with 774 clinics nationwide.

APPENDIX 2: E-MAIL CORRESPONDENCE WITH DR. JUAN FERRERIS, PEDIATRICIAN, SAN ANTONIO, TEXAS (RBCS REFER TO RETAIL-BASED CLINICS)

1. The RBCs focus on areas where patients have insurance and have access to pediatric care, so the main goal of RBCs is NOT to improve access to care but rather how best to profit from this specific healthcare demographic.
2. RBCs use non-pediatric trained providers and in fact don't even use physicians at all except in a cursory "review" or "supervisory" role. Even in that role, it is unusual to have a pediatrician as the "chart reviewer" or supervisor. Also unusual to have pediatric nurse practitioners as the provider.
3. RBCs present themselves as a hybrid model of quasi primary care and quasi urgent care. The point here is to straddle both providers so as to maximize breadth of approach while not really being held to either an urgent care standard of care or a primary care standard of care model.
4. RBC quality of care measurement as it specifically relates to pediatrics is lacking and difficult to measure.
5. RBC clearly seem to provide a convenient place for "some" care that is neither specific nor accountable.
6. When problems in care or f/u occur, the burden of follow up and care goes back to the pediatrician.

My experience has been as follows:

- Some patients that had a "sports physical" never had a hernia or testicular exam and no discussion on risk factors for cardiac/sudden death or diabetes/heart disease issues. These are issues that we as pediatricians address during an annual/sports physical.
- Treatments are typically "adult" type approaches such as three times a day dosing on medications that can be dosed twice a day. For a school aged child this is a big issue, not to mention adherence is problematic with TID dosing versus BID. For example, I commonly see pen v k tid used for treatment of strep. I also commonly see pain medications such as codeine, hydrocodone prescribed for children.
- Parents will call my office asking for a specialist referral for a problem addressed or identified at these clinics which then requires the pediatrician to justify to the ins company reasons for the referral and sometimes we are measured for cost containment or referral patterns by insurance companies. In these situations, we ask patients to come in for our evaluation to determine need for referral and document properly.
- It just seems illogical that at a time when more and more is demanded of primary care physicians for quality, medical home, prevention, board recertification, etc., that RBCs can exist and not be held accountable for any of these same benchmarks.

If these clinics continue to expand without any real benchmarking, quality measurement, proper pediatric oversight, etc., how can we expect that general pediatricians will even continue to exist as a viable model. Who will coordinate the care for these patients? Who will do referrals? Who will follow these patients up? How will we as a society measure the quality of pediatric care? What benchmarks for continuing education and training will we have if no pediatricians can exist because they are increasingly driven out of business?"

APPENDIX 3: LETTER FROM DR. JUAN FERRERIS, ON BEHALF OF THE SAN ANTONIO PEDIATRIC SOCIETY TO THE METHODIST HEALTH SYSTEM (APRIL 2011)

April 27, 2011
Dear Methodist HealthCare:

It is with great sadness that I noted Methodist Healthcare supporting the fragmentation of pediatric care as evidenced by its joint venture with Rediclinic.

As a Primary Care Pediatrician with over 15 years in practice providing a medical home for my patients, it frustrates and saddens me that Methodist finds it a necessity to participate in co branding with the RediClinic.

When one reads RediClinic's mission, it is quite clear that its focus is to offer health screening services such as well child exams, camp and sports physicals as well as acute care diagnostic services. Primary care pediatricians have focused on a medical home concept of care from the outset.

Pediatricians' main goals are well child exams and preventive counseling to children and their parents. Pediatricians use the well child exams as a vital part to the building of a joint family type relationship with the parents and the children. It is this close relationship with the parents and children that then results in the ability of the pediatrician to be pivotal and focused on prevention of significant lifelong issues such as smoking and illicit drug use, abstinence and std counseling, healthy active lifestyles and diet to help prevent or delay the onset of diabetes, hypertension and heart disease.

Pediatricians have always been at the forefront of prevention and screening as well as building relationships with the families through well child exams and brief acute care visits. Lastly, pediatrics and the disease processes in pediatrics are unique and challenging enough to require three dedicated years of training and separate pediatrics board and maintenance of certification. This unique approach to children, their parents, and the training of Pediatricians shows just how critical it is to have general pediatricians care directly for children in a medical home model of care.

With Methodist's approach to co branding with Rediclinic, it gives the community and the primary care pediatricians the impression that Methodist encourages Rediclinic to function in a model that directly challenges the basic unique approach to pediatrics that the pediatric medical home provides.

As per Rediclinic's press release their focus is to offer health screening services in a retail environment:

"Since 1989, RediClinic (formerly known as InterFit Health) has provided people with easy access to high quality, convenient and affordable healthcare services. Today the company is the largest provider of retail health screening services in the United States and is a leader in convenient care. The company also provides health screenings, flu shots and other health-rated services to major employers. For more information, please visit www.rediclinic.com."

The American Academy of Pediatrics also has a specific stance on how these clinics erode the medical home concept and interfere with the unique quality care primary care pediatricians provide.

See the following AAP statement regarding this clinic s and how they threaten the medical home:

First, let's first review the concerns raised by the AAP in abbreviated form:

- Fragmentation of care.
- The possible effects on quality of care. As these clinics have no Board Certified Pediatricians.
- Provision of episodic care to children with special healthcare needs and chronic diseases.
- Lack of access to and maintenance of a complete healthcare record.
- The use of tests for the purposes of diagnosis without proper follow-up.
- Possible public health issues that could occur when patients with contagious diseases are in a commercial, retail environment with little or no isolation.
- Seeing children with "minor" conditions, as these visits are important and provide an opportunity to work with patients and families to deal with a variety of other issues.

This issue is a direct challenge to quality children's healthcare in that erodes the medical home concept. It makes it impossible for General Pediatrics to provide a medical home, since Rediclinic markets general services without a board certified pediatrician, and they are supported by a hospital system that does not provide Board Certified general pediatric oversight. Finally, referrals from these clinics will go to subspecialists not general pediatricians which further erode the central focus of the pediatric medical home and will drive up costs and unnecessary procedures as these children will be referred for more subspecialty care and procedures since the providers in these Rediclinics are not pediatricians.

What is Methodist going to do when we can no longer provide proper care and follow-up since the general pediatricians were not and are not involved in the discussions of this co branding approach and are not at all involved in the care of these children that access these clinics. Who will be there to support the hospitalists and specialists if the General Pediatrician in the community cannot provide a medical home that centers on quality and a uniquely pediatric approach? Maybe Rediclinic has the answer?

As a board certified pediatrician, I believe that we have a lot to offer Methodist Healthcare in this issue by providing open communication of ideas of how to ensure that Methodist cobrands and partners in a way that sends the correct message: quality care centered on children and improved access to that care. Methodist should include board certified pediatricians in discussions on these types of partnerships in order to be sure that the mission remains to increase access to quality healthcare without eroding the quality of the pediatric medical home. These clinics should not examine such young children, provide quick limited physical exams for children given the significant disease processes that can be missed when non-pediatric trained individuals are doing the exam and non-pediatric certified physicians are providing oversight.

Approaches to the Rediclinic/Methodist venture as it currently exists that would be helpful in stressing access to quality pediatric care could be any of the following:

1. Remove the visible Methodist HealthCare marquis so as not to give the perception of Pediatric Specific Methodist oversight which currently is not the case.
2. Rediclinic should limit exposure to children over the age of 16 years of age as Methodist traditionally does for Children's Hospital admissions and procedures in Pediatrics.
3. Rediclinic should not advertise that it can provide well child exams with Methodist as the oversight if there is no Board Certified Pediatric oversight.
4. Methodist Healthcare should involve Board Certified General Pediatricians in out of hospital practice in an effort to avoid these perceptions of conflict and splintering of quality pediatric care now and in their future ventures in pediatric access and care issues."

Chapter 7
Worksite Clinics

ABSTRACT

In this chapter, the evolution and growth of worksite clinics is discussed. Worksite clinics are not a new phenomenon. Prior to the 1980s, many large employers operated onsite company clinics to treat work-related injuries. However, many of these clinics closed in the 1980s and 1990s because of the decline in heavy industry and manufacturing sectors and the reduction in workplace hazards. Recently, there has been a significant resurgence of worksite clinics. The new generation of clinics is markedly different in that their main focus is on primary care, health promotion, and wellness rather than occupational injuries. The authors discuss in-depth the operations, stakeholders, and outcomes of care in worksite clinics. They predict that worksite clinics seem to be well positioned to thrive in a post-reform healthcare environment.

Worksite health clinics appear to be the next big thing, with clearly evident benefits and high satisfaction among employers and their workers. Their presence will increase, and insurers will have to figure out how to treat them. Vendors of clinics already appear to be positioning themselves as network providers, and are likely doing so to take advantage of coming healthcare reforms that will reduce barriers to their use. A worksite clinic's intimate understanding of an employer group suggests it will rank as a high efficiency provider, and insurers should anticipate having to reimburse them at their highest rates. —Rick Byrne, 2009

DOI: 10.4018/978-1-4666-6355-8.ch007

INTRODUCTION

One of the unique aspects of the U.S. healthcare system is employer-sponsored insurance (ESI). Most Americans under the age of 65 obtain their health insurance coverage through an employer, whether that is their own employer or the employer of a family member to whom they are related as a dependent. Companies have traditionally offered healthcare coverage as a benefit to attract and retain top talent. The latest estimates suggest that about 159 million Americans are covered by employer-sponsored insurance (Robert Wood Johnson, 2013). However, the costs of providing that coverage to employees have steadily increased in the last ten years. Costs have grown faster than inflation and now constitute 15% and 40% of the average single and married employee's total annual compensation, respectively (Fuld & Company, 2009). As a result, many employers have dropped or reduced coverage to their employees, while some employees have declined ESI even when offered due to high premium costs. Average annual premiums for employee-only coverage more than doubled from $2,490 in 2000 to $5,081 in 2011. Family premiums have also increased from $6,415 to $14,447 in the same time period. Consequently, the percentage of Americans receiving health insurance through their employer has fallen from 69.7% in 2000 to 59.5% in 2011 (Robert Wood Johnson, 2013).

Facing the hard realities of increasing costs, decreasing profits and reduced overall global competitiveness, American companies have looked for solutions, such as shifting the risk of healthcare coverage to employees through the provision of high-deductible health plans (HDHP) and health savings account (HSAs) (discussed in Chapter 2). Other solutions have emphasized viewing employees as company assets and providing them with valuable alternatives for seeking primary care and other types of services. In that direction, employers are offering worksite clinics that promise to deliver cost-effective healthcare services. The main rationale for these clinics is to help control costs of ESI. Other reasons include improving access and convenience for employees; reducing lost time and absence; improving productivity; improving health outcomes; promoting wellness and encouraging use of screening and preventive services; providing higher quality of care than that received in the community; boosting employee retention, recruitment and morale; redirecting care from expensive, sub-optimal and time consuming settings such as hospital emergency rooms; and serving as the primary locus of healthcare delivery for employees and their dependents (Hochstadt, 2010). A recent report suggested that "[b]y far the strongest motivation for implementing workplace clinics is to contain direct medical costs. In the short term, exerting greater control over direct costs, such as specialist visits, non-generic prescriptions, emergency department (ED) visits and avoidable hospitalizations, is a key employer objective. In the long run, improving population health by preventing and managing chronic conditions is a major objective" (Tu, Boukus & Cohen, 2010), p.2). A survey of employers by the human resources consulting firm Mercer, found that among those offering worksite clinics, 82% were motivated by reducing lost employee productivity, 75% by controlling overall healthcare costs, 73% by managing employees' health risks and chronic conditions, and 50% by attracting and retaining talent (Mercer, 2012). Another survey by Tower Watsons (2012) found that 62% established them mainly to enhance worker productivity, 56% to reduce medical costs, 52% to create a center of health to better integrate all health productivity efforts, 38% to improve access to care, 32% to address occupational health and safety needs, 27% to improve quality of care, 8% to reduce pharmacy costs and 8% to provide concierge service as a perk.

Evolution

It is important to note that worksite clinics are not a new concept. As far back as the 1800's, large railroad and coal mining firms had company physicians that provided occupational health services to workers. These firms were located in remote sites and workers would otherwise have no access to any kind of care. In the 1940's, the Kaiser Steel Company of

California started to provide healthcare to the thousands of workers flowing into northern California to work in the shipyards. Thus the first worksite clinic emerged, and it provided an array of healthcare services, especially occupational health (Thomas, 2011). Other companies operated worksite clinics on-and-off with a main focus on treating work-related injuries. After the 1980's, many clinics were closed because of declines in the heavy industry and manufacturing sectors and reductions in workplace hazards. At the same time, firms in the financial sector for example offered care for minor acute conditions as a perk for high-wage employees and to minimize employees' time away from work (Tu, et al., 2010).

The new iteration of worksite clinics differs from the older ones in that the focus has shifted from occupational health and workplace-related injuries to primary care services, health promotion and wellness. The driving force for the new clinics seems to be cost containment, rather than occupational medicine. For companies with worksite clinics with at least 1,000 employees, 70% of those that have developed clinics after the year 2000 are focused on using them to reduce medical costs, compared to only 49% of those that had installed them prior to 2000. Moreover, only 26% of companies that have post-2000 clinics are motivated by occupational health and safety concerns compared with 54% that had clinics prior to 2000 (Wyatt, 2008).

Recently, that shift has resulted in many employers dropping the use of the term "clinic" and preferring to use "healthy living institute" or "wellness center" (Vesely, 2011). For some, the worksite clinic is just the tip of the iceberg, one element in the larger "employer-managed health" where the "employer is the ultimate determinant of the healthcare status of its employees and dependents" and where "the employer can address the healthcare status of its workforce through a combination of benefit design, direct contracting, preventive measures, and a proactive partnership with the employees to promote general wellness" (Onsiteclinics, 2010).

Growth and Usage

Given the recency of the trend, and the large number of American firms overall, it is difficult to calculate the total number of worksite clinics nationwide. Fuld & Company estimated that about 1,200 firms operated worksite clinics in 2009. Given that many of these are large employers with multiple campuses and multiple clinics, they put the total number at 2,200 clinics. More recent estimates have varied widely:

- A 2011 survey of Benfield Research found that 30% of large employers had a worksite clinic at one or more location, and 7% planned to open one within the next 18 months (Berry, 2012).
- In 2012, Mercer calculated that the prevalence of worksite clinics for employers with 5,000 or more employees increased from 32% to 37% between 2009 and 2012. Another 15% of those large companies were considering adding their own clinics in the next two years. For companies with 500 to 4,999 employees, 15% had clinics and another 11% were planning to add one soon. Overall, about 30% of employers of all sizes had a worksite clinic (Mercer 2012).
- A 2012 study by the Society for Human Resource Management found that only

8% of employers have worksite clinics (Halzack, 2012). Given the other evidence, this percentage seems particularly low.

- A 2012 study by the National Business Group on Health found that 46% of large employers offered at least one worksite clinic, up from 37% the previous year (Halzack, 2012).

Despite the increase in the number of clinics, usage rates have appeared to remain constant. Specifically, the use of workplace clinics among all families stagnated at 3.9% between 2007 and 2010. However, this time period witnessed the economic recession that lead to overall increased unemployment. During that time period, large employers (which typically have worksite clinics) disproportionately shed workers and reduced hiring. Many employees were laid off and therefore lost access to worksite clinics, while financial pressures caused some employers to delay or cancel plans to open new clinics and others with existing clinics to scale down or even eliminate clinics (Boukus & Tu, 2012). The proportion using worksite clinics was 17% among families with workers in the manufacturing sector, 11% among those in public administration and 3.4% among those in the public utilities sector or in wholesale or retail trade. Slight increases in usage were noted among families with employees working for large employers (11.2% in 2010 vs. 10.4% in 2007) and among families with employees working for governmental institutions (9.9% in 2010 vs. 7.0% in 2007) (Boukus & Tu, 2012). More updated estimates on usage rates since 2010 were not available at the time of the writing of this book.

1. OPERATIONS

Services and Care Models

Worksite clinics vary in terms of scope of practice offered, with the variation mainly related to the size of the company and the industry in which it operates. The range of services offered can be summarized by the following categories:

- **Occupational Health:** Treatment of work-related injuries, employment physicals and screenings, travel medicine, and compliance with federal workplace safety regulations.
- **Acute Care:** Ranging from low-acuity episodic care, such as sore throats or sprains, to treatment of more severe symptoms requiring urgent attention, such as exacerbations of chronic conditions.
- **Preventive Care:** Physical exams, immunizations and screening.
- **Wellness:** Health risk assessment follow up, biometric screenings, health coaching, lifestyle management programs and educational programs.
- **Disease management:** Ongoing care for and management of chronic conditions." (Tu, et al., 2010, p.3).

Small companies employing 300-500 employees typically have a worksite clinic staffed by a part-time nurse practitioner. A minimum of 800 to 1,000 employees is needed to sustain a clinic with a full-time nurse practitioner, with a primary care physician visiting the clinic and providing care about two to eight hours per week. Employers with more than 1,000 employees have a large enough patient base to justify the hiring of a full-time primary care physician, and to provide supplemental services such as dental, vision, nutrition, rehab, and wellness (Daugherty, 2012). Overall, there are three models of care. The first one is the "basic primary care" model which is intended to serve only as supplement to primary care physician practices but is occasionally the primary source of care for some employees. Under this model, the worksite clinic is staffed by a part-time nurse practitioner that treats minor injuries and episodic low-acuity illness. It includes some disease management and evaluation of more complex conditions and it offers screenings, health risk assessments (HRAs), and health education. The "comprehensive primary care" model, staffed by at least one primary care physician, is designed to serve as the employees' and their dependents' primary source of primary care. Office hours are extended to evenings but typically not weekends, and services offered may include pharmacy, rehabilitation, vision, dental, dietetics and mental health. Some clinics under this model even offer specialist care on a part-time or full-time basis. The last model is the traditional "occupational health model" that specializes in treating work-related illnesses and promoting health awareness and education. It is typically staffed by a full-time or part-time nurse practitioner (depending on size) that treat treats minor injuries and low-acuity illness and offer screenings, flu shots, health risk assessments, and health education (Daugherty, 2012). Services offered by most worksite clinics include (Benfield Research, 2011):

- **Immunizations:** 89% of clinics
- **Health education:** 82% of clinics
- **Screenings:** 79% of clinics
- **Workplace injury treatment:** 68% of clinics
- **Preventive care:** 66% of clinics
- **Fitness for duty exams:** 63% of clinics
- **Nutrition/weight management counseling:** 53% of clinics
- **Travel medications:** 53% of clinics
- **Primary care:** 47% of clinics
- **Smoking cessation:** 45% of clinics
- **Physical or occupational therapy:** 37% of clinics
- **Maternity support:** 18% of clinics
- **Other (ergonomic evaluations, fitness centers):** 8% of clinics

A survey of families showed that the majority use worksite clinics for minor, routine care, despite their employers' focus on primary care and wellness offerings. Specifically, 63.7% of survey respondents cited vaccination as the primary purpose of their clinic visits, whereas 26.5% cited a new illness or symptom and 10.3% cited prescription refill as the main reason for the visit. Therefore, most families tend to use worksite clinics for episodic, rather than ongoing care. In fact, only 9.3% cited ongoing care of chronic conditions as the primary purpose for their visits, which is far lower than the prevalence of chronic conditions in the general workforce. It is important to note though that while the primary reason may be for a one-time condition, many worksite clinic providers take advantage of the visit to address broader aspects of health and wellness. The authors explained that "employees who go to a clinic with a sprained ankle or a sore throat would undergo blood pressure checks and other screenings at a minimum. Consequently, services such as vaccinations, physical exams- [...] or treatment of new illnesses or symptoms- [...] all can provide opportunities for clinicians to identify health issues beyond the primary reason for the visit" (Boukus & Tu, 2012, p.3-4). Other reasons for visiting the clinic included the treatment of a workplace-related injury (11.3%).

In relation to other non-traditional services, a recent survey of employers indicated that some organizations have hesitated to establish a worksite clinic for fear their employees might consider it an intrusion from their employer into the sensitive area of personal health information (Towers Watson, 2012). However, that concern seems to be waning, as 91% of companies indicated that they offer or plan to offer biometric screening and 61% said that they provide or plan to provide Employee Assistance Programs (EAP) counseling at the worksite clinic (Towers Watson, 2012).

Financial and Staffing Models

There are three main arrangements for companies to operate a worksite clinic: contract with a third-party vendor, contract with a local physician practice or hospital system, and full ownership of the clinic. The model most commonly used is contracting with a vendor (67.2%) (Towers Watson, 2012). Employers outsource clinic operations to vendors that provide comprehensive staffing and management, referred to as "turnkey operations." Running a health clinic is far afield from most employer's core competency, and they prefer to contract with vendors that have expertise in specialized areas such employee data confidentiality, medical malpractice insurance and biomedical waste disposal (Tu, et al., 2010). Under this arrangement, the employer pays for the labor, facility, equipment and supplies, as well as an administrative fee to the vendor. The attractiveness of this model for the employer is that costs are fixed and predictable and the incentives are aligned. The employer's main goal is to provide employees with healthcare services at an average cost that is lower than what traditional medical practices would typically charge. As more employees use the clinic, the employer's savings accumulate. This is also appealing for the vendors because there is virtually no risk with the cost of labor being passed on to the employer (Merchant Medicine, 2013b). Examples of vendors include Take Care Health Services by Walgreens (a retail clinic operator, as discussed in the previous chapter), Quad Med and Concentra. We discuss vendors in more depth in the next section. It is important to note that even when employers outsource clinic management and operations to a third-party vendor, they need to remain engaged in clinic operations and outcomes. Regardless of who manages and staffs the clinic, "the employer ultimately owns the clinic, and strong, ongoing oversight and support by senior leadership are key to the clinic's survival and success" (Tu, et al., 2010).

The full ownership model is a distant second with only 18.8% of employers choosing to directly employ and manage clinic staff (Towers Watson, 2012). Many of these are long-standing worksite clinics that came to existence when vendors were not common yet. Examples of companies that have built successful in-house worksite clinics are Boeing, Quad/ Dow Chemical Company, and Rosen Hotel and Resorts (Tu, et al., 2010; Fottler & Malvey, 2010). An interesting trend is that of non-healthcare companies that developed their own clinics and became so proficient in running them that they started to provide clinic management and staffing as a service to other employers. For example, "... QuadMed, which started as the in-house clinic manager for the printing company Quad/Graphics, now operates primary care clinics for other large employers. Similarly, the Cerner Corp., a health information technology firm, first established a clinic at its Kansas City campus in 2006 and then expanded its onsite-clinic subsidiary, Health*e* Solutions, to provide clinic services for other large employers, including Cisco Systems and Kia Motors" (Tu, et al., 2010).

Only a small minority of employers (4.7%) contract with local health providers to deliver services for their worksite clinics. For some of those, the main reason is to appease local physicians and providers that may be resistant to the idea of an employer competing with their services. For others, especially those in rural and remote areas, the local providers are the only available option as many vendors do not operate there. For example, Perdue Farms, the poultry company with locations in rural and small-town facilities, negotiated preferred provider agreements directly with physicians and other providers in many communities in which it operates. The arrangements are embraced by the providers because they can extend their private practices to the Perdue worksite clinic (Tu, et al., 2010). It is important to note that some health systems in non-rural areas are getting more involved in the worksite clinic model, and some are doing it in collaboration with vendors. Brian Klepper, an officer at worksite vendor WeCare TLC explains: "We are in discussions with a number of hospital systems. And we expect to open our first clinic with a hospital this summer [2013] ...we're going to hospitals and saying, 'Why don't you go after employers with us?' We will build clinics together, drive care that's appropriate, and refer into the hospitals preferentially" (Merchant Medicine, 2013a, p.3).

Staffing

Successful worksite clinics aim to achieve a "trusted clinician" primary care model, which is described as "having the ability to bond with patients, to build a trusted adviser relationship...[a clinician who] can provide compassion, be accessible, and also be very good at motivating employees to do the right thing"(Tu, et al., 2010, p.6). Whether that trusted clinician is a primary care physician or a nurse practitioner depends on the scope of services and the attitudes and preferences of employees. Two corporate medical directors offered polar opposite situations. The first one stated that "[w]e found that having M.D.s was critical to patient acceptance of our [primary care clinic]," whereas the other maintained that there is no need for a "BMW model" of primary care: "I don't think everything has to be done by physicians; great things can be done by NPs [nurse practitioners]. The reason I like NPs is they have to do care planning in school and learn to treat the person as a whole; physicians tend to think about [discrete] problems"(Tu, et al., 2010, p.6). It is important to note that as companies have shifted from an occupational health focus to a primary care and wellness focus, the type of providers and their treatment of patients have had to change too. For example, occupation health nurses were trained to take care of injuries and get the employee out and back to work as fast as possible. A new skill set is now needed to spend more time with employees and treat them as a whole person. Some worksite clinics now hire health coaches and other professionals with varied backgrounds, such as nurses, health educators, nutritionists and exercise physiologists.

Regardless of the model, staffing constitutes about 75% of operating costs. For example, a single non-physician provider with a receptionist who can also serve as a medical assistant will cost about $350,000 per year, while clinics that have full-time physicians and offer additional ancillary services such as laboratory, X-ray, pharmacy, vision and physical therapy, can cost considerably more (Hochstadt, 2010). Peter Hotz, president of Take Care's Employer Solutions division, describes the different staffing situations: "A health center can have a wide variety of staff, judging on the hours of operation [...] We have sites with a single nurse who is a health coach an does a lot of screening and outreach. But we also have sites that have 40 to 50 employees, and can perform full dental, vision, medical and X-ray services. Some are more fitness-oriented, and we can also offer full workplace pharmacies" (Byrne, 2009, p.1).

In worksite clinics, recruitment and retention of primary care physicians in specific, and of all providers in general, is relatively easier than other sites of care. The clinics have some important advantages over typical community-based practices, such as a salaried arrangement, a controllable lifestyle with specific working hours, and the relief of physicians from dealing with malpractice insurance and many other administrative hassles. A medical director suggested the worksite clinics offer providers the opportunity to "get off the hamster wheel...[by] spending time with patients...counseling and not being productivity-incented"(Tu, et al., 2010, p.7). Similarly, Bill Crimmins of Novia CareClinics, a vendor, maintained: "In our world, we offer family practice doctors at $100 an hour, which is in line with what they generally target to make. Rather than seeing five or six patients an hour, we ask them to see three an hour. We want them to dialogue about their conditions, their family background, their nutrition, their exercise, their wellness. All we ask them to do is practice medicine. When they experience what it's like, they start asking for more hours" (Byrne, 2009, p.4). However, these advantages apply only to urban and metropolitan area, as many rural worksite clinics face serious challenges to recruit providers.

Challenges

In operating worksite clinics, companies face a dizzying maze of medical, labor, real estate and data security regulations, at both the federal and state levels. Therefore, it is not surprising that many companies chose to outsource clinic operations to external vendors. One of the most important compliance requirements for workplace clinics at the federal level relate to regulations guaranteeing the privacy of employee health records, as well as regulations governing health savings accounts (HSAs). At the state level, employers must abide by regulations relating to licensure of healthcare facilities and providers, data privacy and access, disposal of biomedical waste, handling of laboratory specimens and storage, and dispensing of pharmaceuticals. As mentioned in previous chapters, some states have corporate practice of medicine laws that restrict or prohibit corporations from providing services through employed physicians, while scope of practice laws for nurse practitioners vary widely by state. This is especially challenging for employers who operate clinics in different states. For example, some states prohibit extending clinic services to non-employees, which makes it difficult to standardize clinic operations and services in different locations (Tu, et al., 2010).

Other non-regulatory challenges for worksite clinics relate to scale and scope of operations. For clinics to be cost-effective, employers should plan and implement the range of services that is needed by the size and the type of its employee workforce. While it makes sense for large employers to invest in a wide array of services such as laboratory, digital radiology pharmacy, dentistry, optometry and physical therapy, for others this might constitute a huge waste of resources because of low utilization. Another challenge relates to getting the employees to actually use the clinic. Employers can't assume that if "we build it, they will come," and therefore have to invest heavily in internal marketing. This can include outreach activities using a variety of methods to connect with different types of employees such as e-mail, newsletters, bulletin boards, fliers, home mailings, health fairs and information sessions. Some companies mandate that new employees receive a tour of the clinic during orientation, and that clinic providers send personalized letters welcoming new employees and encouraging them to use the clinic. It is crucial that the reputation of the clinic is excellent and that customer service is of the highest standards, so that employees will refer others as well as their dependents through word-of-mouth. A clinic director explained: "You need enough people to come in and have a great experience every time [and] talk about it. The No. 1 best way for a new practice [to grow] is [through] word of mouth" (Tu, et al., 2010, p.9).

Some worksite clinics allow dependents of employees to receive services at the clinics, but that presents its own set of challenges. Clinics serving employees and their dependents tend to be larger in size and scope. Moreover, issues of access to the clinic are important, especially in the aerospace and government defense industries where security concerns prohibit non-employees from accessing the building. In the heavy industry and the chemical industry, strong safety concerns apply. Therefore, some employers locate the clinics at the proximity of their campuses, rather than inside the main buildings (Tu, et al., 2010).

2. STAKEHOLDERS

Employers invest in worksite clinics to contain healthcare costs and increase productivity and retention, but need a large workforce with low turnover to make the clinics cost-effective. Employees can benefit from convenient, more affordable and easily accessible healthcare services, but have to get over their skepticism of the worksite clinic first. Vendors are an important player in the worksite clinic industry, and many of them are expanding and assuming a large role. Physician practices, hospital systems and insurance companies are threatened by the model, but many are becoming more involved in it.

Employers

Employers of all sizes, industries and sectors are showing increasing interests in worksite clinics. In this section, we highlight a few examples of employers that have invested in owning and managing their clinics or have contracted with vendors to provide clinic services on their campuses.

In the early 1990's, the Rosen Hotel and Resorts in Florida created its own health insurance plan and established a worksite clinic staffed by two primary care physicians, two nurse practitioners and other support staff. The plan covers employees for free clinic visits with no co-payments, in addition to annual physicals and preventative care, prenatal and baby care, and pharmacy and dental benefits. In addition to primary care services, the clinic has on-site laboratory and X-ray facilities. It is estimated that the plan and the clinic have reduced per-employees costs of care from $2,223 to $850 per year, and have contributed to decreasing turnover rates to less than 15% (Fottler & Malvey, 2010).

Cisco, a large information technology company headquartered in San Jose, California, has 17,000 employees, and a total of 45,000 covered lives. In 2008, it opened the LifeConnections Health Center, a worksite clinic that offers primary care, laboratory and radiology services, a Walgreens pharmacy, vision care, chiropractic medicine, disease management and other services. Cisco also operates a nearby fitness center and day-care center on-site. Sharon Gibson, director of the worksite clinic, describes it as "a primary-care model of a medical home that is extended to include acupuncture, mental health services and health coaching. …Ours is an attempt to get employees engaged" (Vesely, 2011, p.2). The clinic is very convenient for employees to access, as they can use online scheduling to book appointments and are alerted via e-mail when appointments are about to start. Wait times to see a provider are less than five minutes. When the clinic first opened, the company expected between 25% and 30% of those covered to use its services. Three years later, about 43% of the workforce had used it (Vesely, 2011).

Toyota Manufacturing of America operates a large truck factory in San Antonio, Texas. In 2007, Toyota contracted with Take Care Health Systems to operate and manage the factory's worksite clinic. The clinic, called the "Center for Living Well", is a 20,000-square-foot facility that cost about $9 million to build. It serves roughly 7,000 eligible employees, contractors and their dependents and provides a wide range of services such as laboratory, digital radiology and a full-blown pharmacy as well as primary care, dentistry, optometry and physical therapy. Usage rates in 2008 were reported to be about 60% (Fottler & Malvey, 2010; Tu, et al., 2010).

In the public sector, some counties and school districts contract with third-party vendors to provide worksite clinic services to their employees. For example, the school district in Rutherford County in Tennessee has three clinics operated by CareHere. The clinics are staffed by primary care physicians and other personnel, and provide primary care and preventative services to district employees who are on the same insurance plan. They also serve other county employees, retirees and their dependents. Employees schedule appointments by phone or online, and are not charged any co-payments (Fottler & Malvey, 2010).

Employees

Employees who work at companies that provide a worksite clinic are attracted to the clinic for a variety of factors. A recent survey of families who used worksite clinics in 2010 suggested that the major reason for preferring the clinic over other care settings included the fact that the location was more convenient (63.6%), the cost was lower (38.0%), the hours were more convenient (35.1%), there was no need to make an appointment (26.8%) and not having a usual source of care (4.9%) (Boukus & Tu, 2012). In relation to costs, as described in some of the examples above, many companies provide strong financial incentives for their employees to use the clinics. While most employers don't mandate that their employees use the clinics, 70% require no co-payments or offer reduced co-payments for primary care services at the clinics compared to those outside the company doors (Anderson, 2013).

In general, employees tend to be satisfied with the worksite clinics. For example, surveys at Cisco show that 83% view the clinic as a valuable benefit, 80% report higher productivity and less time away from work from using the clinic, and 78% report a less than 10-minute wait to fill a prescription written by a provider at the clinic (Vesely, 2011). However, not all worksite clinics enjoy the same popularity among employees. In some companies, even when employees are aware of clinics, they may hesitate to use them. One of the main reasons behind the hesitation is skepticism of employers' motives for launching the clinics. This is particularly true in organizations with a history of adversarial relationships between management and labor. Moreover, many employees still remember the concept of the "company doctor" whose job was to get people back to work quickly and avoid workers' compensation claims, and that can affect their views of the newly established worksite clinics. Employees can also be concerned about potential misuse of personal health information and they worry that data collected in the clinic will be shared with their supervisors and may have negative consequences such as denial of promotions or job loss (Tu, et al., 2010).

Vendors

There is a large number of well-established vendors that provide management and operation services of worksite clinics. These include atWORK Health Services; MediWell; Care ATC; MinuteClinic; CareHere; Novia CareClinics; Comprehensive Health Services International; OnSiteSolutions; Concentra; QuadMed; HealthSTAT; Take Care; IMC Healthcare and WeCare. Many of these vendors started in occupational health, but have since expanded to other worksite clinics services. Also, some of them operate retail clinics and urgent care centers.

Among these, Walgreens and its recently created employer solutions division is considered the top vendor with nearly 20% share of the market. The Walgreens Health and Wellness division includes Take Care Health Systems, part of Take Care Consumer Solutions (managers of retail clinics) and Take Care Employer Solutions, which manages and operates worksite clinics. The worksite division operates 364 worksite clinics for 183 large (1,000-plus employees) companies, including Lowe's, Scotts Miracle-Gro, Goldman Sachs, Continental Airlines and, as previously discussed, Toyota. The Employer Solutions division was created in 2008 when Walgreens acquired in Whole Health Management, and I-trax, Inc., two operators of worksite wellness programs.

Physicians

While some physicians are excited to join the easier environment of worksite clinics, others in private practice see them as a serious competitive threat. A recent article published in Physician Practice states: "If you think retail walk-in clinics are worrisome, you're going to be thrilled to hear about another new competitor to traditional primary care: onsite clinics run by large employers. While these clinics make a lot of sense for employers, they will make it more difficult for many primary care physicians to stay in business" (Terry, 2009, p.1). Physicians are concerned that the worksite clinics will take away their routine services, such as the easy-to-diagnose and treat colds and infections (referred to as "the bread and butter or primary care"), and leave them with the most complex cases. They are also worried that they are losing their most lucrative commercially-insured patients, and are being left with low-paying publicly-insured and uninsured patients. Bruce Kruger, executive vice president of the Medical Society of Milwaukee County, Wisconsin, suggests: "The initial reaction of doctors is, "I'm going to lose a percentage of my patient base." But the longer-term reality is that you're going to be providing care to a population for which your reimbursement opportunities are much more limited" (Terry, 2009, p.2). Terry concludes: "The screw is [...] turning on reimbursement for routine office visits. When a patient pays little or nothing in an onsite clinic, $59 in a retail clinic, and $100 in a primary-care office, its' a "no-brainer" where the patient is going to seek care"(p.2).

Other opinions suggest that worksite clinics can have synergistic relationships with primary care physicians and their patient-centered medical homes (PCMH). For example, Dr. Bruce Sherman from the Employers Health Coalition of Ohio argues: "Worksite clinics can provide support for community-based PCMHs by serving as a bridge between patients and their primary care physicians. In this capacity, clinic personnel can provide ready access to support for chronic condition management, with point-of-care testing and communication of results to PCMH providers for further action. Additionally, worksite clinic personnel can provide health education and lifestyle counseling to minimize the burden for community clinicians unaccustomed to providing these comprehensive services. In this capacity, worksite clinics can serve as a physical extension of the community-based PCMH. Alternatively, PCMH practitioners may be able to enhance their effectiveness by leveraging worksite clinics to provide readily available services that could pose access and convenience challenges for patient engagement if they were PCMH office based. Such may be the case for lifestyle coaching, monitoring of chronic condition management, or classes. If worksite clinics could provide these services, PCMH office staff would be free for more essential patient care functions, which could have the secondary benefit of increasing PCMH capacity for additional primary care patients. However, any shift of services away from the PCMH may have an adverse impact by diluting the patient–primary care physician partnership" (Sherman, 2010, p.324).

Insurance Companies

The relationship between insurance companies and worksite clinics is uncertain, as most clinics are established by large, self-insured companies. For these companies, a worksite clinic can be administered as a stand-alone benefit, or integrated into an existing company's health plan administration. Some health plans see the savings in members' use of the clinics and agree to waive or reduce copayments when they visit the company clinic. Experts suggest that synergistic ties are obvious: "It brings payers closer to the providers. It makes a lot of economic sense for the folks paying the bills. The direct savings are there because the clinics can contract with physicians at a reasonable cost, and that savings then goes directly to the payer"(Byrne, 2009, p.4). Two recent trends are worth noting. First, some insurance companies are opening worksite clinics for their own employees. For example, Blue Cross and Blue Shield of New Jersey has opened three worksite clinics at its offices and contract with Take Care Health Solutions. Second, other insurers have entered the market as vendors. For example, CIGNA has a worksite health division that operates 22 clinics for employers (Tu, et al., 2010). It remains to be seen what the extent of the involvement of the insurance industry in worksite clinics will be.

3. OUTCOMES

As discussed above, employers establishing worksite clinics are mainly motivated by cost savings and improved employee productivity. However, the Return on Investment (ROI) of worksite clinics has not been thoroughly assessed, and "employers are faced with a confusing dilemma regarding measurement of worksite clinic value, notably from vendors who may provide higher estimates to encourage business development" (Sherman & Fabius, 2012, p.394).

Cost of Care

Worksite clinics can diminish employer healthcare expenditures by providing treatment at lower cost than comparable services provided by community providers, reducing use of higher-cost community healthcare services, improving chronic condition management, and enhancing self-care. The cost of care at worksite clinic is comparable to that at retail clinics, and therefore is less expensive than alternative treatment options such as hospital emergency rooms, urgent care centers and primary care physician offices (Sherman & Fabius, 2012). In addition, in worksite clinics, "...employees can seek prompt treatment of personal health concerns and work-related injuries, enabling worksite clinic personnel to provide timely and efficient care, thereby minimizing delays in care and the need for emergency department use. In a triage role, worksite clinic personnel can have a meaningful influence on subsequent healthcare utilization by making appropriate referrals to high-quality community healthcare services, encouraging greater use of primary care and urgent care services and supporting timely follow-up. For individuals with chronic conditions, ongoing worksite clinic care supporting treatment to evidence-based treatment goals is likely to result in fewer specialist care visits and hospitalizations for avoidable complications. This may be particularly relevant for employers who provide a full continuum of worksite care for occupational injuries" (Sherman & Fabius, 2012, p. 398-399). Others agree with this fact. Tu, Boukus and Cohen suggest that "...what generates savings for employers is the ability to change practice patterns, such as drug prescribing, ordering of tests and procedures, and specialist referrals, along with the potential for early diagnosis and treatment to avoid ED visits, hospitalizations and other costly downstream complications" (p.4). Some of these savings are easily quantifiable while others are not. One expert calculates that for every dollar spent at worksite clinics, employers can save $1.50 to $1.60, and these savings can come in the form of employee retention, higher productivity or other "soft dollars" (Vesely, 2011).

Productivity

Numerous studies have shown that worksite clinics can decrease absenteeism and presenteeism (the act of attending work while sick). Worksite clinics provide prompt treatment of minor acute symptomatic health conditions and work-related injuries and therefore can enhance employee recovery and timely return to work (Grayzel, Finegan & Ponchak, 1997; Zentner, Dellinger, Adkins & Greene, 1995; Goetzel, Anderson, Whitmer, et al, 1998). Moreover, worksite clinic providers have a deep understanding of the emotional, intellectual, and physical work requirements and assessment of the capabilities of employees recovering from illness or injury, and therefore can effectively optimize their accommodation to facilitate their return to work during recovery (Grayzel, et al., 1997; American College of Occupational and Environmental Medicine, 2008). In addition, worksite clinic providers provide treatments that can help better manage acute and chronic conditions. For example, they make treatment decisions that can provide symptomatic improvement without adversely impacting workplace productivity (Bunn, Pikeln, Paralka, et al., 2003; Burton, Morrison, Wertheimer, 2003).

Another important aspect of productivity is reducing the lost time by employees leaving their companies to seek medical care within the community. The literature documents that the proximity of worksite clinics can reduce travel time, resulting in lost work time savings (Scruby, Denham & Larkin, 2001; Prince, Spengler, Collins, 2001).

Quality

There is some evidence that worksite clinics provide high quality care and improve employees' health by promoting patient compliance with evidence-based medicine and treatments to identified clinical goals (Turner, 2010), by implementing quality improvement initiatives (McCarthy & Klein, 2010) and by promoting a better patient-clinician relationship (Atlas, Grant, Ferris, et al., 2009). Moreover, clinics can improve management of chronic conditions such as diabetes, hypertension, and hyperlipidemia, as well as enhance compliance with disease-specific preventive care, which can reduce subsequent healthcare utilization (Bodenheimer, Wagner & Grumbach, 2002).

Cost-Effectiveness and ROI

Few research studies have looked at cost and outcomes for worksite clinics to determine if they are worth the investment. Employers typically assess two types of ROI: "hard ROI," which is limited to savings in direct medical costs, and "soft ROI," which includes productivity gains from reduced absenteeism and reduced travel time. Most experts agree that companies can expect negative hard ROI in the first couple of years, breakeven in the third year, and possible positive ROI in the fourth year and beyond. However, it is important to be realistic, especially with many vendors claiming very ambitious ROIs of 3:1, 5:1 or even 7:1 (Tu, et al., 2010). Some companies, like Toyota, understand that larger savings occur in the longer term. Toyota almost tripled its primary care costs by allowing primary care physicians to take double the time when visiting with patient (20 minutes vs. 10 minutes). However, they more than paid for it by decreasing hospitalization and specialty care costs (Merchant Medicine, 2013a).

A notable exception is the study conducted by Chenewoth and Garrett (2006) that calculated costs of treatment at a worksite clinic with costs of treatment at outside (off-site) clinics, incorporated the cost of decreased productivity of seeking care at off-clinics, and compared those costs to the actual operational costs of running the worksite clinic. The off-site clinics had higher costs of $224,461 than worksite clinics in terms of healthcare costs, and $113,883 higher costs due to lost productivity, which is nearly twice as high as the actual worksite clinic operational costs ($171,332). The authors concluded that it appears the "organization's worksite clinic provides employee healthcare services 2 to 3 times more cost effectively than do off-site healthcare services"(p.84).

However, in their comprehensive review of the literature on ROI of worksite clinics, Sherman & Fabius (2012) found a remarkable lack of information. They asked: "Should employers attempt to replicate the current healthcare system with worksite clinics or actively engage in community efforts to promote the patient-centered medical home? [...] Based on this analysis, the answer is unclear, [...] Although worksite clinics may provide cost-effective services, depending on their level of integration with community practitioners, there is a risk of further fragmentation of care delivery and associated increased healthcare expenditures" (p.401). Similarly, another review study conducted by Cerner investigated whether the ROI numbers of $3-$6 on every dollar spent are realistic and concluded that the evidence on ROI should be interpreted with caution (Gorman, Miller & Kaspin, 2012).

4. FUTURE

Several new trends have recently emerged in worksite clinics. For example, mid-size and small employers who cannot support a worksite clinic on their own are creating shared clinics that can be used by employees of other corporations that are closely located. One company can establish a worksite clinic and make it available to its employees as well as to employees of other organizations under specific arrangements. Alternatively, companies collaborate and co-sponsor a clinic that can be located in a neutral convenient location in an office or manufacturing park (Tu, Boukus & Cohen, 2010). Other employers have invested in mobile clinics to serve their other branches or subsidiaries that are located in remote rural areas (Huff, 2012). And others are using Telehealth to provide better access to their worksite clinics for employees from home. For example, HealthPartners' in Minneapolis, Minnesota operates worksite clinics that have the ability to provide free visits via telehealth to any patient with a capable camera at home, while the University of Pittsburgh Medical Center (UPMC) is using a telehealth program called MyHealth@Work in its urgent care centers for employers that cannot support a worksite clinic. Similarly, Blue Cross and Blue Shield of North Carolina (BCBSNC) Walgreens Take Care Health Systems, and American Well (discussed in the next chapter) started a collaboration to make telehealth services available to BCBSNC employees. The service, called OnlineCareNC, allows employees to receive a healthcare consultation from credentialed nurse practitioners, health coaches or nutritionists via two-way videos, secure text chats or phone calls (American Well, 2012).

Looking towards the future, worksite clinics hold great promise, despite the mixed evidence on their ROI. In a healthcare environment operating under provisions of the Patient Protection and Affordable Care Act (PPACA) mandating changing reimbursement patterns and increased focused on population health, worksite clinics seem to be well positioned to thrive, especially if they extend their services to focus on high-risk employees with chronic diseases, and are proactive in managing diabetes, hypertension and obesity, with case management and education.

REFERENCES

American College of Occupational and Environmental Medicine. (2008). *The Personal Physician's Role in Helping Patients with Medical Conditions Stay at Work or Return to Work*. Elk Grove Village, IL: Author.

American Well. (2012). *Blue Cross and Blue Shield of North Carolina*. Walgreens Take Care Health Systems and American Well Team Up to Provide Telehealth to Workforce.

Anderson, C. (2013). More large employers adding on-site health clinics. *Healthcare Finance News*. Retrieved from: http://www.healthcarefinancenews.com

Atlas, S. J., Grant, R., Ferris, T., Chang, Y., & Barry, M. (2009). Patient–physician connectedness and quality of primary care. *Annals of Internal Medicine*, *150*(5), 325–335. doi:10.7326/0003-4819-150-5-200903030-00008 PMID:19258560

Benfield Research. (2011). *Employer & Coalition Market Overview and Trends — Spring 2011*. Retrieved from: http://www.worksitehealth.org/sites/www.worksitehealth.org/files/assets/Benfield%202011%20On-site%20Clinic%20Data.pdf

Berry, E. (2012). Work-site clinics try to cover employees' medical access gaps. Once limited to major employers that want occupational health services for workers, the clinics are popping up at more employers — and providing more services. *Amednews*. Retrieved from http://www.amednews.com/article/20120618/business/306189965/4/

Bodenheimer, T., Wagner, E., & Grumbach, K. (2002). Improving primary care for patients with chronic illness. *Journal of the American Medical Association*, *288*(15), 1909–1914. doi:10.1001/jama.288.15.1909 PMID:12377092

Boukus, E.R., & Tu, H.T. (2012). *Despite Employer Interest, Workplace Clinic Use Low*. National Institute for Healthcare Reform.

Bunn, W. B. III, Pikelny, D., Paralkar, S., Slavin, T., Borden, S. IV, & Allen, H. M. Jr. (2003). The burden of allergies-and the capacity of medications to reduce this nurden-in a heavy manufacturing environment. *Journal of Occupational and Environmental Medicine*, *45*(9), 941–955. doi:10.1097/01.jom.0000090468.73649.50 PMID:14506338

Burton, W. N., Morrison, A., & Wertheimer, A. (2003). Pharmaceuticals and worker productivity loss: A critical review of the literature. *Journal of Occupational and Environmental Medicine*, *45*(6), 610–621. doi:10.1097/01.jom.0000069244.06498.01 PMID:12802214

Byrne, R. (2009). Worksite Health Clinics Put New Focus On Employee Health. *HealthLeaders-InterStudy's Ohio, Kentucky & Indiana Health Plan Analysis*, *10*(1), 1–5.

Chenewoth, D. H., & Garrett, J. (2006). Cost-Effectiveness Analysis of a Worksite Clinic: Is It Worth the Cost? *AAOHN Journal*, *54*(2), 84–89. PMID:16509183

On Site Clinics. (2010). Retrieved from http://onsiteclinics.org/faqs/#sthash.kqKw1Jxk.dpuf

Commins, J. (2013, July 31). MT Health Clinics Are Cost Effective, Not 'Free'. *HealthLeaders Media*.

Daugherty, A. (2012). Worksite clinics: Which model is right for you? *Advisory Board*. Retrieved from http://www.advisory.com/Research/Marketing-and-Planning-Leadership-Council/Service-Line-Transformation/2012/04/Worksite-clinics-Which-model-is-right-for-you

Fottler, M., & Malvey, D. (2010). *The Retail Revolution in Healthcare*. Santa Barbara, CA: Praeger.

Fuld & Company. (2009). *The Growth of On-Site Health Clinics. On-site clinics are expected to serve over 10% of the under 65s by 2015*. Author.

Goetzel, R. Z., Anderson, D. R., Whitmer, R. W., Ozminkowski, R. J., Dunn, R. L., & Wasserman, J. (1998). The Relationship Between Modifiable Health Risks and Healthcare Expenditures. *Journal of Occupational and Environmental Medicine*, *40*(10), 843–854. doi:10.1097/00043764-199810000-00003 PMID:9800168

Gorman, K., Miller, R., & Kaspin, L. (2012). *Employer Services: Return on Investment*. Kansas City, MO: Cerner Corporation.

Grayzel, E. F., Finegan, A., & Ponchak, R. (1997). The value of in-house physical therapy. *Journal of Occupational and Environmental Medicine*, *39*(4), 344–346. doi:10.1097/00043764-199704000-00014 PMID:9113606

Halzack, S. (2012, October 21). Large employers look to on-site health clinics to reduce costs and absenteeism. *The Washington Post*. Retrieved from http://www.washingtonpost.com/business/capitalbusiness/large-employers-look-to-on-site-health-clinics-to-reduce-costs-and-absenteeism/2012/10/19/305f57ac-1924-11e2-aa6f-3b636fecb829_story.html

Hochstadt, B. (2010). *The Value of On-site Health Centers*. Paper presented at Society for Human Resource Management. New York, NY..

Huff, C. (2012). *Going Mobile: On-Site Clinics Hit the Road for Employee Health Screenings*. Retrieved from http://www.workforce.com/article/20120406/NEWS02/120409962/going-mobile-on-site-clinics-hit-the-road-for-employee-health-screenings

McCarthy, D., & Klein, S. (2010). *QuadMed: Transforming Employer-Sponsored Healthcare Through Workplace Primary Care and Wellness Programs*. Washington, DC: The Commonwealth Fund.

Medicine, M. (2013a). *ConVurgentCare Report*, *6*(3), 1–5.

Medicine, M. (2013b). *ConVurgentCare Report.*, *6*(12), 1–6.

Mercer. (2012). *National Survey of Employer-Sponsored Health Plans*. Author.

Prince, T. S., Spengler, S., & Collins, T. (2001). Corporate travel medicine: Benefit analysis of on-site services. *Journal of Travel Medicine*, *8*(4), 163–166. doi:10.2310/7060.2001.22213 PMID:11703899

Robert Wood Johnson Foundation. (2013). *State-level trends in employer-sponsored health insurance. A state-by-state analysis.* Author.

Scruby, D. J., Denham, S., & Larkin, G. (2001). Economic impact of on-site physical therapy. *Journal of Occupational and Environmental Medicine*, *43*(8), 670–671. doi:10.1097/00043764-200108000-00002 PMID:11515248

Sherman, B.W. (2010). Worksite Clinics and the Patient-Centered Medical Home: Competition or Collaboration? *The American Journal of Managed Care*, *16*(5), 323–325. PMID:20469952

Sherman, B. W., & Fabius, R. J. (2012). Quantifying the Value of Worksite Clini Non-occupational Healthcare Services: A Critical Analysis and Review of the Literature. *JOEM*, *54*(4), 394–403. PMID:22418274

Terry, K. (2009, May 1). Worksite Clinics - The Next Threat? *Physician Practice*, 1-2.

Thomas, L. (2011). *Early Permanente physicians: making do with makeshift facilities.* Retrieved from http://kaiserpermanentehistory.org/tag/sidney-garfield/

Tu, H.T., Boukus, E.R., Cohen, G.R. (2010). *Workplace Clinics: A Sign of Growing Employer Interest in Wellness.* Center for Studying Health System Change.

Turner, D. E. (2010). Worksite primary care: An assessment of cost and quality metrics. *Journal of Occupational and Environmental Medicine*, *52*(6), 573–575. doi:10.1097/JOM.0b013e3181e317b6 PMID:20535088

Vesely, R. (2011). The doctor will see you now—at your office. Workplace health clinics making a resurgence. *Modern Healthcare*, (May): 30.

Tower Watson. (2012). *2012 On Site Health Center Survey Report*. Author.

Watson Wyatt. (2008). Realizing the Potential of Onsite Health Centers. Author.

Zentner, J., Dellinger, C., Adkins, W., & Greene, J. (1995). Nurse practitioner provided primary care: Managing healthcare costs in the workplace. *AAOHN Journal*, *43*, 52–53. PMID:7695807

KEY TERMS AND DEFINITIONS

Cost of Care: The amount in dollars spent on healthcare services within a certain healthcare system.

High-Deductible Health Plans: A health insurance plan that has a high minimum deductible, which does not cover the initial costs or all of the costs of medical expenses.

Quality of Care: The extent to which healthcare services provided to individuals and patient populations improve desired health outcomes.

Return on Investment (ROI): A common profitability ratio calculated by dividing net profit by total assets.

Worksite Clinics: Small clinics located on employers' campuses and dedicated to serving employees by providing primary care services, health promotion and wellness as well as care for occupational injuries.

APPENDIX: THE HELENA CLINIC IN MONTANA (COMMINS, 2013)

The success story of the Helena clinic in Montana suggests that providing easy access to affordable and proactive care is a proven way to reduce the rising costs of healthcare.

One year after its opening in 2012, the clinic has already saved the state of Montana $1.5 million by making available primary care services to about 11,000 employees, their dependents, and pre-Medicare retired state employees. Services provided include health screenings, flu shots, and wellness counseling. The clinics also offer wellness coaches. Russ Hill, the administrator overseeing the Helena clinic for Montana's Healthcare and Benefits Division, explains:

"On staff we have a registered dietician, an exercise physiologist, a behavioral health coach, and a wellness nurse. Those people work with the clinical team to work with our patients who have chronic diseases or even potentially acute diseases. One of the patients was found to have extreme diabetes. He was a walking sugar cube. He came in and said 'I am ready to change everything with my life. I am a smoker. I know I need to lose weight. I know I need to exercise more. Our wellness coaches were able to work with him and develop a program. Rather than 'we are going to start this and you are going to get really sore in the first week trying to do all of this' they developed a year-long process for him to make lifestyle changes. That is a big difference for people to make a real lifestyle change."

Members pay no out-of-pocket costs, as the price of the primary care services is included into the health insurance premiums paid by state employees and their employer, the state of Montana. According to Hill: "We have no out-of-pocket costs for our members. They can get their office visit with their primary care physician. Normally that is $15. Under our plan there is no copayment if you come into the health center. With our normal program we have co-insurance and deductible that applies to lab and X-rays, but we don't have any co-deductible for lab or X-ray [work] that is done at the health center, or ordered by a health center provider. We have a self-funded medical plan and that pays for claims and can also pay for the services at the health center."

The $1.5 million savings figure does not factor in the enhanced productivity from state employees who are less likely to call in sick or have other health-related issues, thanks to their improved health status.

The initial success in Helena has prompted expansion plans. The first clinic was in Helena, and the second one was in Billing, and there are plans to offer 10 more clinics in other locations.

Chapter 8
Online, House Call, and Other Services

ABSTRACT

This chapter focuses on new healthcare services provided online, in the patient home, and elsewhere. Under the umbrella of telehealth, there are three key modes of delivery. First, real time (synchronous) delivery requires a live telecommunication connection and uses phones, video conferencing, and chat sessions. Second, "store & forward" (asynchronous) delivery captures digital media and transmits to it to providers via images, video, audio, x-rays, etc. Third, remote monitoring (synchronous or not) is a combination of real-time and store and forward and it uses connected devices. The author highlights the example of several online care companies such as Hello Health, virtuwell, Zipnosis, and American Well. House call services by nurse practitioners are on the rise again. The author focuses on the example of WhiteGlove, a service that offers access to nurse practitioner care at home or at the office seven days a week. They conclude that many patient visits to the hospital emergency rooms and to primary care physician offices are unnecessary and can be taken care of in a much cheaper and more convenient way through online interactions and house visits.

DOI: 10.4018/978-1-4666-6355-8.ch008

From the halls of the White House to exam rooms around the country, most Americans now realize that their healthcare system is inexorably changing. Rules, processes, and terminology are all in flux. But what will not change, no matter what the acronym of the moment, is the core connection between doctors and the patients they care for. It is for this reason that telehealth – which now uses ubiquitous technologies to facilitate this simple connection – is moving to the fore of physician practices. Telehealth is already breaking down barriers to needed care, while enabling providers to practice in a flexible, convenient manner – generating revenue along the way. — Online Care, 2012

INTRODUCTION

The last few years have witnessed a proliferation of innovations and non-traditional ways of delivering services for minor health conditions, as well as chronic ones. Physicians have started using e-mail messages, video conferencing, online chatting sessions and text messages to communicate with patients and diagnose and treat conditions. New services allow patients to answer a series of questions online and asynchronously receive a diagnosis and prescription from a nurse practitioner. Others allow patients to receive care from the comfort of their homes. In this chapter, we discuss these innovations and assess their impact on primary care delivery in the United States.

1. ONLINE SERVICES

Many patient visits to the hospital emergency rooms and to primary care physician offices are unnecessary and can be taken care of in a much cheaper and more convenient way through online interactions and other technology-enabled visits. This section provides a brief background on telemedicine/telehealth and describes some of the online services that have emerged in the last few years.

Telemedicine and Telehealth

The American Telemedicine Association (ATA) (2013) defines telemedicine as "the use of medical information exchanged from one site to another via electronic communications to improve a patient's clinical health status." It includes multiple applications and services using two-way video, email, smart phones, wireless tools and other forms of telecommunications technology. The Centers for Medicare and Medicaid (2013) defines telemedicine as "the provision of clinical services to patients by practitioners from a distance via electronic communications."

The term telemedicine is often used interchangeably with telehealth. For example, the ATA considers patient consultations via video conferencing, transmission of still images, e-health including patient portals, remote monitoring of vital signs, continuing medical education, consumer-focused wireless applications and nursing call centers to be all part of telemedicine and telehealth (ATA, 2013). Others suggest that the term telehealth refers to a broader definition of remote healthcare that does not always involve clinical services. For example, the Center for Connected Health Policy (2013) defines telehealth as "the use of electronic information and telecommunications technologies to support distance clinical health care, patient and professional health-related education, public health and health administration."

Similarly, the American Academy of Family Physicians (AAFP) defines telehealth as "the use of advanced telecommunication technologies to exchange health information and provide healthcare services across geographic, time, social, and cultural barriers." In that sense, telehealth harnesses technology to bring needed quality medical care into more places, more quickly, and to more patients in need (Reid, 1996).

It is important to note that telehealth is not a new idea. It actually dates back to the late 1950s, when the University of Nebraska first relayed neurological images across campus to medical students using video communications via two-way, closed-circuit television. The advent of the Internet and broadband, high-speed connections have allowed telehealth to become far more accessible, connecting physicians directly with the patients. The prison system has been a pioneer in the use of telehealth. For example, almost 40,000 monthly visits take place involving remotely-located providers and inmates in correctional facilities in Texas (Gartner, 2008).

Under the general umbrella of telehealth, mHealth (mobile Health) is "the use of mobile and wireless devices to improve health outcomes, healthcare services, and health research." It includes the use of smart phones, cell phones, and text messages (U.S. Department of Health and Human Services, 2013. In addition, e-health (electronic health) is the "delivery of health information & care through the Internet and telecommunications" (World Health Organization, 2013). There are three key modes for delivering telehealth. First, real time (synchronous) delivery requires a live telecommunication connection and uses phones, video conferencing and chat sessions. Second, "store & forward" (asynchronous) delivery captures digital media and transmits to it to providers via images, video, audio, x-rays, etc. Third, remote monitoring (synchronous or not) is a combination of real-time and store and forward and it uses connected devices (Smith, 2013).

Until about five years ago, telehealth was a niche industry with narrow applications, such as connecting medical specialists to patients in remote areas. Recently, however, telehealth started to make inroads into primary care by branching into treating low-acuity, episodic illnesses. The first movement in that direction was the announcement in August of 2008 by retail clinic operator My Healthy Access that it had joined forces with a telehealth technology company called NuPhysicia to deploy telehealth carts in a some Walmart stores in Houston. In 2009, UnitedHealth Group and Cisco announced a partnership to build the first national telehealth network called "Connected Care." As a result, "NowClinic" emerged as a new service in retail stores (Merchant Medicine, 2013a). NowClinic was the first service of its kind to allow patients to connect with a physician using secure live chat and even to converse face-to-face using webcams. The service was first offered and is still available in selected neighborhood Rite Aid pharmacies (NowClinic, 2013a). It is also now available as a purely online service from any computer, as discussed later in this chapter.

Online Care and E-Visits

In addition to telehealth applications related to minor conditions in retail settings, other applications started appearing in physician offices, resembling well-established online applications that consumers have used for years, such as buying a book on Amazon.com or booking a plane ticket on Expedia.com. For example, online care (also referred to as e-visits) now allows physicians the ability to deliver live healthcare services to patients through a virtual practice. All what physicians and patients need is an Internet connection, browser, and/or a telephone line. During the visit, physicians can see and talk to the patient through live, web-based videoconferencing, secure chat, and telephone. The physician can diagnose or write prescriptions, as well as share notes with the patient, answer questions, and suggest health assessments and articles. To add more convenience, payment is charged to the consumer's credit card and funds flow directly into the physician's bank account after the visit. Mehrotra, Paone, Martich, et al. (2013) recently described e-visits "in which physicians and patients interact virtually instead of face-to-face. In e-visits, patients log into their secure personal health record internet portal and answer a series of questions about their condition. This written information is sent to the physicians, who make a diagnosis, order necessary care, put a note in the patients' electronic medical records, and reply to the patients via the secure portal within several hours" (p.72). Some physicians are starting to use e-visits as an alternative to face-to-face visits. For example, family physician Barry Bershow in Minneapolis, Minnesota, uses e-visits to review descriptions of symptoms of common ailments patients have emailed him and he follows up by diagnosing the problem and prescribing a treatment. He explains that e-visits work best "for single, relatively simple problems where we have enough information- either from the patient's medical record or from what the patient tells us- to render a sound medical decision" (Mettner, 2009, p.1).

Consumer Attitudes

Patient demand for telehealth services seems to be on the rise. The majority of Americans go online for activities like banking, shopping, and travel, and many feel that they should obtain healthcare services the same way. For example, Manhattan Research estimates that about 80 million patients would like to have online visits with physicians (Zamosky, 2010).

Among patients who have experienced telehealth encounters, satisfaction is high (Heinzelmann, Williams, Lugn, & Kvedar, 2005).

There is an assumption in healthcare that patients prefer to see a provider in a traditional face-to-face way over online care or e-visits. Recent surveys have shown that this belief is, for the most part, wrong. For example, the Cisco Customer Experience Report has shown that 70% of consumers are comfortable with the idea of communicating with doctors using technology instead of seeing them in person. In fact, 19% prefer video chatting, 20% prefer online consultations via instant messages, 21% prefer e-mail consultations, 23% prefer telephone consultations and 20% prefer text message consultations (Cisco, 2013). A recent survey by Harris Interactive showed similar results. About 52% of respondents said they were interested in having a portal to log on and see their health information, 44% were interested in online appointment scheduling, 35% were interested in e-mail correspondence with their provider about their health, and 36% were interested in communication with their providers via an online message platform (Richman, 2013).

Companies and Services

"Hello Health"

One of the first companies to offer online care within the context of a concierge medical practice is Hello Health in Brooklyn, New York. (Concierge medical practices, also called "boutique practices," are discussed later in this chapter. It offers exclusive access to patients for an annual fee. Physicians are typically available after traditional office hours by e-mail or telephone and through house calls, and patients are guaranteed same-day or next-day appointments and a minimum amount of time with the physician per appointment, such as 30 minutes). In a 2008 article in Health Affairs, Hello Health was introduced: "If you want to get a glimpse of what high-tech healthcare could look like one day in the U.S., say hello to 'Hello Health.' Or better still, e-mail Dr. Jay Parkinson, 32, or one of his three clinical associates who run this small primary care medical practice out of sleek offices in Brooklyn, New York. Or even better, you can instant message (IM) or video chat with Dr. Parkinson online through Hello Health's slick Web site. It's a private and secure social network that is the core medium through which this new-age medical practice manages itself and stays in touch with its patients" (Hawn, 2009, p.361). At Hello Health members pay a flat-fee of $35 per month. A quick e-mail to the physician is free, but a chat, instant messaging session or video session cost $50-$100. And an in-person visit to the office or a physician house-call (guaranteed within 24 hours) cost $150-$200. No insurance is accepted, but patients can submit their medical bills to their insurance company on their own. The main medium where these interactions happen is a Facebook-like platform that allows plenty of time for patients to interact with their doctors. The experience of Hello Health patient is described in detail in the article: "Michael Rovner, 38, is a case in point. Rovner, a Brooklyn resident, joined Hello Health as soon as it opened, in part because the firm's offices are two blocks from his house. Prior to Hello Health, he says, 'I'd gone to your typical Park Avenue, very expensive, insurance-only doctor, and I had good care.' But when Rovner left his job last fall to start his own media company-he specializes in launching custom news Web sites-he suddenly found himself without health insurance. Though healthy, he couldn't find any insurer who would cover him for less than $500 a month. 'That's when I started wondering, what am I paying for?' he says. He reasoned that in a perfect world, he might pay $500 a month in health insurance and never go to the doctor because he wouldn't get sick. 'On the other hand, I could pay $35 a month to Hello Health, and [pay] for additional visits only if I need them,' he says. It was clear which course made more sense financially, provided that he never fell catastrophically ill. 'Plus, I loved the whole idea of making your own appointments online, that you can IM with your doctor or you can video chat,' Rovner says. 'I figured if these guys can deliver on the promise, I can't imagine having something more convenient"(Hawn, 2009, p.367).

Today, Hello Health has shifted to licensing its patient management platform to other physician practices. The company's website describes its new focus: "At the heart of Hello Health is our proprietary technology developed by our parent company, Myca Health Inc. The Hello Health platform significantly improves the experience for both providers and patients by reducing paperwork, streamlining processes and leveraging the latest online and mobile communication applications to allow practitioners and patients to engage efficiently and conveniently"(Hello Health, 2013).

"Virtuwell"

Virtuwell, an online clinic, was launched by HealthPartners in Bloomington, Minnesota in October of 2010. HealthPartners is a not-for-profit health care organization that provides health insurance through a health plan and health care services through a large integrated system that consists of six hospitals, more than seventy medical and dental clinics, and a network of contracted providers. The model was recently described in a Health Affairs paper: "Now available to residents of Minnesota and Wisconsin (and newly introduced in Michigan), virtuwell combines rigorous clinical protocols with a carefully designed online user experience and service guarantees. It is accessible at https://virtuwell.com around the clock and offers treatment for about fifty simple conditions such as urinary tract infections, sinus infections, and conjunctivitis. The service uses sophisticated interview algorithms; makes patient- and clinician initiated telephonic interactions available around the clock; and incorporates review by nurse practitioners or physician assistants, who then provide diagnoses and treatment plans, and, if appropriate, prescriptions" (Cournea, Palattao & Gallagher, 2013, p. 386).

The customer experience starts with a visit to the website. A unique feature of virtuwell is that the patient does not need to make any commitment, register or agree to terms upfront. Instead, the process starts immediately with an interview. Kevin Palattao (see Appendix A), Vice President of virtuwell, explains: "One of the things that we studied is that most organizations put their business needs ahead of the consumer's. We wanted to flip this upside down. There's no business benefit for getting at the registration, payment and insurance first. We simply wanted to put the consumer's needs first. We also wanted to give consumers an opportunity to take a test drive without any commitment. Try out the healthcare experience. Learn how the interview process works. People want to get into things before they commit by identifying themselves"(Merchant Medicine, 2011). When the patients visit the site, the first thing that might attract their attention is the "24/7 Online Clinic" and "$45 or less, depending on your insurance" banners. If they click on the large button that says "Start Diagnosis" they are immediately shown 14 categories of medical conditions under the heading, "What do you think you have?" The conditions are acne, bladder Infection, breast Infection, burn & sunburn, chlamydia, gonorrhea & trichomoniasis (exposure), cold, cough & allergy, deer tick bite, ear pain, flu, lice, pinkeye & stye, sinus infection, skin & nail and yeast infection (virtuwell, 2013). For example, if a patient clicks on cold, cough and allergy, they get the following text: "Some common symptoms are sore throat, runny nose, itchy eyes or nose, watery eyes, sneezing, stuffy or blocked nose, congestion, sinus pain and pressure, deep cough and hoarse voice. Conditions We Treat: Bronchitis; Common Cold; Laryngitis; Sinus Infection; Pet Allergies; Seasonal Allergies." If he/she decides to continue, a series of detailed questions that follow a specific protocol for upper respiratory conditions need to be answered. The expert system uses a question and answer interview based on the latest clinical evidence and safety protocols, and takes about 15 minutes. Palattao explains the rationale: "That's a nod to the consumer that we know they took some time to do some research on this already. Our research suggested that most consumers go out and look at up to three Web locations to find information about their conditions. They are trying to triangulate the truth, to find consistency around the information about their condition"(Merchant Medicine, 2011). Some of those interviews end early because the system hits a safety protocol, an answer that indicates the condition is more complicated than the limited-scope menu that virtuwell offers. The system then instructs the patient to contact a physician or, in extreme cases, to call 911. If the interview is completed, the patient is directed to create an account by filling out online forms, including insurance and credit card information, a preferred pharmacy, and consent to treat. The system bills the patient's insurance first and then bills the remaining balance to the credit card provided. After the patient finishes the check-out process, he/she clicks a button that submits the interview to an online nurse practitioner. Sometimes, the nurse practitioner will call the patient with a clarification question. Once the treatment plan is finalized, the patient receives a notice by e-mail or text message, and the prescription, if applicable, is sent to the pharmacy of choice. The average time from beginning to end of the encounter is 30 minutes (Merchant Medicine, 2011).

The software used by virtuwell is based on an algorithmic approach that uses questions and answers to lead the patient through specific clinical protocols. Those protocols are closely aligned with those developed by the Institute for Clinical Systems Improvement. In terms of scope of services, the conditions treated are limited to those generally associated with high diagnostic accuracy and treatment efficacy. In other words, the menu of services focuses on rules-based conditions and treatments. For example, conditions for which the provision of a laboratory test, imaging study, or physical exam is the standard of care are not included. However, for urinary tract infections for example, the published guidelines suggest that a low-risk patient with a typical pattern of symptoms may be safely treated without an exam or laboratory testing (Cournea, et al., 2013).

As of 2013, virtuwell had treated more than 80,000 customers while an equal number have been referred to physicians and other providers because their symptoms were beyond the scope of practice. The majority of patients are female (78%), mostly because females tend to make family health care decisions and because many conditions treated such as urinary tract infections or yeast infections are specific to women. Most patients are 24-45 years of age, and sinusitis, urinary tract infection, conjunctivitis, and viral upper respiratory infections are the most commonly treated conditions. As discussed above, the retail cost of the visit is \$45, up from \$40 when the clinic first opened. Insurance coverage reduces the out-of-pocket fee for many patients, depending on the terms of benefits of their health plans. Only 15% of the patients pay the full fee, while the others rely on their insurance to cover all or part of it (Cournea, et al., 2013).

"Zipnosis"

Also in Minnesota, and just before virtuwell was launched, Park Nicollet Health Services began a one-year pilot with Zipnosis, an online care clinic. Park Nicollet is a not-for-profit, integrated healthcare system located in St. Louis Park, with more than 8,200 employees, and 1,000 employed physicians. Zipnosis was first conceived in 2007 by John Pierce, an MBA student at the University of Minnesota's Carlson School of Management and Steve Claypool, M.D. In 2008, Pearce met Rick Krieger (founder of MinuteClinic, highlighted in Chapter 6) at Carlson's Enterprise Lab. The company was incorporated later that year with Krieger as Chief Executive Officer and Pearce as Chief Operating Officer. Before it won the contract with Park Nicollet, Zipnosis was pilot-tested for three months at St. Olaf

College in Northfield, Minnesota, where students used its services as part of the college's health clinic. Afterwards, the service was offered to the Twin Cities Pipes Trade Service Association, which manages health benefits for 16,000 union members and dependents (Lee, 2010; Newmarker, 2008;).

Similarly to virtuwell, Zipnosis is web-based and was designed to diagnose approximately 30 straightforward conditions such as sinusitis, urinary tract infections, acne, and conjunctivitis that can be reliably identified through a medical history, rather than laboratory testing and/or a physical examination. It uses clinical algorithms built on evidence-based guidelines and patients are led through a series of questions crafted to capture data required for effective clinical decision-making. The main advantage that services like Zipnosis or virtuwell have over traditional e-visits (such as patients sending e-mail messages to their providers) is that the detailed questions allow the provider to get a comprehensive and complete picture of the patient symptoms. When patients send messages only, they are typically very vague, which frustrates providers. Dr. Claypool, co-founder of Zipnosis, explains the situation: "It's very difficult because they go off on tangents and don't describe what you need to know. They'll say they feel bad but won't tell you whether they have a fever" (Newmarker, 2008). With an interview based on specific protocols, no questions are ever forgotten.

Zipnosis uses mostly physician assistants employed by Park Nicollet's urgent care clinics. Unlike virtuwell, when patients log in to Zipnosis.com, they have to create a new account first. Then they read over their HIPAA (Health Insurance Portability and Accountability Act) notice related to privacy, see an explanation of what to expect, and pay a $25 fee. While the fee is lower than that of virtuwell, Zipnosis does not accept any insurance plans in order to keep administrative costs down (Ford, 2011; Mettner, 2011). The obvious drivers behind Zipnosis, like other online care clinics, are convenience and affordability. Pearce sought to create a healthcare service that was "ridiculously convenient" (Ford, 2011, p.17). He clarifies: "There is nothing that can hold water to what we are doing. We can lower the cost of healthcare and still make it profitable for clinicians" (Lee, 2010). He also boasts: "Zipnosis has proven we dramatically shift the cost curve in healthcare. We've taken a 2 hour, $200 urgent care visit and made it 5 minutes and $25.00 using Zipnosis online"(Business Wire, 2013). Jon Bylander, M.D., chair of urgent care at Park Nicollet, and the lead physician for the Zipnosis pilot project, explained: "What led us to try this was basically a sign of the times. Patients want to be able to communicate with their providers electronically, so the market forces are right for change in this area; this isn't going to be a fad that fades" (Mettner, 2011, p.2). Zipnosis proved to be a success and the one-year contract became more permanent. In 2013, the company announced that its services are becoming available in 11 states: Alaska, Colorado, Connecticut, Kentucky, Maryland, Massachusetts, Minnesota, New York, Rhode Island, Washington and Wisconsin. The company states that it has successfully treated over 12,000 patients, delivering close to $2 million in direct healthcare savings to patients and employers. Its plan is to provide those services to millions of patients and hundreds of millions in savings across the country. Moreover, Zipnosis now licenses a "Powered by Zipnosis" package to other providers seeking a customized virtual care offering (Business Wire, 2013).

It is important to note that in the summer of 2012, Park Nicollet ended its relationship with Zipnosis and started one with virtuwell. Then, in 2013, Park Nicollet and HealthPartners merged, while Zipnosis established a relationship with Fairview Clinics in Minneapolis (Kevin Palattao, e-mail correspondence, 2014; Fairview; 2014; HealthPartners, 2014).

"American Well"

American Well is an industry leader in virtual visits and online care. Founded by Drs. Ido and Roy Schoenberg, it offers complete telehealth services such as software, services, and access to clinical services. The platforms are provided to health plans, employers, or delivery networks. In 2008, the company introduced the Online Care Suite, after partnering with IBM to build the security platform, and with Microsoft to integrate the virtual visit platform with Microsoft's HealthVault online consumer health platform (Merchant Medicine, 2011). The Online Care Suite software connects physicians with patients for live, on-demand video visits over the internet and handles the required administration, security, and record keeping (American Well, 2013).

American Well defines the services that it provides as follows: "Online medical care is medicine built for the way you live today. It's a simple, affordable service that lets you see a physician whenever, however, wherever you want to online or by mobile app. All our doctors are local- licensed in your state of residence and the service is as secure as an in-office visit. Your visit is scheduled for 10 minutes-the amount of time needed to handle most medical issues. Of course you can add more time should you need to. Once you're connected, your doctor can review your history, answer your questions and at their discretion diagnose, treat and even prescribe medication. If you receive a prescription, we'll send it straight to your pharmacy" (American Well, 2013). The convenience is emphasized by describing the situations in which a patient may need a service of this kind: "I feel like I should probably see a doctor, but can't really fit it into my over-booked schedule; I'm flying tomorrow and can't get out of work; It's difficult for me to get a doctor's appointment; I'm not sure if I should go to the ER or not; My doctor's office is closed and I don't want to go to an urgent care clinic or hospital; I just moved and don't know any doctors in my area; I just need a second opinion; I'm between jobs and have no coverage; I have a question about a loved-one's health and would like some advice." The conditions treated are similar to other convenient care services such as acute bronchitis, cough acute sinusitis, acute pharyngitis, acute cystitis, urinary tract infection, abdominal pain, diarrhea, fever, acute conjunctivitis, painful urination, influenza, respiratory infection, headache and strep throat (American Well, 2013).

The company contracts its services to an impressive list of clients: Ascension Health; BlueCross BlueShield of Louisiana; BlueCross BlueShield of Massachusetts; Blue Cross and Blue Shield of Minnesota; BlueCross BlueShield of North Carolina; BlueCross BlueShield of Western New York; HMSA; Massachusetts General Hospital; OptumHealth; Patient Advocates; Rite Aid; Tufts Medical Center; U.S. Department of Veterans Affairs; ValueOptions and WellPoint. For example, Blue Cross and Blue Shield of Minnesota calls its service "Online Care Anywhere." The service is available to members in all except six states, and it links patients to board-certified physicians using video or secure text chat. The physician offers a diagnosis, a prescription if needed, and follow-up care, and the service costs $45 per episode (Online Care Anywhere, 2013).

Other Services

Other services offered by various companies follow the same two models described above: asynchronous diagnosis by a non-physician provider following detailed online survey questions, or live chat by video, text, or phone with a physician, resulting in a diagnosis. For example, Teladoc calls itself the "first and largest provider of telehealth medical consultations in the United States". Founded in 2002, the company has 4.5 million members. It contracts with employers and health plans to provide the service to their employees/members. Similar to other models, the patient logs-in online or calls Teladoc by phone and explains his/her symptoms. Within 24 minutes, they are contacted by phone by a board-certified internist, state-licensed family practitioner, or pediatrician. The physician talks to the patient and reviews the symptoms. The average consult duration is 13 minutes, but there is no limit to the length of time. A diagnosis is made and the prescription (if applicable) is sent to the pharmacy. Depending on their employer/health plan, the patient's credit card is charged the appropriate co-pay. Teladoc reports 97% member satisfaction and that 90% of patients stated that their issues were resolved by the physician who contacted them (Teladoc, 2014). Similarly, and as previously mentioned, UnitedHealth first started offering a service called "NowClinic" in First Aid pharmacies. Today, its OptumHealth division offers the service to members, dependents and children older than two in 21 states. It allows them to receive healthcare services from local providers through secure webcam, chat, or phone. Providers diagnose, prescribe medications (non-controlled substances only), and offer educational content and self-care plans (NowClinic, 2013b). Other similar services provided by other companies include memd.com, and carenamd.com (discussed later).

In addition to the models described above, some new and different services are appearing. For example, QuickCheck Health is a "test at home, treat online" service with a pending patent. A consumer purchases a QuickCheck Health rapid home test at a local drugstore for about $7.50 per test. There are a number of tests such as urinary tract infection, strep throat, flu, cholesterol, A1c, Lyme disease, Mono, sexually transmitted diseases, pregnancy, pink eye, yeast infections and others. The patient administers the test at home and is given a result code. This result code provides proof of a positive test. The patient then goes to the company's website or calls and enters the code. He/she finds out the result of his/her test immediately at no charge. If positive, the patient can begin an online clinic visit. The visit fee is $35, eligible for coverage by most insurance companies. A clinician reviews the visit, and if appropriate, a prescription is sent to the pharmacy within as little as 5 minutes (QuickCheck Health, 2014). QuickCheck Health has a great potential given that as many as 13% of primary care consultations could be substituted by the home diagnostic and support package, which is a fifth of the cost of a face-to-face consultation (Linklaters, 2011).

Another service offered is 'itriage,' which is a decision support tool to research problems, take action, and improve care. The free smart phone application allows users to check their symptoms; learn about possible causes; research medications; determine if a trip to the hospital emergency room is necessary, or if an urgent care center or retail clinic might be a more appropriate; locate and compare nearby care options, and choose a medical provider (itriage, 2014). A more technologically advanced service is Scanadu. The company provides mobile applications and devices that let people track their vital signs at home. It claims to be "taking your smartphone to med school." Scanadu is developing two consumer health devices: Scout and ScanaFlo. Scout is designed to collect data on vital signs, including pulse, heart rate, respiratory rate, blood pressure, temperature, and even emotional stress. This will be possible by just holding a smart phone against the temple for 10 seconds. Scanaflo is a home urine test kit that will test for levels of glucose, protein, leukocytes, nitrates, blood, bilirubin, urobilinogen, specific gravity, and pH, as well as test for pregnancy. Both devices have not received FDA (Food and Drug Administration) approval yet (Scanadu, 2014).

Quality Assurance

Critics have argued that providing healthcare services in an online format can compromise quality of care and patient safety. The online care industry is adamant that its services are provided according to the most thorough protocols that have been developed by physicians using evidence-based medicine. Dr. John Misa, Park Nicollet's chief of primary care, defends Zipnosis: "This is not medicine by algorithm. This is medicine by Park Nicollet clinicians" (Lee, 2010, p.2).

One of the main concerns relate to misdiagnosis. Many providers argue that since there is no face-to-face physical examination, providers may miss some serious conditions, or mistake a condition for another. For example, around the time virtuwell and Zipnosis appeared, Dr. Benjamin Whitten, president of the Minnesota Medical Association, stated that "written information and checklists can't replace seeing a patient in person. I see the absence of a direct communication as a shortcoming and a potential problem" (Lee, 2010, p.1). Similarly, Robert Coffield, a West Virginia-based specialist in healthcare compliance and regulatory law questioned: "What can a doctor do over video versus in person? Will they overstate [a diagnosis], or miss something? There are no guidelines telling doctors 'this is how far you can go, but not beyond that.' What kind of liability does [AmericanWell] have?" in the event a doctor in Wyoming makes a misdiagnosis by video of a Honolulu patient?" (Hawn, 2009, p.363).

While these concerns are legitimate, online clinics address only problems that are common and easy to diagnose. Moreover, a service like virtuwell has developed hundreds of safety protocols to ensure on-line care is safe. They argue that the virtuwell interviewer never gets too busy or distracted and always asks all the right questions needed for an accurate diagnosis and treatment plan. For example, if a virtuwell patient indicates that he/she has had burning or frequent urination for more than ten days, the virtuwell interview ends and the patient receives a thorough explanation of why the interview was stopped, what virtuwell practitioners worry about and the standard of care they should expect for their unique presenting symptoms. The patient is strongly encouraged to visit a physician. A box on the screen explains that symptoms lasting more than seven days can be a sign of a more complicated infection and need a urinalysis or examination of the abdomen and kidneys. Similarly, if a pediatric patient has a sore throat and no other symptoms, the virtuwell visit stops. The patient is then asked to visit a physician because the child may have strep, which requires a throat culture to diagnose.

Other concerns relate to possible over-prescribing of antibiotics. Both virtuwell and Zipnosis, for example, review antibiotic prescribing for common conditions such as viral upper respiratory infection or sinusitis, and make sure that it is within the guidelines. Rebecca Hafner-Fogarty, M.D., chief medical officer of Zipnosis explains: "When we initially reviewed the Zipnosis sinusitis visits, we found that there were episodes where the clinician prescribed antibiotics outside the guidelines. We gathered this information and presented it in aggregate form to the clinicians. We also reviewed our guidelines with them and added reminders to our sinusitis pages" (Mettner, 2009, p.2). Since these are new services, many of the approaches used are being constantly revised. Developed by a physician-led organization, virtuwell takes quality and safety seriously. And, they've been transparent about their results. In a February 2013 Health Affairs paper, virtuwell explains their results for antibiotic appropriateness for adults with acute bronchitis. Using NCQA's HEDIS methodology, virtuwell delivered a 94.2% effectiveness rate compared to the 22% national average. And upon review, those who did get antibiotics inappropriately, got them from a venue other than virtuwell. Palattao credits the virtuwell approach, especially how its nurse practitioners engage and educate consumers about the differences between viral and bacterial infections and when antibiotics work versus effective over-the-counter options. In another example, virtuwell providers noticed that patients were not responding appropriately to questions related to the appearance of their skin. So they changed the questions and added sample images showing different types of lesions. They also allowed patients to upload images of their own skin to give the provider more information. Another advantage of the online experience is that every element of the patient encounter is documented and audited so when discrepancies occur, it is easy to identity the reason (Mettner, 2009).

Despite these assurances, many experts agree that there is a need for an entirely new national infrastructure that regulates online care. Coffield suggests: "We'll have to build out a whole new interstate network of health information particularly as it applies to use of patient data and provider licensing"(Hawn, 2009, p.367). Hawn (2009) adds that "the health sector needs a modern-day information network analogous to what the banking industry built, for national- and now, global-banking via automated teller machines (ATMs)"(p.367).

Impact on Primary Care Physicians and Retail Clinics

The services provided by online clinics have obvious overlap with those traditionally provided by primary care physicians in their private offices. Therefore, it is not surprising that many of those physicians consider the online clinics a serious competitive threat that can cannibalize their services. In a recent article, Don Fluckinger, News Director for the website "Search Health IT", asks rhetorically: "Could you blame physicians for shuddering at the thought of their health system employers contracting - no, outsourcing - after-hours care to a telemedicine clinic provider who brought its own physicians to the table?" (Fluckinger, 2013). It is important to note that when some health systems have made these services available to their patients, they have emphasized their after-hours availability. For example, Franciscan Health System in Tacoma, Washington, has a partnership with carenamd.com, an online clinic service. When Franciscan's brick-and-mortar primary care clinics close, the phones auto-forward calls to Carena' office, which is staffed with receptionists and healthcare providers ready to take phone and video calls to treat patients (Fluckinger, 2013a). As a result, the demands on on-call physicians on weeknights and weekends have dropped dramatically.

It is not clear what the specific effect of online services on retail clinics will be. It is obvious though that online services are even more convenient and cheaper than care delivered in supermarkets or drugstores. Therefore, it seems inevitable that these services will be in direct competition for patients in the next few years. Innovators observing some saturation in the retail clinic market have decided to bypass retail and jump directly into online care. Merchant Medicine explains: "HealthPartners has an extensive network of urgent care centers. Like most health systems, HealthPartners did extensive research around retail clinics and other limited-scope concepts. And their answer to the "limited-scope" movement has been to leapfrog retail medicine in favor of on-line and telephonic visits [through virtuwell]" (Merchant Medicine, 2011, p.3). Similarly, HealthPartners President and CEO Mary Brainerd stated "We've changed ourselves to say, 'We can't be just about seeing patients in exam rooms, we need to be about 'Call, click, come in.' In developing virtuwell, "we gave ourselves the challenge of 'out-MinuteClinic-ing' MinuteClinic, and ended up creating some online capabilities for care received through a nurse practitioner for routine, inexpensive acute health conditions" (Stempniak, 2013, p.4).

Challenges

When providing telehealth services, healthcare organizations need to comply with the Health Insurance Portability and Accountability Act (HIPAA) guidelines for securing personal medical data. Online exchanges with patients involving transfer of private personal, diagnosis and disease information can create several risks for providers. For example, although patients give consent to have their medical information distributed outside the closed online provider system, HIPAA requires that providers save it and archive it as part of the official medical record. As a result, many providers have put in place modern Electronic Health Records (EHRs) that protect records behind secure firewalls, and that automatically save the patient information (Hawn, 2009). For example, e-visits taking place within a secure portal, require the patient to supply a user name and password. As a result, the email exchanges and any other ancillary data are automatically imported and saved into the patient's EHR (Mettner, 2009)

Another possible challenge relates to geography. While online care does not recognize state borders or physical boundaries, healthcare providers such as physicians and nurse practitioners are licensed in their individual states, which can limit the geographic expansion of telehealth companies. For example, when virtuwell and Zipnosis first emerged, they were limited to the state of Minnesota and its specific rules and regulations. In order to expand their services to other states, they needed to contract with providers that are licensed to practice in those states. Representatives from virtuwell commented on this issue in a recent article: "[…] for online care to deliver on its potential, a reexamination of the regulatory environment is required. Following the launch of the service in Minnesota and Wisconsin, we have routinely received inquiries from large employer groups, with employees located in other states, about when the service might be available nationally. We will soon extend the service to consumers in a number of additional states, despite the fact that variations in state regulations governing a service such as virtuwell have presented barriers to doing so. Statutes in many states appear to discourage a service such as virtuwell in allowing legal prescribing only during a face-to-face clinical encounter or when an existing clinician-patient relationship exists. Some state statutes require clinicians to be located in the same state as the patient, or require the involvement of an in-state supervising physician. We acknowledge and support the importance of regulations addressing abuses associated with healthcare in online environments, such as unsafe and irresponsible online pharmacies. In that sense, however, we also believe that it is useful to consider how the evolution of care innovations tends to prompt review of existing regulations. For example, we applaud the trend toward multistate licensing strategies for clinicians-a trend that recognizes how thoughtfully applied technological advancements can break down outmoded or unnecessary geographic barriers" (Cournea, et al., 2013, p.390).

Another key hurdle affecting online services relates to reimbursement by pubic health insurance plans. As discussed above, some private health plans such as UnitedHealth, Aetna, Cigna and WellPoint have been among the first companies to offer online care services to their members. These companies realize the significant cost savings that an online encounter presents over care at the hospital emergency room, urgent care center, primary care physician, or even retail clinic. Among those payers, the requirements for covering e-visits are: The e-visit must be initiated by the patient; the patient must agree to pay for the encounter if their insurer does not; and the physician cannot take longer than 24 hours to respond to the patient's initial e-visit request. Also, as mentioned above, a physician who is licensed in one state can conduct e-visits only with patients who permanently reside in that state. It is important to note that e-visits are reimbursed at a different rate than in-person clinic visits, which is $35. In order to be covered, an e-visit should bring new information into the patient's history and should involve medical decision-making. For example, physicians treating patients in an office setting cannot send the patient lab results or answer follow-up questions by e-mail or video and call it a billable e-visit. There is some disagreement about whether the $35 reimbursement fee is appropriate, as some experts argue that e-visits are sometimes as time consuming and complex as regular office visits (Mettner, 2009).

Public insurance players have been late to the join the trend. However, it is important to note that despite some resistance, online care has not been subject to the same regulatory pushback that the retail clinic industry faced during its emergence (see Chapter 6). The main reason relates to medical societies and their lobbying efforts. While some online care services, especially the asynchronous ones, have focused on non-physician providers, many online care services have been available for physicians as an extension to their private office practices. Therefore, physician professional associations have not been as vocal in their resistance to online care. Retail clinics, on the other hand, had excluded physicians from direct patient care at the expense of nurse practitioners and physician assistants, and as a result have received strong opposition from physicians (Merchant Medicine, 2013a).

When it comes to public reimbursement, CMS (Centers for Medicare and Medicaid) makes a distinction between asynchronous care (care that is not provided in real time such as diagnosis after the patient logs out, e-mail messages and text message) and synchronous care (care that is provided in real-time interactions between patient and provider such as video conferencing). For a long time, CMS had reimbursed only for synchronous care services, so email or secure messages were not covered. CMS is actually reimbursing for telehealth in 41 states and have only reimbursed for asynchronous communication in rural settings (Merchant Medicine, 2013a). Recently, this seems to be changing, as companies such as virtuwell (which provides asynchronous care) have earned some favorable treatment. Kevin Palattao from virtuwell explains: "CMS has been cautious about paying for online care. But we met with them and showed them how we re-invented the diagnosis and treatment process to address quality and safety concerns. They asked lots of good questions that demonstrated thoughtful consideration. I think they were impressed because within one day or two, we got approval to add virtuwell to our Medicare-cost products, the first in the country" (Personal interview, 2013). Representatives from virtuwell recently argued that "the fee-for-service Medicare program and state Medicaid plans have much to gain by considering how to use online care delivery such as ours to lower costs for common conditions" (Cornera, Palattao & Gallagher, 2013, p.390). There is evidence that changes are starting to take place at the state level. There are currently 122 bills presently proposed by state and federal governments related to telemedicine. Mississippi and Maryland are the only two states governments to have successfully passed telemedicine reimbursement laws. Others states are expected to soon follow their example (Fluckinger, 2013b).

Research

Given the recency of the online care trend, there is a paucity of peer-reviewed research that evaluates the quality outcomes and weighs the potential costs savings in these settings. In this section, we summarize the few studies that have been published in the last few years. In 2010, Adamson and Bachman conducted a descriptive pilot study of patients using the Internet for online care ("e-visits") at the Department of Family Medicine at the Mayo Clinic in Rochester, Minnesota. Patients signed up for the service and were able to use the online portal for consultations with their primary care physician. The 4,282 patients included in the study made 2,531 online visits in a two-year period. Most of the visits were made by women during working hours. Uploading photographs was available for patients, but only 2% of visits took advantage of that feature. Billings were made for 1,159 patients and 16% of the visits replaced traditionally non-billable telephone protocols with billable encounters. The e-visits made office visits unnecessary in 40% of the cases. The patient conditions required the scheduling of a face-to-face appointment with a physician in 13% of the cases. The authors concluded that "the extent of conditions possible for treatment by online care was far-ranging and was managed with a minimum of message exchanges by using structured histories. Processes previously given as a free service or by nurse triage and subject to malpractice (protocols) were now documented and billed" (Adamson & Bachman, 2010, p.704). Another study from the Mayo Clinic matched costs of care for online visits with those in a standard drop-in visit in a conventional medical office setting during a six month period (Rohrer, Angstman, Adamson, et al., 2010). The results showed that the median standard costs for an online visit was $161 compared to $219 for same-day acute visits, and that the adjusted odds of being a cost outlier was lower for the online visit group than for the standard visit group.

More recently, Mehrotra and his colleagues evaluated the characteristics of patients that used e-visits and office visits for sinusitis and urinary tract infections (UTIs) at four primary care practices. E-visits accounted for almost 7% of visits for these two conditions, and patients most likely to use e-visits were those 18-44 years of age and those that lived more than 10 miles away from the clinics. Income was not a factor in e-visit use (Mehrotra, Pa-one, Martich, et al., 2013a). In another study, the same group of researchers examined test ordering, antibiotic prescribing, preventative care, follow-up care and costs at those same e-visits and office visits. The results showed that physicians were less likely to order a UTI-relevant test at an e-visit (8%) vs. an office visit (51%). There was no difference between the two types of visits in how many patients had a follow-up visit either for that condition or for any other reason. Physicians were more likely to prescribe an antibiotic at an e-visit for both sinusitis and urinary tract infections (UTIs), but the antibiotic prescribed at either type of visit was equally likely to be recommended by guidelines. Moreover, physicians were less likely to order preventive care in e-visits for both conditions. The costs calculations showed that e-visits were less expensive. For example, UTI visits costs were $74 for e-visits vs. $93 for office visits. The authors commented on what these results mean for quality and costs of care at e-visits: "Our findings refute some concerns about e-visits but support others. The fraction of patients with any follow-up was similar. Follow-up rates are a rough proxy for misdiagnosis or treatment failure and the lack of difference will therefore be reassuring to patients and physicians. Among e-visit users, half will use an e-visit when they have a subsequent illness in the next year. Patients appear generally satisfied with e-visits. On the other hand, antibiotic prescribing rates were higher at e-visits, particularly for UTIs. When physicians cannot directly examine the patient, physicians may use a "conservative" approach and order antibiotics. The high antibiotic prescribing rate for sinusitis for both e-visits and office visits is also a concern given the unclear benefit of antibiotic therapy for sinusitis" (Mehrotra, et al., 2013b, p.73).

Lastly, researchers from HealthPartners examined claims data to compare costs for episodes of care delivered by virtuwell compared with care delivered in retail clinics, physician offices, urgent care centers, and hospital emergency rooms for patients with acute sinusitis, lower genitourinary system infections, and conjunctivitis (Cournea, et al., 2013). Virtuwell patients were slightly younger (mean age of 37.3 years of age vs. 40.9 years for patients in other settings), and a greater percentage were female (83.4% versus 76.9%). In terms of costs, acute sinusitis episodes treated through virtuwell cost $78.90 less, genitourinary system infections episodes cost $127.61 less and conjunctivitis episodes cost $69.00 less than the same episodes treated in the other settings. On average, per episode treatment costs were $88.03 lower for virtuwell-treated episodes. More specific analyses indicated that virtuwell treatment cost $20–$30 less than retail clinic visits, $80–$142 less than physician office visits, $82–$124 less than urgent care center visits and $159–$469 less than hospital emergency room visits. Since online services such as virtuwell are available around the clock, the authors assessed whether they can lead to increased demand. Patient surveys showed that 90% of virtuwell visits replaced face-to-face visits, whereas in the other 10%, the patient would have adopted a "watch and wait" approach or used home care. Therefore, those 10% of visits represent possible additional use. However, the authors noted that "given the cost of a virtuwell visit, we estimate that this slight increase in utilization reduces the cost differential between virtuwell- and non-virtuwell- treated episodes by about 10 percent"(p.388), which suggests that the virtuwell costs savings are only slightly reduced by over-utilization. Moreover, the study looked at inappropriate antibiotic prescribing for acute bronchitis, and found that antibiotics were appropriately avoided in 94.2% of the cases. These rates are higher than the national benchmarks. Patient satisfaction surveys in the same study indicated that 99.5% of patients felt that the service was easy to use, 94.2% would highly recommend the service to friends and family; 95.9% received enough information in their treatment plans and 92.7% had confidence and trust in the quality of care received. Moreover, patient indicated that on average, virtuwell saved them 2.5 hours per visit (Cournea, et al., 2013).

Despite the scarce evidence and the small sample sizes used in the above studies, care delivered in online clinics and through e-visits seems to follow clinical guidelines, and costs are significantly lower than other settings of care. While the assumption that online clinics will over-prescribe antibiotics persists, the emerging data suggests that belief might be wrong. Future research should clarify many of these issues.

Future

According to BCC Research, the telemedicine technology market is expected to grow from $3.8 billion in 2010 to $11.3 billion in 2016, with a CAGR (compound annual growth rate) of 19.8% over the next five years, whereas the telemedicine service market is expected to grow from $5.9 billion to $16 billion during that same time period (BCC Research, 2012). Experts agree that telemedicine/telehealth in general, and online care and virtual visits are here to stay, and will only continue to grow as consumers, providers, payers, and employers continue to embrace these innovations.

In a 2012 book titled "The Creative Destruction of Medicine: How the Digital Revolution Will Create Better Health Care," Dr. Eric Topol argues the digital age and new technologies will enable a radical revolution that will transform American medicine from its traditional outdated practice to a new efficient and innovative system (Topol, 2012). Large scale data intensive biological repositories, and advances in information and sensor technology and their impact on medical practice are discussed in detail. Phenomenal innovations such as those in wireless biosensors, dynamic imaging, electronic health records and genomics will result in massive benefits for preventative services, cost reduction and quality improvement. Based on these advances, Dr. Topol imagines what the individual medical record of the future will look like: "Simply put, everything should be in it. This will inevitably require cloud-based storage: the data sets will be huge, at terabytes of data per individual, to encompass a record that starts prenatally and extends to the end of an individual's life. All of the actual imaging data should be incorporated to allow physicians to view the files directly rather than having to only rely on the report. The size of the typical files have been quantified by the Federal Communications Commission [...] It will include one's DNA sequence along with all major forms of digital imaging. It must also include data for all radiation exposure, as the risk is cumulative over one's entire life. Collectively, with a national or, even better, international public health monitoring capability, we will be able to determine such environmental effects of radiation exposure on increased risk of cancer, and particular genomic variations that predispose particular individuals to ill effects of radiation exposure at even low doses" (Topol, 2012, p. 151). He also envisages the effects of the changes on physicians and office visits: "These new models are just the beginning of where medicine can go when it is wireless, connected to an Internet on steroids, and capable of tracking comprehensive physiologic metrics and even some forms of digital imaging. Data never previously available to both patients and physicians are now streaming. With the individual's biologic and DNA sequence data in the EHR [Electronic Health Record] and the patient's PHR[[Personal Health Record], indicating all pharmacogenomic interactions, and with this information shared with the patient's pharmacist, prescriptions will eventually have a whole new look of precision. The need for in-person office visits will be substantially reduced over time, along with those to emergency rooms. Those physicians who can emerge as the medical digerati will have a decided advantage-their accurate data on outcomes, quality, and cost will be posted on the Web and automatically updated on a frequent basis. House calls of yesteryear will be making an incredible comeback, but done through the Web" (Topol, 2012, p. 181).

2. HOUSE CALL SERVICES

Physician House Calls

House calls by physicians and other providers are an ancient idea in healthcare delivery. Before the 1940s, the majority of physician encounters in the United States took place in patient homes (Kao, Conant, Soriano &McCormick, 2009). House calls allowed physicians to build a strong relationship with their patients as they were able to see them in their own environment where they are the most comfortable. A physician from Kentucky in the early 20th century wrote about his encounters treating patients in their homes: "I recall an experience I had one winter day with the thermometer near zero and about five inches of snow on the ground. I was called about eight miles from home and found a young farm boy with a well-marked case of appendicitis with apparent abscess formation. I called a very fine, competent surgeon from Henderson, Kentucky, to come prepared to operate in the home. . . . The patient being satisfactorily anesthetized, the surgeon removed the appendix and sutured the wound in about forty minutes. After [the] operation, the surgeon got in his buggy and started home, a distance of about twenty-five miles. I spent the night with the family and saw the patient daily for several days. He made a very rapid and satisfactory recovery. Some years later the family had a son operated on in a hospital with modern skill and care. A few days later this son died. Sometime after the death the good old mother stated to me, 'If he had been home where you and me could have cared for him, I believe he would have gotten well.' I am sure the son had better care than he could have in the home. Some people manifested such explicit confidence and esteem of me, it made me love them and realize how great my obligation to them" (Herritt, 2012, p.175).

As hospitals and physician offices started thriving and as transportation improved, more and more patients traveled to seek their care, and fewer physicians made house calls. Only 1% of physician encounters in the 1980s were house calls (Kao, Conant, Soriano &McCormick, 2009). However, recent evidence suggests that house calls are making a comeback (Leff & Burton, 2001). As Medicare made it easier for physicians to get paid for house calls, the trend has peaked. Starting in 1998, Medicare increased reimbursement for a house call by nearly 50%. Between 1998 and 2004, house calls to seniors on Medicare increased by 40%. In that same time period, the amount of house calls completed by geriatricians increased by 92%, compared with 41% for family practitioners and 59% for internists, while family practitioners continue to have the lion's share of house calls (Landers, Gunn, Flocke, et al., 2005).

There are some differences however between house calls of today and those of the old days. First, the majority of recent house calls are for people who are home-bound due to multiple chronic conditions, such as diabetes, heart disease or Alzheimer's, rather than for the general population. These patients are very limited in their ability to visit their physicians on a periodic basis to make sure that their chronic conditions are kept under control. Another difference is that today's technology allows physicians to check patients in their homes using state-of-the-art portable X-ray machines, laptop-based tests and EKGs (electrocardiogram), compact ultrasounds, and other small diagnostic devices that were not available in the 1930's and 1940's.

Nurse Practitioner House Calls

A more recent trend has been for house calls made by nurse practitioners. These tend to focus on patients who are elderly, chronically ill-children, people with disabilities and with psychiatric conditions (Lavoie-Vaughan, 2013). For example, in 2004, Scharmaine Lawson-Baker, a nurse practitioner, opened the first nurse practitioner house call practice in New Orleans. She describes a part of a day in her practice:

7:30 am: I arrive at the office, and check my schedule. I inspect my medical bag for adequate gauze, alcohol pads, and Otoscope tips, before checking my email again.

8 am: The Office Manager gives me a quick rundown of the patients who will be home today. She also tells me about any specific instructions for the house call, such as who is leaving their door open, who wants me to enter through the carport while ignoring the Pit Bull, and who has asked that I grab the mail from the mailbox on the way in.

8:45 am: I drink a protein shake while on a conference call with an NP (nurse practitioner) who is starting her first house call practice. She has a few questions about how to sell her vision to her new collaborating physician.

9 am: I'm at my first home. Even though I was told to just walk in, I always announce that I am entering, ring the bell, or knock on the door prior to going into the home. One must always remember that when you enter someone's home, it is *their* territory and it must be respected. This is an important pearl that must never be forgotten. It is the hallmark distinction between a traditional clinic visit and a house call.

9:45 am: I stop to get gas and some bottled water for the tiny ice chest I keep in my care. I always try to be prepared for the balmy N'awlins climate. While the gas is pumping, I use these few minutes to update the business Facebook and Twitter accounts, check-in at the office, and call my next patient to let her know I am 15 minutes out. I also scroll through lab results and messages on my iPad.

10 am: I arrive at the next home and immediately snatch the mail from the mailbox. I head towards the front door that is almost hidden behind the most beautiful Crape Myrtle ever imagined. Even though the patient is bedbound from debilitating Rheumatoid Arthritis, she has her sitter prepare my favorite cup of mint tea and Lorna Dune cookies as a small thank you for bringing the mail. We review her labs and I electronically prescribe her heart medicines before it's time to go. With Gino the Persian cat lightly whisking his tail past my calf, I reach across the bedrail for a warm hug before dashing off to the next patient. I love house-calls because you get to interact with the entire family and the environment, which often includes pets.

10:30 am: I get to the home of a new patient and there are so many people in the home it is reminiscent of a family reunion. I am warmly greeted and offered lunch with a cold Sprite. I politely decline the lunch, but sip on the Sprite while gathering the patient history from the family. The patient is unable to speak secondary to his recent cerebral vascular accident (CVA). The family is extremely grateful for my visit because the patient has vehemently refused to go to his usual primary care provider. The family found our services on the internet, and his appointment was scheduled within 48 hours. I love supportive families because they make my job easier. They work together with me to develop a focused and deliberate plan of action to ensure speedy recovery to optimal health for their beloved patriarch" (Amirault, 2012, p.1-2). Lawson-Baker has founded a consulting company called Housecall Course, which trains nurse practitioners on how to start a house-call practice (Housecall Course, 2013).

WhiteGlove

Another recent trend mentioned in the "Preface" section of this book is WhiteGlove Health. In contrast to other house call services, this service was first started to focus on episodic, low-acuity conditions, rather than chronic ones. The company has taken the concept into a new level by offering individuals and families of all ages yearly membership in return for "access to high quality, affordable routine care at home or work, 365 days a year, 8am to 8pm." The care is typically provided by a nurse practitioner.

WhiteGlove Health is offered on a membership basis for individuals and for employees of certain companies with specific health plans. A customer becomes a member by registering online or by phone for $35 per month ($88/month for families). If the customer needs medical attention on any day of the year, he/she can request an appointment via phone or online. Within hours, a nurse practitioner visits him/her at work or at home. During the visit, the nurse practitioner diagnoses and treats the customer and, for no extra charge, provides him/her with most of the generic medications that are prescribed on the visit. He/she uses an iPad to write medical notes. In the past, a Well-Kit with foods, beverages, and over-the-counter remedies was provided, but that service has recently been discontinued. At the end of the visit, the customer is asked to fill a quick satisfaction survey on the iPad. Customers also have secure online access to their information including their medical history, lab results, visit history, etc. Each visit costs $35. Alternatively, employees of companies that contract with Aetna/Humana in Texas are offered the service as a health benefit at no annual cost. Employer membership fees are $300 per member.

The scope of care provided by WhiteGlove Health when it first opened was similar to that of a retail clinic. Merchant Medicine (2011) described it as "a mobile MinuteClinic and more, providing primary care and urgent care services, using nurse practitioners" (p.1). The "Get Well" service provided care for routine conditions such as sore throats, common cold, coughs, sinus infection, seasonal allergy, earache, swimmers ear, pink eye, upper respiratory infections, bronchitis, flu, urinary tract/bladder infection, nausea, vomiting, diarrhea, as well as minor burns, cuts, and rashes. The "Stay Well" service helped customers maintain their health and prevent illness by providing vaccines, allergy tests, cholesterol panel tests, complete blood counts, diabetic panel tests, glucose screening, pregnancy tests, strep tests, etc. Recently, however, WhiteGlove Health expanded its scope of services. It now offers "Complete Health Solution" which "provides a comprehensive suite of technology-enabled health and wellness services - including biometrics, wellness coaching, acute care, telemedicine, chronic care, and on-site services" (WhiteGlove, 2014).

WhiteGlove Health started in major Texas metropolitan cities only (Austin, Dallas/Fort Worth, Houston and San Antonio), but has since expanded to Phoenix, Arizona and Boston, Massachusetts. The company was founded in 2006 by Austin entrepreneur Bob Fabbio and William Rice, M.D. In 2011, it had 469,000 members (Hawkins, 2011) and it currently provides services to 130 employers (WhiteGlove, 2014). Fabbio describes how the company was founded: "I literally had lunch with myself and concluded I was too young to retire. I knew I didn't want another high-tech venture. I wanted to launch a service business that was focused on a large, messy market, that had complex subject matter, and could leverage my technology background. Essentially, a complex, messy service industry that was in need of disruption"(Merchant Medicine, 2011, p.1). Soon after, Fabbio got sick and had to go to the physician office. He added: "Between driving to a 9 a.m. appointment, waiting in the waiting room, waiting for the doctor, waiting for labs, waiting to be discharged, driving to the pharmacy, and waiting for a prescription, and then going to the grocery store, it was 2 o'clock in the afternoon by the time I got home. I realized this was the messy, complex service business that was ready for disruption. It was healthcare. We quietly went to work signing up members in the early going. We initially thought the market was busy soccer moms and busy professionals. But it became immediately apparent that if we were going to grow this rapidly, we needed to figure out how to sign up large groups of members." (Merchant Medicine, 2011, p.2). As part of the research for this book, we interviewed

Dr. William Rice in March of 2013 (See Appendix A).

To date, there has not been any research that evaluates WhiteGlove Health or similar services. The company provides some examples of the benefits that contracted employers have reaped. For example, for an unnamed law firm with 46 employees, WhiteGlove "has prevented 30% of the routine medical care visits that would have normally taken employees away from work for 3-4 hours at a time. The resulting productivity improvement has helped the firm maintain excellent service to their clients and continue to bill at a level the business needed." At an information Technology (IT) Service company with 122 employees, "The WhiteGlove service has eliminated the hassles of getting routine medical care as well as lowering the employees' out-of-pocket expenses. With each WhiteGlove visit saving employees between $40 and $160 dollars and the company paying for their membership fees, it has been like giving the employees a raise. With no claims filed against the company's health insurance plan for the WhiteGlove visit and most of the Rx medications that are prescribed during the visit, they are hopeful to negotiate better rates next year. The company has benefited from employees who are away from work less and the employees are thrilled to have a great new benefit for themselves and their dependents." At a plastics manufacturer firm with 98 employees "WhiteGlove showed them how the combination of a high deductible healthcare plan with WhiteGlove's service could reduce their costs while providing their employees with a better routine medical care experience that costs the company and the employees less. This combination reduced their overall healthcare costs by 37% over their previous plan and their employees love the WhiteGlove service." Finally, at a commercial printing with 77 employees "WhiteGlove collects biometric information on each employee and dependent by providing wellness assessments that are included as part of its corporate membership program. This information is aggregated and provides the company with the visibility they need to put effective wellness programs in place to prevent surprise claims. As a result of their wellness programs, they haven't had a single surprise claim in the last 12 months" (WhiteGlove Health Case Studies, 2014). It is important to note that these claims have not been evaluated by an objective third party.

3. OTHER SERVICES

In addition to the innovations discussed in the previous sections, some other new services are also worth highlighting. While not in the same category of cheaper and more affordable care, an interesting trend witness in the last few years is that of free-standing emergency rooms. As the name suggests, these are walk-in facilities that are structurally separate from a hospital, but that provide emergency care to consumers. They are equipped to diagnose and stabilize cardiac arrests, stroke symptoms, breathing problems and trauma, and they provide many urgent care services. However, their scope of service is more limited than a traditional emergency room. Patients requiring hospital admission or surgery are typically transported by ambulance to nearby facilities. Many of the free-standing emergency rooms are owned by hospital system, by joint ventures between hospital and private companies, or by private investors. While providing easy-to-access convenient care, especially in areas where no other emergency services are available, they don't represent a low-cost alternative. In fact there has been recent controversy surrounding these facilities. Patients have been shocked to receive expensive medical bills that they were not expecting, as many confuse them with urgent care centers.

For years, concierge or boutique medicine practices have provided affluent patients with prime medical services for high annual fees. In some practices, patients could get same-day appointments and are guaranteed low wait times at the office and long visits with the provider for about $2,500 or more per year. A recent development called "direct primary care" (DPC) borrows the concierge concept but makes its cheaper so that it is more affordable and accessible to many patients. Dave Chase, a DPC observer describes the trend: "Direct primary care is essentially concierge medicine for the masses. It's a retainer-based primary care that is completely free of insurance. You pay for it like a gym membership: a monthly fee no matter how much you use it" (Merchant Medicine, 2013b, p.1). Patients pay about $50 per month and are guaranteed virtually unlimited access to their physician. For example, "One Medical Group," which has six locations in New York, charges its members $200 per year in return for same-day appointments, online scheduling and short wait times. The company describes it model: "As a group of physicians, we got tired of practicing medicine in a broken system. Instead, we listened to our patients and built a totally new medical group designed specifically to meet your needs. From on-time appointments to longer visits, you'll experience healthcare designed around you, not the other way around" (One Medical Group, 2014). While some physician practices have individually offered DPC services, the recent growth of this small industry has been fueled by the introduction of some large companies such as Davita Healthcare Partners, Iora Health, Qliance and MedLion (Merchant Medicine, 2013b).

Another service that has many similarities with concepts that we have already discussed in this book is that of the "medical mall." The last 20 years have witnessed the growth of medical malls, where traditional retail space malls are repurposed to create a mixed-use medical/retail facility. This model presents several advantages for healthcare consumers such as convenient locations, ample parking, extended hours, easy access to non-medical services, and the available of primary care and specialty services in a one-stop healthcare experience. For physicians and other providers, the medical mall allows them expanded clinical and office space, better visibility and brand recognition in their market, and potential increase in patient referrals. Services typically offered in these settings include primary care, psychology, acute care rehabilitation/physical therapy, screening/wellness/health education, elder services, women's health, health department clinic/administration, cosmetic dermatology/laser clinic dialysis, surgery, podiatry, laboratory, imaging and substance abuse. A recent descriptive study concluded that medical malls "have a great deal of *potential* to improve access to care, transform the patient experience, reach low income individuals, and help "save" the American mall" (Uscher-Pines, Mehrotra, Chari, 2013, p.7).

On the other end of the spectrum, mobile health clinics providing services on the road have been in increasingly wide use in the last few years. For example, the Family Van in Boston, Massachusetts is a "mobile health program designed to increase access to health and improve healthy behaviors by providing free culturally and linguistically appropriate health services to our clients". It serves communities with disproportionately high rates of preventable diseases, poor health status and high use of hospital emergency room and is staffed by health educators, a registered dietician, and counselors, who provide health screenings, offer oral and written information to encourage patients to improve their health and follow healthy lifestyles (The Family Van, 2014). A recent study showed that the services provided allowed patients with high blood pressure to reduce their systolic and diastolic blood pressure by 10.7 mmHg and 6.2 mmHg in, respectively. These changes were linked with 32.2% reduction in the relative risk of myocardial infarction and 44.6% reduction in the relative risk of stroke. The savings from the reduction in blood pressure and patient-reported avoided emergency department visits produced a Return on Investment (ROI) of 1.3 (Song, Hill, Bennet et al. 2013). Other vans provide similar services to homeless people who have no access to fixed clinics (Post, 2007).

4. CONCLUSION

The healthcare industry is ripe for innovations being delivered in examination rooms, online, in patient homes or on the road. These innovations have "no status quo to defend, no arcane rules [to] follow" and their "…goal is to dramatically improve the experience and quality of care for everyone" (Iora Health, 2014). If these trends indicate anything, they suggest that the current healthcare system is broken, and that entrepreneurs, providers, hospitals and other players will continue to tinker to provide solutions that advance value, convenience and access.

REFERENCES

Adamson, S. C., & Bachman, J. W. (2010). Pilot study of providing online care in a primary care setting. *Mayo Clinic Proceedings*, *85*(8), 704–710. doi:10.4065/mcp.2010.0145 PMID:20516427

American Telemedicine Association. (2013). *What is Telemedicine?* Retrieved from http://www.americantelemed.org/learn

American Well. (2013). Retrieved from http://www.americanwell.com/howItWorks.html Last accessed 1/3/14

Amirault, B. (2012). *Day in the Life: Running a nurse practitioner house-call practice*. Retrieved from http://www.bartonassociates.com/2012/11/16/nurse-practitioner-day-in-the-life-1/

Business Wire. (2013). *Zipnosis Announces Service in New Markets*. Retrieved from http://www.businesswire.com/news/home/20130118005961/en/Zipnosis-Announces-Service-Markets#.UsbhnvRDuSo

Care, O. (2012). *Growing your practice through telehealth*. Retrieved from: http://www.mackstudiopro.com/projects/client/AmericanWell/undocumented/videoLibrary_corpSite_v11_NewSite/pdf/OnlineCare_GrowingYourPracticeWithTelehealth.pdf

Center for Connected Health Policy. (2013). *What is Telehealth?* Retrieved from http://telehealthpolicy.us/what-telehealth

Cisco. (2013). *Customer Experience Report for Health Care*. Insight Express.

Fairview Clinics. (2014). Retrieved from https://fairview.zipnosis.com/

Courneya, P. T., Palattao, K. J., & Gallagher, J. M. (2013). HealthPartners' Online Clinic For Simple Conditions Delivers Savings Of $88 Per Episode And High Patient Approval. *Health Affairs*, *32*(2), 385–392. doi:10.1377/hlthaff.2012.1157 PMID:23381532

Family Van. (2014). Retrieved from http://www.familyvan.org/about/

Fluckinger, D. (2013a). Telemedicine clinics: Could they cannibalize primary care practices? *Search Health IT*. Retrieved from http://searchhealthit.techtarget.com/feature/Telemedicine-clinics-Could-they-cannibalize-primary-care-practices

Fluckinger, D. (2013b). Telemedicine reimbursement transcending party politics in some states. *Search Health IT*. Retrieved from http://searchhealthit.techtarget.com/healthitexchange/healthitpulse/telemedicine-reimbursement-transcending-party-politics-in-some-states/

Ford, J. (2011). Online healthcare: A new wave in convenience. *Advance for NPs & PAs*, *2*(4), 17. PMID:21661286

Gartner Industry Research. (2008). *Case Study: A Texas Telemedicine Program Offers Lessons for Governments and Care Delivery Organizations Worldwide*. Retrieved from http://telehealth.utmb.edu/news/Gartner%20case_study_a_texas_telemedic_157582.pdf

Hawkins, L. (2011). WhiteGlove seeks to raise $32.5 million in 'Dutch auction' IPO. *Austin American Statesman*. Retrieved from http://www.statesman.com/news/business/whiteglove-seeks-to-raise-325-million-in-dutch-auc/nRZg9/

Hawn, C. (2009). Take Two Aspirin And Tweet Me In The Morning: How Twitter, Facebook, And Other Social Media Are Reshaping Health Care. *Health Affairs*, *28*(2), 361–368. doi:10.1377/hlthaff.28.2.361 PMID:19275991

Hello Health. (2013). Retrieved from http://hellohealth.com/about-myca/

Iora Health. (2014). Retrieved from http://www.iorahealth.com/

HealthPartners. (2014). Retrieved from https://www.healthpartners.com/public/care/family-of-care/parknicollet/

Heinzelmann, P.J., Williams, C.M., Lugn, N.E., & Kvedar, J.C. (2005). Clinical Outcomes Associated with Telemedicine/Telehealth. *Telemedicine and eHealth*, *11*(3), 329-47.

Herritt, B. J. (2012). The House Call: Past, Present and Future. *UTMJ*, *89*(3), 175–177.

HouseCall Course. (2013). Retrieved from http://advancedclinicalconsultants.org/the-housecall-course/

Itriage. (2014). Retrieved from http://about.itriagehealth.com/for-consumer/what-is-itriage/

Kao, H., Conant, R., Soriano, T., & McCormick, W. (2009). The Past, Present, and Future of House Calls. *Clinics in Geriatric Medicine*, *25*(1), 19–34. doi:10.1016/j.cger.2008.10.005 PMID:19217490

Landers, S. H., Gunn, P. W., Flocke, S. A., Graham, A. V., Kikano, G. E., Moore, S. M., & Stange, K. C. (2005). Trends in house calls to Medicare beneficiaries. *Journal of the American Medical Association*, *294*(19), 2435–2436. PMID:16287953

Lavoie-Vaughan, N. (2013). *House Calls as a Practice Venture. Nurse Practitioner and Physician Assistant Advanced Web.* Retrieved from http://nurse-practitioners-and-physician-assistants.advanceweb.com/article/house-calls-as-a-practice-venture-2.aspx

Lee, W. (2010, May 19). Online medicine in a hurry. *Minnesota Star Tribune*.

Leff, B., & Burton, J. R. (2001). The future history of home care and physician house calls in the United States. *The Journals of Gerontology. Series A, Biological Sciences and Medical Sciences*, *56*(10), M603–M608. doi:10.1093/gerona/56.10.M603 PMID:11584032

Linklaters. (2011). *Encouraging sustainable innovation in health*. White Paper. Retrieved from http://quickcheckhealth.com/encouraging-sustainable-innova/

Medicaid.gov. (22013). *Keeping America Healthy-Telemedicine*. Retrieved from http://www.medicaid.gov/Medicaid-CHIP-Program-Information/By-Topics/Delivery-Systems/Telemedicine.html

Medicine, M. (2011). *ConvUrgent Care Report*, *4*(4), 1–4.

Medicine, M. (2013). *ConvUrgent Care Report*, *6*(5), 1–6.

Medicine, M. (2013b). *ConvUrgent Care Report*, *6*(8), 1–5.

Mehrotra, A., Paone, S., Martich, G. D., Albert, S. M., & Shevchik, G. J. (2013). A comparison of care at e-visits and physician office visits for sinusitis and urinary tract infection. *JAMA Internal Medicine*, *173*(1), 72–74. doi:10.1001/2013.jamainternmed.305 PMID:23403816

Mehrotra, A., Paone, S., Martich, G. D., Albert, S. M., & Shevchik, G. J. (2013a). Characteristics of patients who seek care via eVisits instead of office visits. *Telemedicine Journal and e-Health*, *19*(7), 515–519. doi:10.1089/tmj.2012.0221 PMID:23682589

Mehrotra, A., Paone, S., Martich, G. D., Albert, S. M., & Shevchik, G. J. (2013b). A Comparison of Care at E-visits and Physician Office Visits for Sinusitis and Urinary Tract Infection. *JAMA Internal Medicine*, *173*(1), 72–74. doi:10.1001/2013.jamainternmed.305 PMID:23403816

Mettner, J. (2009). The Doctor Is In (Your Inbox). E-visits can be an efficient way to practice, but they have been slow to catch on. *Minnesota Medicine*. Retrieved from http://www.minnesotamedicine.com/PastIssues/PastIssues2009/January2009/PulseInbox-January2009.aspx

Mettner, J. (2011, April). Virtual Visits Two Twin Cities-based online diagnostic services are bringing relief to patients—and providers. *Minnesota Medicine*. Retrieved from http://www.minnesotamedicine.com/Default.aspx?tabid=3736

Newmarker, C. (2008). MinuteClinic co-founder launches e-medicine startup. *Minneapolis/St. Paul Business Journal*.

NowClinic. (2013a). Retrieved from https://www.mynowclinic.com/riteaid/about_us/overview/

NowClinic. (2013b). Retrieved from https://www.mynowclinic.com/patient/faq/

Online Care Anywhere. (2013). Retrieved from http://www.onlinecareanywheremn.com/howitworks.php

Post, P. (2007). *Mobile Healthcare for Homeless People: Using Vehicles to Extend Care*. National Healthcare for the Homeless Council. Retrieved from http://www.nhchc.org/wp-content/uploads/2012/02/mobilehealth.pdf. Last accessed 1/4/14

Reid, J. (1996). *A Telemedicine Primer: Understanding the Issues*. Billings, MT: Innovative Medical Communications.

BBC Research. (2012). Retrieved from www.bccresearch.com

Richman, D. (2013). H*arris Interactive: Consumer trends in retail medicine*. Paper presented at Retail Clinician Education Congress. New York, NY.

Rohrer, J. E., Angstman, K. B., Adamson, S. C., Bernard, M. E., Bachman, J. W., & Morgan, M. E. (2010). Impact of online primary care visits on standard costs: A pilot study. *Population Health Management*, *13*(2), 59–63. doi:10.1089/pop.2009.0018 PMID:20415617

Rohrer, J. E., Angstman, K. B., Adamson, S. C., Bernard, M. E., Bachman, J. W., & Morgan, M. E. (2010). Impact of online primary care visits on standard costs: A pilot study. *Population Health Management*, *13*(2), 59–63. doi:10.1089/pop.2009.0018 PMID:20415617

Scanadu. (2014). Retrieved from http://www.scanadu.com/

Smith, K. (2013). *Telehealth: Management of Patient Outcomes and Protecting the Continuity of Care*. Paper presented at Retail Clinician Education Congress. New York, NY.

Song, Z., Hill, C., Bennet, J., Vavasis, A., & Oriol, N. E. (2013). Mobile Clinic In Massachusetts Associated With Cost Savings From Lowering Blood Pressure And Emergency Department Use. *Health Affairs (Project Hope)*, *32*(1), 36–44. doi:10.1377/hlthaff.2011.1392 PMID:23297269

Stempniak, M. (2013, October). Retail Clinics: Threat or opportunity? *Hospital and Health Networks*.

Teladoc. (2014). Retrieved from http://www.teladoc.com/

Topol, E. (2012). *The Creative Destruction of Medicine: How the Digital Revolution Will Create Better Health Care*. New York: Basic Books.

U.S. Department of Health and Human Services. (2013). *"What is mHealth?"*. Retrieved from http://www.hrsa.gov/healthit/mhealth.html

Uscher-Pines, L., Mehrotra, A., & Chari, R. (2013). On call at the mall: A mixed methods study of U.S. medical malls. *BMC Health Services Research*, *13*(1), 471. doi:10.1186/1472-6963-13-471 PMID:24209495

Virtuwell. (2013). Retrieved from https://www.virtuwell.com/

WhiteGlove Health. (2014). Retrieved from http://www.whiteglove.com/

WhiteGlove Health Case Studies. (2014). Retrieved from http://www.whiteglove.com/images/stories/documents/case-study-fully-insured.pdf

World Health Organization. (2013). *E-health*. Retrieved from http://www.who.int/trade/glossary/story021/en/

Zamosky, L. (2010, June 7). The doctor's in-box. *Los Angeles Times*. Retrieved from http://www.latimes.com/health/la-he-doctor-emails-20100607,0,639147.story#ixzz2pIdYp0mP

KEY TERMS AND DEFINITIONS

House-Call Services: Services provided for minor conditions in the patient's home or workplacc.

Online Services: Healthcare services provided electronically in real time (synchronous) or through "store & forward" (asynchronous) delivery via images, video and audio.

Telehealth: The use of advanced telecommunication technologies to exchange health information and provide healthcare services across geographic, time, social, and cultural barriers.

Telemedicine: The use of medical information exchanged from one site to another via electronic communications to improve a patient's clinical health status.

APPENDIX 1

Kevin Palattao, Vice President of Patient Care Systems for HealthPartners & Vice President, Virtuwell

Kevin Palattao is credited with the vision behind virtuwell, but he's quick to deflect that praise preferring to talk about all of the smart people on the virtuwell team that collaborate to make it what it is today. As part of research for this book, we interviewed him by phone in March of 2013. He describes himself as "a dreamer, who wants to do good things and leave a positive legacy." Palattao is the son of an MD and RN, so "it can be a blessing or a curse" he laughs. He has been in health care most of his life and has listened to stories growing up about how difficult it was to practice medicine and health care which has deeply impacted him.

He was a Political Science major at the University of California-Berkley, and then worked in physician offices in billing. About 23 years ago, he started working at HealthPartners in Minneapolis, when technology was just emerging. He has a healthy disregard for the status quo, and an "affinity for process design, removing unnecessary steps." He became a Minnesota quality award evaluator based on the Malcolm Baldridge approach.

In his current role as Vice President of Patient Care Systems, he is the interface between clinicians and information technology, understanding what the consumers expect and what physicians expect and identifying new processes and technologies that make diagnosis and treatment more reliable and more empowering for consumers.

Palattao says that HealthPartners has been developing clinical protocols for more than 20 years, as well as nurse protocols under physician supervision. They were one of the first organizations in the country to hire midwives and nurse practitioners.

In 2009 he did a fellowship and worked on a project to reduce cost and increase quality and satisfaction. HealthPartners is focused on the Triple Aim of the Institute for Healthcare Improvement (IHI) of improving the patient experience of care (including quality and satisfaction); improving the health of populations; and reducing the per capita cost of health care. All of those experiences inspired him to pursue the virtuwell project and take existing consumer and medical pieces, and re-arrange them to reinvent the diagnosis and treatment process to directly deliver on the Triple Aim. He selected Chief Marketing Officer Andrea Walsh to sponsor his fellowship project and who helped guide the idea through executive leadership and the board of directors. They loved the idea and demonstrated their support by funding it. As an integrated delivery system, they wanted to improve quality and deliver an exceptional experience all at an affordable price. Virtuwell won hearts and minds because here was a way to deliver needed savings for everyone in a manner that everyone loved. The business proposal and innovation was to start from the consumer's point of view and then blend proven clinical practices with a refreshingly simple online and mobile platform, and best-in-class customer service to save consumers time and money.

Palattao explains the process of designing virtuwell:

"At HealthPartners, we already knew how to deliver safe and evidenced based care. What we wanted to do differently was engage consumers in a completely different way. We wanted to create something simple, fresh, empowering, approachable and trustworthy. Those are attributes not frequently associated with traditional health care. We wanted to modernize the diagnosis and treatment process to feel more like the way the rest of the world was operating (e.g. airlines, banking, travel, auto, consumer goods)…simple, safe, and affordable.

Palattao discusses the quality of care standards for virtuwell:

"As a not-for-profit integrated care system, quality and safety is paramount. We believe in and work hard to facilitate expert discussions around evidenced based care. And we share our results transparently. When we started design, we were well aware of examples of unscrupulous Internet pharmacies. So we felt compelled to take a leadership position with virtuwell to help define what constitutes a safe and effective standard of care in virtual medicine. This is precisely why we chose to launch with a limited menu set. In fact, we selected conditions that behave well to rules. The conditions we treat can be reliably and accurately diagnosed with a thorough medical history and in some cases augmented with an uploaded photograph. These are the same types of medical interviews you'd expect in a doctor's office but we do them online. And, consumers can pace themselves through the process making this an amazingly empowering experience. Our published results on antibiotic appropriateness and clinical resolution rates suggest we're helping lead the way in this new era of virtual medicine."

As for the business model, he says "it is too early to call, we have been in operation for only 3 seasons. It is volume sensitive, but we believe it can stand on its own once greater levels of market awareness are achieved. The model has demonstrated great appeal to health plans, employers and consumers. We believe this will be even more attractive to consumers who shift to high deductible and HSA plans."

Assessing the online care industry, Palattao notes: "If you look at the trend of how people use the Internet and mobile to communicate with each other, it compels us to ask 'why not in health care?' The notion that you have to go somewhere to solve a problem and tether yourself to one person does not apply anymore. Team based care models that are engineered for quality and simplicity like virtuwell are very appealing to consumers who are looking for around the clock help from a trusted health care brand where access and quality isn't limited to an individual practitioner. And as scientists continue to map the human genome, we believe that diagnostic techniques and treatments will continue to become more precise. And virtual medicine models will continue to play an important role in the health care ecosystem. Moreover, I can't recall ever meeting a doctor who didn't dream of being able to spend more time with her patients. With real cost pressures and access being universally poor in the U.S. we believe that virtual medicine can relieve pressure from primary care practices by taking on the easy things and creating space for those who really need to be seen in person. Is this disruptive? Of course. But, it's healthy disruption and pushes us to continue re-inventing and advancing primary care."

APPENDIX 2

Dr. Bill Rice, WhiteGlove Co-Founder

Dr. Bill Rice is the co-founder and previous chief medical officer of WhiteGlove Health (he founded the company with Mr. Bob Fabbio). After he left WhiteGlove, he became senior vice president of clinical innovation for St. David's Health Care in Austin, Texas.

Dr. Rice's background is in emergency medicine, but he has been involved in several start-up companies such as RevolutionHealth and Stat Healthcare. He authored a book entitled "American Healthcare 2008, Opportunities for Disruptive Improvement." As part of the research for this book, we interviewed him by phone in March of 2013.

Dr. Rice describes the initial focus of WhiteGlove as being on 'soccer moms' and convenience. The main value proposition was to see patients within two hours, provide them with a 24-hour supply of chicken soup and crackers and three days of medicine, send the rest of the medications to the preferred pharmacy, and a follow-up call the next day. Initially, the service was hard to market directly to consumers, so WhiteGlove decided to target self-insured large employers to convince them that "little Johnny's earache is costing them $700 in the emergency room." The founders insisted on staying away from Fee For Service (FFS) with insurance companies because they did not want to be part of the existing system of volume-based incentives. Instead, they offered companies a low-cost capitation model with an annual membership and a flat rate of $25 copayment per visit (increased to $35 later). As companies started to sign up, many employees called the nurse practitioner to be seen at work, which was a selling point for employers to save money and time and improve productivity. About one third of the visits were for employees at work, while the rest were for spouses and children at home.

Dr. Rice explains the technological aspects of the service: an end-to-end system was built from scratch, including web-based patient scheduling, clinical documentation, as well as a patient portal with laboratory results and medication information. The system allowed WhiteGlove to provide useful information to companies that were interested in knowing how many of their employees had a certain chronic disease such as hypertension.

Some of the most important challenges faced were regulatory in nature. For example, in Texas, which is where the service was first offered, nurse practitioners could not practice independently and needed to operate under physician supervision. However, the regulations applied only to office settings, not mobile settings. So they had lawyers involved and figured out that they could have one medical director for every three nurse practitioners seeing patients in the field. Another challenge related to the safety of the providers in the patient homes. WhiteGlove performs a real-time sex offender/background check for every patient that calls the service. Moreover, if the provider and the patient are of the opposite gender, a third person is required to be present at the time of the visit. Nurse practitioners carry mace sprays in their bags and have the option of pressing a panic button if they perceive a potentially dangerous situation. Other issues related to supplies and transportation. They needed to find out how many medications were needed in the car at any point in time, and how to transport blood samples from patient homes to laboratories.

One way WhiteGlove ensures high quality of care is by hiring good nurse practitioners with experience. Because they are on their own with no help from any physician, they need to have a deep clinical experience and need to be independent and self-assured. Moreover, diagnoses and antibiotic usage rates are consistently tracked, and periodic quality review meetings including the chief medical officer, chief nursing officer and providers take place.

The future of WhiteGlove lies in a new value proposition focusing on elderly patients in order to reduce hospital readmissions. In a pilot program with Medicare patients, readmission rates were reduced by 90% using phone calls and home visits by nurse practitioners.

Section 3
Future Developments

Chapter 9
Hospital Systems and Healthcare Reform

ABSTRACT

In this chapter, the author addresses the degree of involvement of large hospital systems in convenient care models. These systems are not known for being nimble and innovative, as many are inhibited by fixed budgets and low tolerance for risk. However, they have recently joined the trends and developed their own retail clinics, urgent care centers, and online clinics. In fact, several hospital systems now have a "convenient care strategy" to reduce demand on their overwhelmed emergency rooms and better serve their patients. These strategies also help the systems better position themselves to deal with recent regulatory provisions. Implications of the Patient Protection and Affordable Care Act (PPACA), such as value-based purchasing and bundled payments are discussed in depth. The authors propose that hospital-based convenient care models that are appropriately aligned and integrated with the new arrangements will embody excellent opportunities for hospital systems to provide easy-access entry-points for new patients, to substitute expensive traditional care settings with less costly alternatives, and to deliver high quality and expedient care that will keep patients in their network.

What is all this [healthcare reform] stuff about? It's about all the stuff we were supposed to be doing the past 10 years, but yet the market is saying get market share, get volume. — Larry Goldberg, CEO, Loyola University Health System in Maywood, Illinois (in Dunn, 2010)

INTRODUCTION

The disruptive innovations described in the previous chapters have mostly originated from outside the traditional healthcare organization circles such as hospitals and hospital systems. As discussed, retail clinics were imagined by a dissatisfied patient turned innovator, urgent

DOI: 10.4018/978-1-4666-6355-8.ch009

care centers first started with physician entrepreneurs, and online care can be credited to a young MBA student. Large hospital systems are not known for being nimble and innovative, as many are inhibited by fixed budgets and low tolerance for risk. However, as innovations start spreading, hospital systems notice them and occasionally decide to join the trend, often prompted by regulatory forces. In this chapter, we discuss the extent of involvement of hospital systems in convenient care models in the last decade or so. We also discuss the major provisions of the Patient Protection and Affordable Care Act (PPACA), and its implications on how hospital systems position themselves in terms of convenient care offerings. Table 1 summarizes our previous and current research on hospital-related retail clinics. In 2009, prior to the passage of PPACA, we conducted a first wave of eight in-depth interviews with executives in hospital systems that have a relationship with retail clinics. We have reported the results of that work in two papers (Kaissi, 2010a; Kaissi 2010b). In 2011, with PPACA just signed into law, Merchant Medicine, a consulting company that we are partnered with, conducted a survey of 20 executives from health systems operating retail clinics. The findings were reported in two recent papers (Kaissi & Charland, 2013a; Kaissi & Charland, 2013b). Lastly, early in 2013, we conducted another wave of thirteen interviews with hospital executives with convenient care relationships, as well as convenient care executives, researchers, and other experts in the field (see Key Informants section). This chapter will draw heavily on the results of these recent interviews, as well as synthesize our and others' published research in order to examine how the retail clinic strategy fits with hospital system response to PPACA.

Table 1. Summary of author's research on hospital-related retail clinics

Nature of Research	Year conducted	Publications
Qualitative: Interviews with 8 health system executives	2009	Kaissi (2010a) Kaissi (2010b)
Quantitative: Survey of 20 health system executives	2011	Kaissi & Charland (2013a) Kaissi & Charland (2013b)
Qualitative: Interviews with 13 health system executives and convenience care experts	2013	

1. HOSPITAL SYSTEM INVOLVEMENT

Urgent Care Centers

As discussed in Chapter 5, urgent care centers first appeared in the 1970's and 1980's when some physicians, partly concerned about surpluses in their profession, decided to venture into a new form of care that is delivered outside hospitals and traditional medical practices. However, it did not take long for hospitals to catch up and to start buying urgent care centers or developing their own. Unfortunately, that trend was short-lived as many hospitals treated urgent care centers like another department without a good understanding of their retail nature. As a result, most urgent care centers lost money and closed. The second boom came in the mid-1990's and continued till today, mainly driven by hospitals systems, private equity firms and some health insurance companies. The rationale for hospital systems operating urgent care centers is to generate downstream revenue and market share by increasing referrals to hospitals and their affiliated physicians. Moreover, since many emergency room visits can take place at urgent care centers, hospitals have tried to relieve their busiest emergency rooms by providing an alternative to patients without losing them to another system or urgent care operator. Some of the top hospital systems operating urgent care centers in the United States in 2013 are Aurora Urgent Care in Wisconsin, Intermountain InstaCare in Utah, Carolinas HealthCare in North Carolina (highlighted later in this chapter), CentraCare in Florida, St. John Providence in Michigan, Norton Immediate Care in Kentucky, Health Partners in Minnesota, and Advocate Health in Illinois, among others (Merchant Medicine, 2013). Currently, hospital systems own about 27% of the nation's 9,000 urgent care clinics nationwide (Gold, 2012). It is important to note that some hospital systems design their urgent care centers as "Type-B" emergency rooms, rather than as typical urgent care centers. Type-B emergency rooms are not open 24 hours a day, 7 days a week, and provide a more limited scope of practice than Type-A ones, which are regular emergency rooms that are open 24/7.

Retail Clinics

When retail clinics emerged and started to expand their footprints in supermarkets and drugstores, retailers and investor-owned companies were driving the growth, while hospital systems were watching from the sidelines. In fact, the retail clinic trend represents a classical example of a disruptive innovation that was introduced by new organizations to replace existing services offered by established organizations such as hospitals and their associated physician offices. According to disruptive innovative theory discussed in Chapter 4, incumbent organizations with sustaining innovations are driven out by new organizations with disruptive innovations and tend to disappear and cease to exist. Disruptive innovations in any industry tend to sneak in from below. These are typically introduced by newer and smaller companies that gradually improve their products and services until they finally meet the demands of the vast majority of users and drive the dominant companies out. However, retail clinics as a disruptive innovation seem to follow a slightly different path. While they were originally introduced by new organizations such as retailers and investor-owned companies, hospitals have joined the trend and got involved in the disruptive innovation five or six years after its appearance.

One of the first alarm sounds in the hospital industry came from a 2004 article entitled "Are you ready for big-box healthcare?" by industry expert and healthcare executive Preston Gee. In the article, published in Health Leaders, a widely read hospital executive publication, Gee asked: "What keeps hospital CEOs up at night? […] what might make the blood drain from a provider CEO's face is this thought: What if the mass merchandising giants like Wal-Mart, or Target got into the healthcare delivery business in a big way?"(p.1) He also warned: "What is happening all around the industry is the migration of high-margin business from traditional inpatient settings (hospitals and health systems) to more retail-oriented enterprises. This mass exodus leaves healthcare executives in a position of being in one of two camps: 'the haves or the have nots.' The 'haves' group consists of healthcare executives with a plan in place, sound strategies to execute the plan, and committed resources to compete aggressively and successfully. In essence, they are prepared to stave off the rapid evacuation of high-margin services from their facilities. The 'have nots' do little more than watch in dismay and disdain as their business exits their facility and migrates to more market-savvy competitors, all the while tied up in the paralysis of their own provincialism. So what can be done? First, healthcare executives need to focus their attention on a different competitive target. For the last five to 10 years, the focus has been on the wrong competitor. The established health system across the valley, or the large hospital across town is not the greatest threat anymore. The more menacing, would-be-market-share thief is the hungry, agile and entrepreneurially oriented new competitor that understands retail transactions and consumer desires" (p.4).

In subsequent articles, Gee reminded that "retail health clinics are a harbinger of what lies on the healthcare horizon" (2007a) and advised hospitals to "compete with retail clinics and the rise of moi-medicine, or risk drowning in the wave of change" (2007b). Similarly, in a two-series article entitled "Retail Clinics- Friend or Foe of the Hospital," industry expert Mary Kay Scott (2008a) inquired "… why are multi-billion dollar hospital systems interested in these relatively small-time operations? In short, it's because there are strategic, operational, and learning opportunities for hospitals in the retail clinic space. Forward-thinking hospital managers are looking for ways to capture the upside of retail clinics and mitigate the potential future loss of patients and earnings they represent"(p.1). In 2008, *Frontiers of Health Services Management*, one of the official journals of the American College of Healthcare Executives (the body representing more than 30,000 hospital and health system executives), dedicated a full issue to retail clinics. The articles featured health system executives, physicians and nurses that commented on their experience of starting their first hospital-based retail clinics, with recommendations and suggestions for the rest of the field (Pollert, Dobberstein, Wiisanen, 2008; Fenn, 2008; Lin, 2008; Newbold & O'Neill, 2008).

Before too long, other hospital systems seemed to have heard the message and were engaging in the retail option. For example, Aurora Healthcare System in Wisconsin opened retail clinics in order to serve its non-urgent patients far more quickly and economically than emergency rooms. AtlantiCare in New Jersey opened retail clinics mainly to create some barriers to entry and to prevent Minute Clinic from coming to their market. Sutter Health in Northern California wanted to keep patients in its network, so it "named its clinics Sutter Express, leveraging a strong brand name, differentiating itself from other clinics, emphasizing the clinics' hospital roots, and highlighting the advantage of a common EMR [Electronic Medical Record]" (Scott, 2008a). Geisinger Health System in Pennsylvania located its retail clinics 10-plus miles from its hospital locations "in an explicit effort to bring new patients from a broader area into its network"(Scott, 2008a). Similarly, Alegent Health of Omaha opened a clinic about 20 miles away from its hospital base, because "it couldn't yet justify a full service hospital in this small (but growing) bedroom community, but wanted to establish a foothold for its brand in a promising market"(Scott, 2008a).

In addition, the health systems engaging in the retail clinic model were seeking to expand their continuum of care and controlling referrals to their own physicians, emergency rooms and hospitals (Laws & Scott, 2008; Tu & Boukus, 2013). Building on their recognizable community brand, they began to compete head-to-head with the major for-profit retail clinic operators. Given that a significant number of patients were worried about staff qualifications and misdiagnoses in the retail clinic setting (Leppel, 2010), hospital systems were in an excellent position to ensure quality and patient safety (Lin, 2008). Some the most prestigious hospital systems in the country such as the Mayo Clinic, Geisinger Health System, Sutter Health and Intermountain Healthcare developed their own retail clinics, while others such as the Cleveland Clinic, HCA, Oshner and Allina Health affiliate with retail clinic operators (Fenn, 2008; Fottler & Malvey, 2010; Kaissi, 2010 (a); Lin, 2008; Newbold & O'Neil, 2008; Pollert, et al., 2008). In fact, the percentage of retail clinics that are owned by hospital systems increased from 9% in 2007 to 18% in 2010 (Laws & Scott, 2008; Tu & Boukus, 2013). In their book entitled "The Retail revolution in healthcare", Malvey and Fottler suggested that hospital systems can be classified as potential winners/losers in the retail clinic movement, depending on their ability to collaborate with, become subcontractors for and extend services of retail clinics (Fottler & Malvey, 2010). Appendix A highlights the example of Bellin Health in Green Bay Wisconsin, which owns and operates five retail clinics, and helps other health systems across the country set up their own.

The general reasons that drove retail clinic growth, as previously discussed, were overcrowding in hospital Emergency Rooms (ERs), a growing primary care physician (PCP) shortage, reduced patient access to care due to increased insurance costs, and growing consumer demands for convenience, reliability and affordability (Lin, 2008, Fottler & Malvey, 2010). Our analyses revealed an additional number of strategic drivers that were considered by hospital systems deciding to operate retail clinics (Kaissi, 2010a):

- Increasing market share through enhanced referrals to physician offices and hospitals
- Growing closer to consumers and to the community
- Experimenting with non-traditional ways of delivering healthcare
- Branding the health system
- Beating the competition to be the market leader
- Providing a "release valve" for overcrowded emergency rooms and PCP offices

Also, since retail clinics serve predominantly younger patient populations, hospitals "want to catch this young demographic now. Before they're getting married and having babies, hospitals want to recruit a new generation of brand advocates who will result in downstream revenue for years to come" (Aiello, 2013, p.2).

Our subsequent quantitative research involving 20 hospital systems that own retail clinics confirms that they were overall satisfied with the performance of the clinics in relation to these strategic priorities: 79% of the hospital executive respondents indicated that their organizations were strongly satisfied/satisfied with improved access, 69% were strongly satisfied/satisfied with increased referrals, 74% were strongly satisfied/satisfied with defense against competitors and 79% were strongly satisfied/satisfied with increased brand exposure (Kaissi & Charland, 2013a).

Hospital systems have historically acted as large bureaucratic entities that focus on traditional care provided within the four walls of the hospital or physician office. Their involvement in retail clinics represents a strategic move that has been rarely witnessed before. The two common models of operations between hospital systems and retail clinics include a partnership/affiliation between the retail chain and the hospital system, or full ownership of the retail clinic by the hospital system. Under a partnership, the retail chain owns and operates the clinics and makes decisions about the location of the clinics and the hiring of the clinicians, while the hospital system provides physician supervision, marketing and support for referrals. With ownership, the hospital system owns the clinics, decides on the location of the clinics, employs the clinicians, and pays rent to the retail chain for the space provided (Kaissi, 2010a). Burns and his colleagues concluded that hospitals have responded to retail clinics in three different ways: make (i.e. creating their own clinics), ally (i.e. partnering with retailers) or deny (ignoring retail clinics all together) (Burns, Guy & Helmchen, 2011). The Advisory Board Company (2012) defines the models in slightly different ways:

- "**Full operations model:** Under this model, used by Wal-Mart, health systems lease space for a clinic within the retail store. The clinics are typically branded as "The Clinic at Wal-Mart operated by XXX Health System." However, the retail giant is somewhat prescriptive in terms of where the health system name can and cannot appear. You probably wouldn't see a health system's signage on the exterior of a Wal-Mart, for instance.
- **Physician oversight model:** Under this model, used by Minute Clinic, the health system partners provide physicians who oversee MinuteClinic-employed nurse practitioners, a model that asks for a much smaller investment from the health system. As such, the affiliation is not marketed extensively—the health system typically features its name on a plaque within the clinic and the affiliation is highlighted on any provider referral lists that are given to patients.
- **Enhanced access practice model:** Rather than establishing retail clinic partnerships, some health systems are choosing to offer retail-like access within their existing physician practices. Access expansion strategies include offering evening and weekend appointments, walk-in availability, e-visits, and "fast-track" clinics for a specific set of low-acuity conditions. Practices may dedicate providers to these "enhanced access" options or may incorporate them into the regular care team's workflow."

One of the retail clinic operators that have been most aggressive in partnering with hospital systems is CVS' Minute Clinic. In 2012, the company had 20 partnerships with hospital systems nationwide. These partnerships included Advocate in Chicago, Allina in Minneapolis, Carolinas Health System in Charlotte, Barnabas Health in New Jersey, Catholic Healthcare West in Phoenix, Catholic Healthcare West in Las Vegas, Cleveland Clinic in Cleveland, Cleveland Clinic in South Florida, Emory Healthcare in Atlanta, Henry Ford Health in Detroit, Indiana University in Indianapolis, Inova in Northern Virginia, Ohio Health in Columbus, OH, St. Vincent's in Jacksonville, U Mass Memorial in Central Massachusetts, HCA/TriStar in Nashville, Atlantic Health in Morriston, Hackensack University Health in Hackensack, UCLA Health System in Los Angeles and Florida Hospital in Orlando (Aiello, 2013; Merchant Medicine, 2012; Rodak, 2012). Moreover, Minute Clinic has affiliation with physician practices such as UT Medicine, the academic medical practice of the School of Medicine at The University of Texas Health Science Center at San Antonio. Under this agreement, for example, UT Medicine physicians serve as medical directors for the retail clinics, and the two entities collaborate on patient education and disease management initiatives. If patients need a level of care that is not provided at Minute Clinic, they are transferred to UT Medicine clinics (Alexander, 2012).

As previously mentioned, some nationally-known and other less well-known hospital systems directly own retail clinics. The mean number of retail clinics owned by a hospital system is 3.1, and most of the systems own one (30%) or two clinics (30%). Three main management structures are typically used to run the owned clinics: management by the hospital system medical group (40%); management by the hospital system outpatient services group (35%); and management by a group within hospital system administration (25%). The retail venues chosen consist mainly of "big box retailers" such as Walmart, Shopko or Meijer (70%), with other venues including standalone drugstores (15%), grocery stores such as Albertson's or Cub Foods (10%) or drug store chains (5%) (Kaissi & Charland, 2013b).

Early adopters of retail clinics among hospital systems entered into this strategy with the assumption that it is a straight-forward business model that will generate significant revenues and lucrative down-stream referrals at a relatively low cost. However, they soon realized that many significant operational, financial and promotional resisters exist. Our 2009 research suggested that physician resistance and skepticism topped the list of challenges (Kaissi, 2010a). As discussed in chapter 5, several physician groups have raised serious concerns about retail clinics (Paddock, 2007). These concerns relate to the potential for fragmentation of care, especially for patients with special healthcare needs and chronic conditions, and to the possibility of compromised quality and patient safety, particularly when patients present with serious conditions that may be beyond the scope of practice of nurse practitioners and physician assistants. Not surprisingly, physicians felt threatened by the competition presented by retail clinics, as these tend to attract their easy-to-treat patients and leave them with the most complex patients. To alleviate physicians' fears, some hospital systems spent considerable time and energy educating them about the retail clinic model and convincing them that it does not compete with their core business. Some of the systems that we interviewed in 2008 approached the local physician association while others held long meetings with the primary care physicians to share the operating model with them. Once the physicians were on board, hospital executives involved them in the care provided in the clinics by sending them their patients' medical charts electronically or by fax after the retail clinic visit. Other forms of involvement included hiring physicians as medical directors providing oversight to the clinics. These physicians appreciated the potential to increase their revenue, without having to actually deliver any clinical services. Physicians typically earn $100/hour to provide supervision for retail clinics (Kaissi, 2010a).

Moreover, many of the retail clinics were facing serious financial struggles which led to clinic closures in some markets. One medical director of a clinic explained: "The margin of profitability is very narrow, if you are seeing 25-30 patients per day then you need to hire a second clinician, which is very expensive. No one is going to make a lot of money from this business" (Kaissi, 2010a). A related concern has to do with marketing and the difficulty to change public perceptions. While the number of retail clinics had grown exponentially by 2009, many people still did not understand what these clinics do and what services they offer, while others were very skeptical about their quality of care (Leppel, 2010). In addition, staffing, recruitment and retention of mid-level providers proved problematic for some systems. The non-challenging and limited nature of the services provided made it hard to keep the providers motivated and engaged. In order to deal with this issue, some systems had their nurse practitioners work one or two days per week at a family clinic in order to keep them challenged and satisfied (Pollert, et al., 2008).

Subsequent research conducted in 2011 showed that many of these issues were still relevant among hospital system owners of retail clinics (Kaissi & Charland, 2013a). Executives from these systems indicated moderate to low levels of satisfaction with physician support and backing (47%). Moreover, 63% indicated they were dissatisfied/strongly dissatisfied with profitability of the clinics, 53% were dissatisfied/strongly dissatisfied with patient volumes and 42% were dissatisfied/strongly dissatisfied with response to marketing initiatives. Additional analyses revealed that only 5 out of 20 hospital systems had their retail clinics operating at financial breakeven (Kaissi & Charland, 2013b).

More recent interviews offer mixed results. An executive at a retail clinic chain with relationships with hospital systems offered this explanation: "Historically the challenges were external: how to make consumers aware of the model, how to get retailer to want to have clinics and to give us good space, how to contract with payers, and resistance from some in the medical community. They had to deal with many external hurdles. Today, many of these obstacles haven been diminished or are being eliminated. Consumers are accepting of the concept, payers have been contracting with retail clinics, and retailers want the clinics. And physician resistance has dissipated. The basic value proposition of quality, convenience and affordability is very attractive to consumers and payers. But the business model is still challenging. You have to process a lot of patients at a relatively low margin. So how do you turn it into a sustainable business? We are providing value; there is no question about that. But the question is how to create a sustainable, efficient model? So while the challenges in the past were external, todays' challenges are more internal in nature. We have invented a new business, and even though we have served about one million patients, we are still inventing the business every day" (Web Golinkin, personal interview, 2013).

In addition, staffing remains an important issue. As competition for nurse practitioners and physician assistants continue to intensify, their salaries continue to climb. One executive of a health system that owns clinics summarized: "The major challenge is finding an adequate number of mid-level providers. There is a lag in supply, and an increase in the number of clinics hiring them. Also, the challenge is also to keep them, as many of them want broader scope of practice and are trained to do so much more." Tracking downstream referrals and revenues also continue to worry hospital system executives. An executive in a hospital system partnering with retail clinics recently warned: "One area that we haven't managed well with retail clinics is hardwiring of downstream referrals. We have provided them with our physician referral line, but what we need is to go ahead and schedule the appointment with our physician while the patient is still at the clinic, and track that patient down, call them a day before the visit, and if they don't show up to the visit and call them to follow-up and reschedule. We need better capturing of downstream business to quantify the benefits and return on investment. Just co-branding is not sustainable" (Mark Clayton, personal interview, 2013). This represents a serious issue for many cost-conscious health executives who continuously have to justify the investment in retail clinics by showing potential increased referrals and profits.

Online Services

As discussed in Chapter 8, online services first appeared when business entrepreneurs created Zipnosis and other companies offering e-visits and asynchronous care. Surprisingly, hospital systems joined the trend much faster than they did with other innovations such as retail clinics. For example, in 2010, Park Nicollet engaged with Zipnosis for a one year-trial period (Newmarker, 2008; Lee, 2010), while Health Partners created its own product in the form of Virtuwell (Cornera, Palattao & Gallagher, 2013). Around the same time, some of the primary care practices that are part of the Mayo Clinic started offering e-visits (Adamson & Bachman, 2010; Rohrer, Angstman, Adamson, et al., 2010). Pioneer hospital systems were probably less hesitant to embrace these models vs. other models partly because online care could be designed around physicians, and not just non-physician providers.

2. PROVISIONS OF THE PPACA

The Patient Protection and Affordable Care Act (PPACA), signed by president Barrack Obama on March 23rd, 2010, is the most significant piece of legislation in the history of American healthcare. Never before has a healthcare-related policy been so fiercely debated, widely beloved, and vehemently opposed. The provisions of the act aim to expand coverage, control healthcare costs, and improve the healthcare delivery system, and therefore have many substantial implications on the way hospital systems provide healthcare services and the way they get paid for those services.

As explained in Chapter 1, the American healthcare system is plagued with problems related to the cost, access and quality of care. When compared to other developed countries, it is significantly more expensive. The percentage of the Gross Domestic Product (GDP) spent on healthcare services is 17.9, and the average cost per person per year is at $8,608 (World Bank, 2013). While most other rich nations provide 100% coverage to their citizens, the American healthcare system leaves about 50.2 million without insurance (the "uninsured"), and an additional 25 million with inadequate insurance (the "underinsured") (Kaiser Family Foundation, 2013). Numerous studies comparing countries on quality outcomes have documented the serious issues in the American system, especially when it comes to life expectancy at birth and various preventative services. To address some of these issues, the Patient Protection and Affordable Care (PPACA, also known as Healthcare Reform or Obama-Care in the United States) was passed in 2010. Of the hundreds of the provisions contained in the act, many will directly or indirectly affect hospital systems.

The major aspect of the act includes a variety of provisions that aim to address the coverage gap. These include the "individual mandate," the "employer mandate," Medicaid expansion, health insurance exchanges, and coverage of young adults. The "individual mandate" requires all citizens and legal residents to have qualifying health coverage or pay a tax penalty of the greater of $695 per year up to a maximum of three times that amount ($2,085) per family or 2.5% of household income (Patient Protection and Affordable Care Act, 2013). Beginning in January 2014, all individuals who are not exempt must maintain "minimum essential coverage" for themselves and their dependents which is defined as any exchange plan (explained later), any employer plan, Medicare, Medicaid, or other government-sponsored plan. Exemptions apply for individuals who are uninsured for less than three months of the year; who have very low income, making coverage unaffordable; who are not required to file a tax return because their income is so low; who would qualify for Medicaid but their state has chosen to not expand it (explained later); who are a member of a federally-recognized Indian tribe; who participate in a healthcare sharing ministry; who are members of a recognized religious sect with religious objections to health insurance; who are incarcerated; and who are not lawfully present in the United States (Centers for Medicare and Medicaid, 2013b, PPACA, 2013). The rationale for the individual mandate is explained by the federal government: "When an uninsured person requires urgent-often expensive-medical care but doesn't pay the bill, everyone else ends up paying the price in the form of higher insurance premiums. That's why the healthcare law requires all people who can afford it to take responsibility for their own health insurance by getting coverage or paying a penalty. In the absence of the requirement, some individuals would make an economic and financial decision to forego health insurance coverage and attempt to self-insure, which increases financial risks to households and medical providers." By requiring everyone to buy health insurance coverage, the act prevents individuals from taking advantage of the system by only signing up for insurance when they are sick (PPACA, 2013). The individual mandate was ruled as constitutional by the Supreme Court of the United States in June of 2012.

The "employer mandate" requires employers with 50 or more full-time employees to offer coverage for their employees or pay a penalty (PPACA, 2013). There are two types of penalties: a heavy penalty and a light penalty. Employers that do not provide health coverage and end-up having employees enroll in a marketplace insurance exchange must pay a heavy penalty, while employers that provide coverage that is not considered "affordable" and end-up having employees enroll in an exchange must pay the light penalty. These penalties are not tax-deductible:

- **Heavy Penalty:** The employer must pay a $2,000 penalty for each full-time-equivalent (FTE) employee over 30 whether or not they enroll in the exchanges. For example, a firm with 80 full-time-equivalent employees would pay $100,000.
- **Light Penalty:** The employer must pay a $3,000 penalty only for employees who actually enroll in the exchanges. For example, if only six employees opt out of the employer-offered insurance and enroll in the exchanges instead, a firm with 80 full-time-equivalent employees would pay $18,000.

The Department of Labor (2012) explains that the employer mandate is intended to "expand access to affordable health coverage," while the Small Business Administration

(2013) comments that it will offset part of the cost of the Marketplace premium tax credits.

In addition, the act calls for all states to expand Medicaid, the public program for the poor, in order to reduce the number of uninsured Americans by providing access to affordable coverage for people that qualify based on income levels. Before PPACA, Medicaid covered pregnant women and children under age six with family incomes at or below 133% of the federal poverty level (FPL), children under 18 with family incomes at or below 100% of the FPL, certain low-income parents or caretaker relatives, and low-income elderly people with disabilities. The expansion applies to all individuals under age 65 (children, pregnant women, parents, and adults without dependent children) with incomes up to 133% of the FPL ($15,856 for an individual or $26,951 for a family of three in 2013). Since Medicaid is a state-based program, the federal government will fund 100% of states' cost increases related to expansion between 2014 and 2016. This funding will gradually drop, eventually reaching 90% by 2020. Originally, PPACA intended to punish states that did not expand Medicaid coverage by withholding their federal Medicaid dollars. However, the Supreme Court of the United States ruled in 2012 that this provision was overly coercive for the states, and therefore made Medicaid expansion optional for each state. By the end of 2013, 28 states and the District of Columbia had opted to expand Medicaid and 23 had declined (Kaiser Family Foundation, 2013a).

The American Health Benefit Exchanges and Small Business Health Options Program (SHOP) Exchanges will allow individuals and small businesses with up to 100 employees to purchase health insurance coverage in a newly created healthcare marketplace, in which prices and benefits are easily explained and compared. The purpose of this provision is to lower the cost and increase the quality of health insurance through competition and transparency while making insurance plans easily accessible to consumers. According to the Department of Health and Human Services (HHS, 2013) "the insurance exchange will pool buying power and give Americans new affordable choices of private insurance plans that have to compete for their business based on cost and quality." Plans will be sold side-by-side in an online exchange, which will enhance competition as standardized comparison mechanisms will allow consumers to easily compare characteristics and coverage-levels. Exchanges are intended to be similar to airline and hotel bookings' websites such as Travelocity or Expedia. They will include resources to help users such as a subsidy calculator, a toll-free telephone hotline, and "navigators" to help use resources and make decisions about plans. In terms of regulatory requirements, exchange plans will be categorized by actuarial value into Platinum, Gold, Silver, or Bronze ranking and will delineate standard benefits, allowing for easy cross-plan and cross-category comparison. Platinum plans must cover at least 90% of the actuarial value of care, Gold plans 80%, Silver plans 70% and Bronze plans 60%. The exchanges have been made available first to individuals and small businesses starting October of 2013, while medium-sized businesses will be given access by 2015, and all businesses will have access by 2017. They can be implemented by states, the federal government, or by state-federal partnerships. Under state-run exchanges, the individual states control marketing, insurer participation in the exchange, exchange fees, and regulations, but all state exchanges must be approved by the federal government. As of May 2013, 27 states had opted for federally-facilitated exchanges, 16 states and the District of Columbia had opted for state-based exchanges, and 7 states had established partnerships with the federal government to run their exchanges (Kaiser Family Foundation, 2013b).

The last provision of PPACA relating to insurance coverage states that young adults under age 26 will be allowed to receive coverage under their parents' existing health insurance plan (PPACA, 2013). Young adults have the right to stay in a parent's plan or to get back into that plan if the following conditions are met: the parent has coverage through an employer or buys family coverage in the individual market; the parent's health plan provides "dependent coverage"; and the young adult cannot have a job that offers coverage, unless the parent's plan is either a plan purchased in the individual market or a plan that did not exist before March 23, 2010 (Families USA, 2011).

As a result of these various provisions, it is expected than an additional 32 million Americans will have insurance coverage by the year 2019, and that the number of underinsured could decrease by 70% (Schoen et al., 2011). This will have major implications on all providers of healthcare services, especially hospital systems and their physicians. As individuals find themselves with coverage or with more adequate coverage, demand for primary care, emergency and specialty services will exponentially increase. However, the supply of physicians in general, and of primary care physicians (PCPs) in particular, is not likely to meet those expected demands, as discussed in Chapter 2. It is well documented that a shortage of about 46,000 PCPs will be observed by the year 2025 (Bodenheimer & Pham, 2010). In addition to PPACA, several other factors have contributed to this expected shortage on the supply and demand side. On the supply side, a stagnant number of American-trained physicians, an increase in female physicians, an aging of the physician workforce and significant income gaps between primary care and other specialties have resulted in insufficient numbers of PCPs and of PCP hours worked. On the demand side, an aging population and an increase in obesity and chronic diseases have created unprecedented needs for physician services. PPACA includes some provisions that address impending PCP shortages such as increased scholarships loan repayment programs for medical students choosing primary care, as well slight increases in reimbursement rates for PCPs. However, most experts agree that these provisions are modest at best, and do not even come close to closing the primary care workforce gap (Iglehart, 2010; Porter, 2012; Perman, 2012).

In addition to the general provisions discussed above, PPACA includes some sections relating directly to hospitals and other providers. To help reduce costs and improve quality of care, two new payment systems will be implemented: value-based purchasing and bundled payments. These systems will aim to tie public (and private) reimbursement to performance, a clear contrast to previous fee-for-service systems that paid hospitals for the quantity of services delivered. Under value-based purchasing, hospitals will be reimbursed for reporting and meeting specific standards related to efficiency, patient satisfaction, and clinical quality metrics (Centers for Medicare and Medicaid, 2013). Under bundled payments, providers will receive a single reimbursement for an episode of care, beginning three days before admission to the hospital and ending thirty days after the patient is discharged. Hospitals and physicians, who previously received separate payments for each service and procedure, will now share one "capitated" payment, regardless of patient utilization (Centers for Medicare and Medicaid, 2013). Therefore, greater accountability and financial risk will be required by providers, who will see their role shifting from treating individual patients in hospitals or physician offices to managing "population health" through integrated programs that allow the system to oversee, and be financially responsible for, a patient's entire continuum of care. As a result, several hospital systems have engaged in new organizational structures referred to as Patient-Centered Medical Homes (PCMHs) and Accountable Care Organizations (ACOs) (American Hospital Association, 2010). In a PCMH model, physicians and other caregivers that are part of one healthcare team are financially rewarded for improving outcomes and reducing costs through well-coordinated care activities. The central tenets of a PCMH as defined by various physician professional associations include:

- "Ongoing partnership between the primary care physician and patient that encourages patient engagement and emphasizes the patient's shared responsibility for care.
- Physician-directed medical practice in which the provider leads the healthcare team in coordinating proactive and holistic care centered around patient needs.
- Whole-person orientation of care in which the provider communicates with all referral sources throughout the patient's life cycle.
- Coordination of care in which the provider embraces all elements of the complex healthcare system and uses information technology, health information exchange, and patient registries.
- Quality and safety focus that includes continuous quality improvement, adherence to evidence-based guidelines, and active performance reporting driving behavior change
- Enhanced access to care to anticipate open scheduling, expanded hours, and communication among the care team.
- Restructured payment system that recognizes provider performance and added value by rewarding providers for performance and for systematizing the necessary coordination and communication activities, such as enhanced patient communication and remote patient monitoring" (McDaniel & Dishman, 2012, p.3).

An ACO is a network of hospitals and physicians that share responsibility for providing coordinated care to patients in order to reduce unnecessary spending and enhance quality of care. The PPACA requirements for an ACO is that it is willing to become accountable for the quality, cost, and overall care of at least 5,000 Medicare fee-for-service beneficiaries assigned to it for at least three years; it defines processes to promote evidence-based medicine and patient engagement and report on quality and cost measures; and that it uses an alternative payment mechanism, including bundled payment or shared savings, to encourage financial and clinical accountability (PPACA, 2013). In 2013, there were 488 ACOs operating under different models.

In summary, PPACA creates unique challenges for American hospital systems: an unprecedented increase in demand for primary care and specialty services without a real increase in PCP supply, and a new reimbursement system that will reward efficiency and performance, penalize waste and incentivize access, care coordination and population health.

3. HOSPITAL SYSTEMS' RESPONSE TO PPACA

Prior to the passage of PPACA, many hospital systems struggled to provide care for an increasingly large population of uninsured and underinsured patients that could not afford to pay for their care. At the same time, the public and private reimbursement systems favored these hospitals by paying them for the quantity of services they provided (fee-for-service) without any real concern for quality of care. This situation created interesting strategic and operational dynamics in which many hospital systems used revenue from payments by privately and publicly insured patients to subsidize some of the uncompensated care that they provided for patients without insurance. In addition, the shortage of primary care physicians and the lack of care alternatives created a real access problem for millions of patients as they faced overwhelmed physician offices and overcrowded emergency rooms. With the passage of PPACA, many of these dynamics are starting to shift, and while some problems are being resolved, others are left untouched, and new difficulties are starting to surface. To deal with the new healthcare landscape, hospital systems have been busy at work designing new strategies and changing their day-to-day organizational practices.

PPACA will require hospitals to take on substantial financial risks for population health management, with specific implications such as increasing access, focusing on primary care and post-acute providers and others along the continuum of care; dedicating resources and expertise to reduce cost and increase value, better coordinating services and reducing readmissions; investing in health information systems and robust analytics programs to track large amounts of data on care quality and costs and assess risk and price services (Dunn, 2011). Interestingly, hospital systems were already starting to think about the implications of the impending reforms before it passed. For example, one respondent from our 2009 interviews noted that "reform will have a positive effect. There are incentives to provide greater access. Retail clinics are part of the reimbursement formula. There is a push for more use of non-traditional providers. New evidence shows that retail clinics provide better value for the dollar, and reform will focus on value"(Kaissi, 2010b).

Experts suggest that while the partnership model represents the least amount of risk for the hospital system, the ownership model has the greatest potential for achieving integration goals and better positioning the organization for PPACA. A health system executive with an affiliation with a retail clinic chain clarifies this issue: "Affiliations with co-branding are not viable or sustainable, because the exit clause is just 90-days. So a safer place for them to be overtime is with a health system that is growing its convenience care strategy. To be honest, we currently see that retail clinic players do not provide significant quantifiable benefit to the health system. Yes, there is brand awareness, which is good, they are so good at managing their scope of care with mid-level providers and physician supervision, but there are very few referrals, and not much benefit for [our system]. We would like to maintain the relationship with co-branding, it doesn't help us much but it doesn't hurt us. So status quo is OK, but not an increased cost. Since in the future, under population health, low-cost and efficient access points will make a lot of sense. It will be cheaper for us to provide the care than in primary care offices. But we need the clinics to be part of our network, our system. If the joint venture is going to cost us much, and if [retail clinic operator] decides to work with our competitor instead, we will probably give up the relationship."

Pollack, Gidengil and Mehrotra (2010) examined the relationship between retail clinics and Patient-Centered Medical Homes (PCMHs), a crucial "mechanism to better co-ordinate care, improve quality, decrease costs, and revitalize primary care" under healthcare reform (Pollack, Gidengil and Mehrotra (2010: 998). Briefly, the PCMH concept emphasizes improved access though open scheduling and enhanced hours, is staffed by a team of providers led by a personal physician; and focuses on coordination of the patient's care among providers using electronic health records and other decision-support systems. They concluded that the greatest potential exists under an "integrated model" where retail clinics are owned and operated by existing healthcare providers. They described the case of the Heritage Valley Health System in Pennsylvania which operates three retail clinics in nearby Wal-Mart stores: "The nurse practitioners who staff the retail clinics are employees of Heritage Valley. Each retail clinic is linked to a primary care practice and the larger health system through a shared electronic health record, which gives the retail clinic provider access to the patient's medical history. The nurse practitioners at the retail clinic collaborate with physicians in the linked practice, and their notes are cosigned by physicians in the practice. Nurse practitioners may work at both the retail clinics and the linked primary care practices. Lastly, visits to the retail clinic accrue to the larger physician group, which mitigates any negative impact of retail clinics on aggregate primary care physician revenue." (Pollack, et al.,2010). They concluded that when hospital systems run medical homes and own the retail clinics, the clinics represent a natural extension to the medical home. For example, the PCMH will rely on the retail clinics to attend to simpler conditions as well as to extend hours and convenience. Moreover, retail clinic visits can be used to encourage patients to receive chronic care management or preventive services.

Under the "hybrid model" where hospital systems and their practices affiliate with the retail chain, some potential for collaboration between the retail clinic and the medical home exist, although several barriers are also in place. If the health system and the retail clinic share the same electronic medical record, the nurse practitioner or physician assistant treating the patient would have access to the patient's history, including medications and allergies, whereas the physician in the medical home could review the patient's retail clinic records. However, retail clinic use under this model may represent lost opportunities for patients to strengthen their relationship with the medical home, and the medical home may lose revenue from acute care visits at retail clinics (Pollack, et al., 2010).

In summary, "the appeal of retail clinics for many hospitals is their ability to provide patients increased access to high-quality, low-cost care -the top goals under healthcare reform" (Rodak, 2012). There are six ways hospitals can align a retail health strategy with PPACA goals:

1. Increase access to care: By partnering with retail clinics, hospitals can increase patients' access to healthcare services

and hospitals' access to patients. A retail clinic strategy allows hospitals to extend the hospital's reach to its entire region, thus allowing it to manager its patients' health more effectively, which is a key goal under PPACA

2. Coordinate care: Retail clinics can help systems care for patients throughout the continuum of care, which allows the system to build an integrated network of hospitals, providers, ambulatory surgery centers and retail clinics. If hospital systems manage to connect their electronic health record systems to the retail clinics', they can transfer patients' medical information between different sites of care, such as between retail clinics and primary care physicians, and therefore improve coordination of care.
3. Connect patients to primary and preventive care. By connecting patients to primary care and preventive care through retail clinics, hospital systems can help improve population health, which is one of the aims of PPACA. For example, Dr. David T. Feinberg, CEO of UCLA Hospital System which is affiliated with Minute Clinics argues: "I don't think of it as retail, I think of it as pre-primary care. From a health reform standpoint, [retail clinics] allow a lot of people with insurance and new people who will get insurance to access care and ultimately get into care appropriately so they have an ongoing relationship with a primary care provider." (Rodak, 2012). This is especially true that many patients who visit retail clinics do not have a primary care physician relationship (as discussed in Chapter 6).
4. Increase convenience. By providing a convenient service to patients, hospital systems affiliating with retail clinics can encourage patients to engage in their health- a critical part of meeting the PPACA goal of improved population health.
5. Become patient-centered. By having retail clinics, hospital systems can switch from being provider-centric, to being patient-centric, a key change for competing and surviving under PPACA.
6. Improve quality. By lending their names and proving physicians to act as retail clinic directors, hospital systems can ensure quality of care provided in these clinics is of the highest standard. This is especially important as hospitals are getting paid on performance and quality.

Similarly, hospital systems seem to be interested in opening urgent care centers for the same reasons. As previously discussed, the short-term goals for most hospitals are to recruit patients into the system, boost referrals, generate downstream revenue through follow-up care, keep patients out of the emergency room and boost patient satisfaction. However, longer-term goals that are more aligned with PPACA provisions are also seriously considered. As health insurance plan will start paying providers to keep patients healthy and out of the hospital, urgent care centers will increasingly a crucial role as an inexpensive and convenient alternative to hospital emergency rooms. Bob Gilbert, president of MedStar ambulatory services suggests that urgent care clinics hold a promise to be "vehicles for managing the health of populations" (Gold, 2012). However, other experts were more cautious. Tom Charland, walk-in industry consultant advises: "We're still in the very early stages of this trend. I think we're going to see a lot more hospitals opening urgent care centers, either their first one or you're going to find hospitals who might have one or two opening more. [...] Things like understanding how to locate an urgent care clinic in the right retail complex, keeping the wait times down, offering people to book their appointments online- hospitals have yet to prove that they can do that effectively"(Gold, 2012).

It is important to note that, in their attempts to strategically prepare for PPACA's impact, many hospitals have engaged in several convenient care strategies at the same time, rather than focusing on just retail clinics or urgent care centers. For example, Presbyterian Health System in New Mexico restructured its organization and created a "Convenient Care Division" in 2012. The system owned and operated seven urgent care centers, but was considering the addition of retail clinics, worksite clinics, telehealth services, mobile vans and house call services. Lauren Cates, Senior Vice President of Market Development and Operational Planning, heads the new division. She explains the organizational strategy: "[PPACA] has positioned convenience care very well as a concept in an organization, especially for integrated care and bundled payments. You need to have a breadth of services to meet patients when and where they need them. Patients want flexibility, so you have to create access points on the patients' terms" (Personal Interview, 2013). The Carolinas Healthcare System in North Carolina operates twenty urgent care centers, has an affiliation with twenty Minute Clinics, and provides worksite occupational health and wellness services. Stephen Jones, Vice President of the Carolinas HealthCare System Medical Group who operates their urgent care centers and employer worksite services proposes: "With healthcare reform, access is becoming key, making sure patients are getting the right care, at the right place, at the right cost, especially as part of a larger health system focused on population health. Patients need alternatives from going to higher cost ED's for low acuity care. By creating move convenient lower cost alternatives the result is savings to the patient and the overall system. In North Carolina, we will see an increase with the Affordable Care Act as more patients have access to insurance looking for quality care. This is another reason why there is continued increase of convenient and accessible models. The access to these clinics should be within 5-10 minute drive to anyone who lives in the area" (Personal Interview, 2013).St Davids' Health in Austin was affiliated with RediClinic to co-brand six retail clinics in H-E-B stores, has joint-venture relationships with urgent care centers, operates free-standing emergency rooms and is considering the addition of other services such as WhiteGlove Health. Mark Clayton, Senior Vice President of Business Development, expounds: "It's all about access points, and no one strategy can address that. There are a variety of settings/structures, and alignment. There is a need for a network of access points that meet three goals: provide a stream of business into the health system, manage care effectively (right care at the right time in the right place) and position the system for clinical integration and managing population health. [Convenient care] services will make sense under the Affordable Care Act. We will have to reposition our health system to offer low cost alternatives that are clinically integrated. But regardless, many people don't want a primary care physician even if they have a great health pan. We should provide to them episodic, convenient, low cost access points. For example, they are healthy, they get their annual screening through their employers. If they have minor conditions, they go to convenient care access points, and then if they have any symptoms they can get a referral from the urgent care center to the specialists" (Mark Clayton, personal interview, 2013).

Other health systems are combining convenient care strategies to better organize for PPACA provisions. The University of Pittsburgh Medical Center (UPMC) operates nine urgent care centers. It also provides worksite services such as wellness, health coaching, employee assistance, FMLA (Family Medical Leave Act) administration, disability administration and consulting for about 55,000 employees. In 2011, UPMC introduced a new program, called MyHealth@Work, which provides healthcare services for smaller employers that cannot support an on-site clinic. Under the new program, employees are able to engage with a provider off-site using a telehealth system that is setup on site. Providers emphasize health, wellness and preventative care. As a result, UPMC Health Plan members have increased their compliance in 12 of 18 preventive and condition management area, which will be crucial under PPACA (Merchant Medicine, 2013). Similarly, Franciscan Health System in Tacoma, Washington contracted with Carena Inc., to provide phone and video calls for their employees and patients after-hours. Franciscan's strategy was mainly prompted by the aggressive Pacific Northwest's healthcare environment which is rapidly moving to accountable care organizations (ACOs) and other global-payment models. The health system sought tools for population health management that can keep costs down. Cliff Robertson, M.D., Franciscan's chief operating officer, elucidated: "We really looked at it as a way to expand capacity for our primary care network. More importantly, we saw it as a tool that was vital as we transition from a fee-for-service reimbursement model into a risk-based model. [We looked] at this virtual primary care as a tool that we would absolutely need if we were to manage a population of patients in a more cost-effective, lower-cost setting" (Fluckinger, 2013).

In summary, the provisions of the PPACA have created unprecedented incentives for healthcare providers such as hospital systems and physicians. In the old world of fee-for-service payments, hospital systems and physicians operated in silos. Hospitals worried that urgent care centers, retail clinics, worksite clinics and online services might cannibalize its high-profit emergency room visits, whereas physicians separately worried that these same services might snip patients away from their practices. In the new world of global payments and accountable care organizations (ACOs), hospitals, physicians and other providers will have to work hand-in-hand to manage the health of their populations, reduce costs and improve quality. Convenient care models that are appropriately aligned and integrated with the new arrangements will embody excellent opportunities to provide easy-access entry-points for new patients, to substitute expensive traditional care settings with less costly alternatives, and to deliver high-quality and expedient care that will keep patients in the network.

4. CONCLUSION

After apparently missing out on the early stages of the convenient care trend, hospital systems appear well positioned to capitalize on it as they navigate the challenges created by PPACA. In fact, while many hospitals are still trying to understand the economic and business realities of the new model, they may have numerous cost-saving advantages over independent operators, since "they can leverage their existing infrastructure (technology, protocols, and electronic records), assets, physician referral networks, brands, and insurance carrier relationships" (Scott, 2008b, p.3). Given the recency of the policy change (PPACA) and its gradual implementation in the last three years and expected continued implementation over the next five years, much remains to be seen about how hospital systems will continue to address the trend.

REFERENCES

Adamson, S. C., & Bachman, J. W. (2010). Pilot study of providing online care in a primary care setting. *Mayo Clinic Proceedings*, *85*(8), 704–710. doi:10.4065/mcp.2010.0145 PMID:20516427

Aiello, M. (2013). *Hospitals, Don't Fear Retail Health Clinics. Join Them.* HealthLeaders Media.

Alexander, A. (2012). MinuteClinic, UT Medicine San Antonio form clinical affiliation. *Drug Store News*. Retrieved from http://www.drugstorenews.com/article/minuteclinic-ut-medicine-san-antonio-form-clinical-affiliation

Bodenheimer, T., & Pham, H. H. (2010). Primary care: Current problems and proposed solutions. *Health Affairs*, *29*(5), 799–805. doi:10.1377/hlthaff.2010.0026 PMID:20439864

Burns, L. R., David, G., & Helmchen, L. A. (2011). Strategic Response by Providers to Specialty Hospitals, Ambulatory Surgery Centers, and Retail Clinics. *Population Health Management*, *14*(2), 69–77. doi:10.1089/pop.2010.0021 PMID:21091376

Centers for Medicare and Medicaid. 2013. Retrieved from http://www.cms.gov/Medicare/Quality-Initiatives-Patient-Assessment-Instruments/hospital-value-based-purchasing/index.html?redirect=/Hospital-Value-Based-Purchasing/

Centers for Medicare and Medicaid Services. (2013b). *HHS Final Rule and Treasury Notices on Individual Shared Responsibility Provision Exemptions, Minimum Essential Coverage, and Related Topics*. Retrieved from http://www.cms.gov/Newsroom/MediaReleaseDatabase/Fact-Sheets/2013-Fact-Sheets-Items/2013-06-26.html?DLPage=1&DLSort=0&DLSortDir=descending%20and%20a%20guidance%20

Courneya, P. T., Palattao, K. J., & Gallagher, J. M. (2013). HealthPartners' Online Clinic For Simple Conditions Delivers Savings Of $88 Per Episode And High Patient Approval. *Health Affairs*, *32*(2), 385–392. doi:10.1377/hlthaff.2012.1157 PMID:23381532

Dunn, L. (2010). Quotes on Healthcare in the Midst of Reform. *Top (Madrid)*, *10*.

Dunn, L. (2011). From Treating the Sick to Managing Community Health: Hospitals' New Role in Managing Population Health. *Becker's Hospital Review*. Retrieved from http://www.beckershospitalreview.com/hospital-management-administration/from-treating-the-sick-to-managing-community-health-hospitals-new-role-in-managing-population-health.html

Families U. S. A. (2011). *Understanding the New Health Reform Law: Fact Sheet*. Retrieved from http://www.familiesusa.org/assets/pdfs/health-reform/coverage-for-young-adults.pdf

Feder, J. L. (2011). Charting A Life-and-Health Cycle And Expanded Primary Care Options For Patients In Wisconsin. *Health Affairs*, *30*(3), 387–389. doi:10.1377/hlthaff.2011.0062 PMID:21383347

Fenn, S. (2008). Integrating Retail clinics into the Hospital System. *Frontiers of Health Services Management*, *24*(3), 33–36. PMID:18435359

Fluckinger, D. (2013). Health Systems involvement in online care Telemedicine clinics: Could they cannibalize primary care practices? *Search Health IT*. Retrieved from http://searchhealthit.techtarget.com/feature/Telemedicine-clinics-Could-they-cannibalize-primary-care-practices

Fottler, M., & Malvey, D. (2010). *The Retail Revolution in Healthcare*. Santa Barbara, CA: Praeger.

Gee, P. (2004). *Are You Ready for 'Big Box' Healthcare?* HealthLeaders Extra.

Gee, P. (2007a). Compete with retail clinics and the rise of moi-medicine, or risk drowning in the wave of change. *Healthcare strategic management, 25*(2), 4-5, 16.

Gee, P. (2007b). Retail Clinics' Influence on Healthcare. *HealthLeaders Media Corner Office,* 29.

Gold, J. (2012). Hospitals Gamble On Urgent Care Clinics To Keep Patients Healthy. *Kaiser Health News*. Retrieved from http://www.kaiserhealthnews.org/Stories/2012/November/08/urgent-care-clinics.aspx

Healthcare.gov. (2013). *What if someone doesn't have health coverage in 2014?* Retrieved from https://www.healthcare.gov/what-if-someonedoesnt-have-health-coverage-in-2014/

Iglehart, J. K. (2010). Health reform, primary care, and graduate medical education. *The New England Journal of Medicine*, *363*(6), 584–590. doi:10.1056/NEJMhpr1006115 PMID:20660398

Kaiser Family Foundation. (2013). Retrieved from http://kff.org/uninsured/

Kaiser Family Foundation. (2013a). *Status of State Action on the Medicaid Expansion Decision*. Retrieved from http://kff.org/health-reform/slide/current-status-of-the-medicaid-expansion-decision/

Kaiser Family Foundation. (2013b). *State decisions for creating health insurance exchanges*. Retrieved from http://kff.org/health-reform/slide/state-decisions-for-creating-health-insurance-exchanges/

Kaissi, A. (2010a). Hospital- Affiliated and Hospital-Owned Retail Clinics: Strategic Considerations and Operational Challenges. *Journal of Healthcare Management*, *55*(5), 324–337. PMID:21077582

Kaissi, A. (2010b). The Future of Retail Clinics. *The Health Care Manager*, *29*(3), 223–229. doi:10.1097/HCM.0b013e3181e93149 PMID:20686393

Kaissi, A., & Charland, T. (2013a). How Satisfied are Hospital Systems with their Ownership of Retail Clinics? *Journal of Healthcare Management*, *58*(2), 143–153. PMID:23650698

Kaissi, A., & Charland, T. (2013b). Hospital-Owned Retail Clinics in the United States: Operations, Patients and Marketing. *Primary Healthcare*, *3*(1), 1–5.

Laws, M., Scott, M.K. (2008). The Emergence Of Retail-Based Clinics In The United States: Early Observations. *Health Affairs*, *27* (95), 1293-1298.

Lee, W. (2010, May 19). Online medicine in a hurry. *Minnesota Star Tribune*.

Lin, D. Q. (2008). Convenient Care Clinics: Opposition, Opportunity, and the Path to System Integration. *Frontiers of Health Services Management, 24*(3), 3–11. PMID:18435355

McDaniel, R. D., & Dishman, E. (2012). *Patient-Centered Medical Home. A Foundation for Delivering Better Care, Better Health, and Better Value*. Sage Growth Partners LLC.

Medicine, M. (2013). *ConvUrgent Care Report, 6*(12), 1–6.

Medicine, M. (2013). *ConvUrgentCare Report, 6*(2), 1–4.

Newbold, P., & O'Neil, M. J. (2008). Small Changes Lead to Large Effects. *Frontiers of Health Services Management, 24*(3), 23–27. PMID:18435357

Newmarker, C. (2008). *MinuteClinic co-founder launches e-medicine startup*. Minneapolis: St. Paul Business Journal Afternoon Edition Newsletter.

Patient Protection and Affordable Care Act. (2010). Retrieved from http://www.healthcare.gov/law/full/index.html

Perman, C. (2012) *Healthcare reform's major hurdle: doctor shortages*. Retrieved from http://www.cnbc.com/id/36036747/Health_Care_Reform_s_Major_Hurdle_Doctor_Shortages

Pollack, C. E., Gidengil, C., & Mehrotra, A. (2010). The growth of retail clinics and the medical home: Two trends in concert or in conflict? *Health Affairs, 29*(5), 998–1003. doi:10.1377/hlthaff.2010.0089 PMID:20439897

Pollert, P., Dobberstein, D., & Wiisanen, R. (2008). Jumping into the Healthcare Market: Our Experience. *Frontiers of Health Services Management, 24*(3), 13–21. PMID:18435356

Porter, S. (n.d.). Provision in healthcare reform law gives primary care financial boost. *AAFP New Now*. Retrieved from http://www.aafp.org/online/en/home/publications/news/news-now/practice-management/20100903primcarebonus.html

Rodak, S. (2012). How Can Retail Health Help Hospitals Meet Health Reform Goals? *Becker Hospital Review*. Retrieved from http://www.beckershospitalreview.com/strategic-planning/how-can-retail-health-help-hospitals-meet-health-reform-goals.html

Rohrer, J. E., Angstman, K. B., Adamson, S. C., Bernard, M. E., Bachman, J. W., & Morgan, M. E. (2010). Impact of online primary care visits on standard costs: A pilot study. *Population Health Management, 13*(2), 59–63. doi:10.1089/pop.2009.0018 PMID:20415617

Scott, M.K. (2008a, January 4). Retail clinics- Friend of Foe of the hospital- Part I. The opportunity for hospitals to win with a retail clinic model. *HealthLeaders Media*.

Scott, M.K. (2008b, January 18). Retail clinics- Friend of Foe of the hospital- Part II. Tools to assess the potential impact on patient and physician populations, economics, and brand. *HealthLeaders Media*.

The Advisory Board Company. (2012). *Member asks: How can we set up a retail clinic partnership?* Retrieved from http://www.advisory.com/Daily-Briefing/2012/11/13/Member-asks

Tu, H. T., & Boukus, E. R. (2013). Despite rapid growth, retail clinic use remains modest. *Center for Studying Health System Change Research Brief*, *29*, 1–7.

United States Department of Labor. (2012). *Technical Release No. 2012-01: Frequently Asked Questions from Employers Regarding Automatic Enrollment, Employer Shared Responsibility, and Waiting Periods*. Retrieved from http://www.dol.gov/ebsa/newsroom/tr12-01.html

U.S. Small Business Administration. (2013). *Employers with 50 or more employees*. Retrieved from http://www.sba.gov/content/employers-with-50-or-more-employees

World Bank. (2013). Retrieved from http://data.worldbank.org/indicator/SH.XPD.PCAP

KEY TERMS AND DEFINITIONS

Healthcare Reform: A common term referring to the provisions of the Patient Protection and Affordable Care Act signed into law in March of 2010.

Hospital System: A healthcare organization that owns and operates several hospitals and other types of healthcare delivery organizations.

Online Services: Healthcare services provided electronically in real time (synchronous) or through "store & forward" (asynchronous) delivery via images, video and audio.

Patient-Centered Medical Home: A care delivery model whereby patient treatment is coordinated through their primary care physician to ensure they receive the necessary care when and where they need it, in a manner they can understand.

Retail Clinics: Small clinics located in general merchandise or drug stores and offering a limited scope of diagnostic and treatment services for common medical conditions.

Urgent Care: Healthcare provided on a walk-in, no-appointment basis for acute illnesses or injuries that are not life-threatening.

APPENDIX: BELLIN HEALTH FAST CARE

Bellin Health, based in Green Bay, Wisconsin, is a not-for-profit hospital system of 117 primary care physicians, 41 employer-based clinics, a 220-bed community hospital, a critical-access hospital, a psychiatric hospital, and a hospice. It serves a market of 600,000 patients.

The system adopted as a strategy a "life-and-health cycle" approach that emphasizes prevention and minimization of acute, hospital-based inpatient care. It focuses on engaging its patient population in new innovative ways and deliver services that allow patients to easily access appropriate care at the lowest cost (Feder, 2011).

About eight years ago, Bellin Health created "Fast Care" which owns and operates three retail clinics in the Wisconsin area. Fast Care clinics are affiliated with Bellin's medical practices and are connected through a system of electronic health records.

It then added "Fast Care Development" which is a consulting arm that supports other health systems to develop their own retail clinics. To date, Fast Care Development has helped open 35 hospital-based retail clinics in nine states, making Bellin Health the sixth largest retail clinic operator in the country.

Stephen Lazzari, Director of Fast Care Development, who we interviewed for this book in early 2013, explains Bellin Health's involvement in retail clinics and its consulting arm:

"We are a very large employer and we have self-funded insurance. About 7-8 years ago, we noticed that our own employees were showing up in our emergency rooms for minor episodic conditions. So we started conversations with Shopko, who were already aware of the retail clinic model. Shopko had room in their store, so we put the model together and were very pleased with the results as episodic care in the emergency room started to decrease. The community embraced it so we added 3 retail clinics and created "Fast Care." Then we were approached by two health systems: ThedaCare in Appleton, and Froedtert Health System (Medical College of Wisconsin in Milwaukee). They asked us to help them with starting retail clinics. So we put together a model and recommendation. That was the birth of "Fast Care Development" as a brand. And then we grew out of Wisconsin into 9 states and more than 30 clinics. Our model is growth of 15 clinics per year. We don't have as many sites as CVS, but we always look for a health system to own and operate the retail clinics, not just as an affiliate but as an owner. The way our model works is that we find a health system and a retailer. We build the clinic, provide the furniture and equipment and negotiate the contract between the hospital system and retailer. It is a "turn-key" arrangement. We give the hospital system a marketing and business development platform. We work with local businesses to inform them about the clinics. We want them to send their employees to the clinics instead of the emergency room. Then the hospital system takes over, puts their own director and staff in the clinic and deliver care the way they know. We give them the latitude to create their own menu of services, because the primary care physicians need to buy in and not see the clinic as a threat. We want the retail clinic to help bring patients to the primary care physicians, because the retail clinic is not a medical home."

While most hospital systems in the country have seen their costs steadily increase in recent years, Bellin reports flat costs. It estimates that its retail clinics have delivered care outside regular business hours to 250,000 patients since their opening. If those patients had sought care in emergency rooms, they would have cost the system an additional $52.9 million.

By providing numerous easy access points into the system, Bellin Health creates opportunities to bring care to people who would otherwise not seek it out. For example, of the patients that were treated at Fast Care clinics, 50% are new to the health system, and 35-40% have no primary care physician. Therefore, the clinics help patients create a primary care physician relationship that is critical to their care. George Kerwin, president and chief executive officer of Bellin Health, summarizes the model: “We’re improving health at a cost factor that is relatively flat. Instead of costs skyrocketing and health deteriorating, we’re experiencing just the opposite” (Feder, 2011, p.389).

Chapter 10
The Future

ABSTRACT

In this chapter, the author evaluates the convenient care models on convenience, costs, access, and quality. The models studied receive high scores on convenience, costs, and quality when compared to hospital emergency rooms and primary care physician offices, despite issues related to possible fragmentation of care. However, improving access to care, especially among uninsured and underserved populations, does not seem to be an advantage offered by convenient care. The author posits that the American healthcare system appears to be at a tipping point, with rising consumerism, demands for price and quality transparency, and regulatory forces that are forcing providers to focus on value over quantity. He envisages that the race between hospital systems under legislative pressures and giant retailers spotting strategic opportunities will accelerate innovations and enable convenient care models to move from the margins to become the mainstream way of providing preventative services, treating minor conditions, and managing some chronic conditions.

Retail clinics are the most critical intersection between healthcare delivery and a retail-like experience. Healthcare has been long overdue in embracing a retail-like approach in terms of convenience and access to patients. We're beyond the stage where it might be a fad, a trend; it's a proven and established healthcare delivery model that is here to stay, and should be considered as part of hospitals' larger entry point strategy. —Matt Montgomery, Senior Vice President -Healthcare Division, Buxton (in Rodak, 2012)

INTRODUCTION

The convenient care models that are discussed in this book still do not represent how the majority of Americans receive their primary care services today. Compared to the total number of primary care physician visits and non-emergent emergency room visits, the number of urgent care center visits, retail clinic visits, worksite visits, e-visits and house calls remains minute. However, the evidence that we showcased strongly suggests that these trends are rising, and that they will

DOI: 10.4018/978-1-4666-6355-8.ch010

continue to grow at an unprecedented rate in the next few years. The growth will likely be propelled by rising consumerism; continued dissatisfaction with traditional models; new technologies; and regulatory forces that emphasize cost savings. In this chapter, we review the evidence of the impact of convenient care models on access, cost and quality of care in the American healthcare system at large and we make some predictions about their future forms and roles.

1. EFFECTS OF ON CONVENIENCE, COST, QUALITY, AND ACCESS

While urgent care centers and worksite clinics have been around for a long time, other innovations such as retail clinics, online services and house-call services have just emerged in the last decade. Therefore, the scientific evidence relating to their convenience, quality of care outcomes, costs of care, and access to services is scarce at best. However, as we reviewed in Chapters 5-8, research findings seem to point in some general directions. When assessing that research, the main frame of reference is comparisons with hospital emergency rooms and primary care physician offices (Tables 1 and 2).

Urgent care centers are conveniently located in strip malls with easy access and parking, and provide care after-hours on weeknights and weekends. Wait times tend to be shorter than hospital emergency rooms, but can be longer than some primary care physician offices. Given the walk-in nature of these centers, wait times can fluctuate and patients might end up waiting for more than one hour. As a result, patient satisfaction is higher than for emergency rooms, but patients are sometimes hesitant to refer others to the centers. Urgent care centers that have managed to predict peak hours and to reduce their cycle time (from admission to discharge) to less than 60 minutes tend to be preferred by patients. Despite limited evidence, urgent care centers seem to score higher on quality of care scores for minor conditions than hospital emergency rooms, but have similar scores to primary care physician offices. As for costs of care per visit or per episode of treatment, urgent care centers are much less expensive than hospital emergency rooms and slightly less expensive than physician offices. Urgent care centers tend to be located in high-density suburban areas serving patient populations with private health insurance. For some of these patients who do not have a primary care physician and who visit urgent care centers, access is improved. However, specifically for patients living in rural areas, and for uninsured patients living in all areas, urgent care centers have not improved availability and access to

Table 1. Convenience, quality, cost and access grades for convenient care models in comparison to hospital emergency rooms

	Convenience	Quality	Cost	Access
Urgent Care Centers	A	A	A	B+
Retail Clinics	A+	A+	A+	B
Worksite Clinics	A+	A+	A+	B
Online & Other services	A+	I*	A+	A

*Given the lack of evidence, we chose to give an "I" Incomplete Grade

Table 2. Patient satisfaction, quality, cost and access grades for convenient care models in comparison to primary care physician offices

	Convenience	Quality	Cost	Access
Urgent Care Centers	B	A	A	B+
Retail Clinics	A+	A	A+	B
Worksite Clinics	A	A	A	B
Online & Other services	A+	I*	A+	A

*Given the lack of evidence, we chose to give an "I" Incomplete Grade

care. Given the relatively high visit price, urgent care centers are not especially attractive to uninsured or underinsured populations.

Retail clinics are also conveniently located in drug stores and grocery/general merchandise stores, are open after-hours on weeknights and weekends, provide a menu of services with prices, and have low average wait times. Therefore, patient satisfaction scores are very high in these settings, although some patients complaint about waiting longer than expected and not seeing a physician. For the minor conditions treated by retail clinics, there is strong evidence that providers adhere strongly to clinical guidelines and strict standards, and that patients receive appropriate preventative care and do not need to see another provider after the retail clinic visit. These outcomes are better or as good as those in primary care physician offices, and much better than those in hospital emergency rooms. As for continuity of care, the evidence is mixed but some research has suggested that retail clinics may reduce subsequent visits to the patient's physician and undermine care coordination. Costs of care per visit/episode are much lower at retail clinics than physician offices and hospital emergency rooms. Similar to urgent care centers, retail clinics tend to be located in areas with high socio-economic status, rather than deprived areas. Therefore, while they improve access for some insured patients, there is no evidence that they make it easier to uninsured and underinsured patients. Also compared to about 5,000-9,000 urgent care centers, there are only 1,500 retail clinics nationwide, which does not contribute to mass access to services.

Worksite clinics are conveniently located in employees' workplaces, and provide services during work hours with short waiting times. Most employees are satisfied with care, even though there is hesitance to use the clinics in some companies. Care provided for minor conditions, as well as for chronic disease management is of high quality, while costs for the employee and for the provider are much lower than the alternatives. Worksite clinics naturally improve access to employed individuals, but do not benefit uninsured populations that may be unemployed, self-employed, or employed by companies that cannot afford to provide coverage or health services.

Care provided through online clinics is extremely convenient and is available for patients 24 hours per day/7 days per week, which leads to high patient satisfaction scores. Evidence about quality of care evidence is especially scant, with some research showing similar preventative care and follow-up care in e-visits vs. physician offices. Cost of care is much lower than costs in hospital emergency rooms and physician offices, even though there is evidence of some over-prescribing of antibiotics. Unlike urgent care and retail clinics, online clinics are available virtually "anywhere." While most online care services have been offered to specific populations that are part of certain companies or health plans, some services provided at very low costs ($25 per visit) may be more accessible to uninsured patients, assuming that these have access to a phone/the Internet. An important observation relates to cost of care in these convenient care models. The data suggests that cost per visit/episode is generally lower than that in primary care physician offices and hospital emergency rooms. However, they can be more expensive overall if they lead to increased unnecessary utilization and fragmentation of care. A portion of convenient care consumers say that they might have not sought care anywhere if convenient care was not available. Therefore, it is possible to think that from the healthcare system's perspective, a retail or urgent or online visit represents "increased utilization" that would not have occurred otherwise. The extent of this increased utilization is not well understood, and some suggest that the patients delaying care and seeking home remedies may end developing more serious conditions that will cost the system more in the long run.

In summary, the convenient care models studied receive high scores on convenience, costs and quality when compared to hospital emergency rooms and primary care physician offices, despite issues related to possible fragmentation of care. However, improving access to care, especially among uninsured and underserved populations, is not an advantage offered by convenient care (Tables 1 & 2). Given that the majority of the uninsured population will be receiving coverage under the Patient Protection and Affordable Care Act (PPACA), this might be less of an issue in the near future.

Predictions

The American healthcare system appears to be at a tipping point. Consumerism is rising, demands for price and quality transparency are increasing, and regulatory forces are forcing providers to focus on value over quantity. Moreover, as the growth in high-deductible health plans and health insurance exchanges accelerates, and as more and more employers reduce or eliminate their employer-sponsored health plans, the business model will shift from wholesale to retail. Individual consumers will go online one-by-one and shop for health plans and care, instead of insurance companies selling to one large employer for thousands of employees (Commins, 2014a). In this new healthcare reality, traditional healthcare providers such as hospitals and physician will have to rethink their roles and business models, and new convenient care models will continue to emerge.

We predict that the lines between the models of delivery will blur, and more cross-over will take place between services provided in urgent care centers, retail clinics, online, at home or on the road. We also predict that the new American healthcare system will have new levels of delivery that can provide higher quality care at lower costs. Hospital systems will play an increasingly important role in driving and sustaining convenient care models, in the context of patient-centered medical homes, accountable care organizations, and other structural arrangements that can survive under global payments. While we discussed the convenient care models in separate chapters for ease of illustration, we strongly believe that new hybrid models will continue to emerge. The forces that will propel those models are already in place, as urgent care, retail clinic and online care operators are already involved in providing worksite clinics for example. The diversification of offerings will be especially true as more hospital systems embrace the innovations and have deliberate convenient care strategies, and as large companies like Wal-Mart and Walgreens aspire to play a larger role in primary care. As for the healthcare system at large, provider shortages and escalating costs will require the development of a new three-tiered delivery system (Jacobsen, Jazowksi, 2011). The first tier of care will consist of basic retail clinics, online clinics, urgent care centers, worksite clinics, house call services and other convenient care services providing preventative services, vaccinations, and treatments for acute, episodic, minor conditions. Care in this first line of defense will invariably be provided by non-physician providers, under indirect physician supervision and oversight. The second tier of care will consist of primary care physician offices, as well as advanced retail clinics, advanced urgent care centers, worksite clinics, and ambulatory surgery centers, providing care for complex uncertain chronic conditions and same-day surgeries. Most of the care provided in this tier will require a physician, even though some of it (such as chronic disease monitoring) can be provided by experienced non-physician providers. The last tier of care will consist of specialist physician practices, hospital emergency rooms and in-patient hospital care providing complicated surgical procedures, intensive care and immediate treatment or trauma and other life-threatening conditions

The intriguing question about the future of convenient care relates to who will be the main driver of change and innovation: hospital and health systems or large retailers? As discussed in Chapter 9, regulatory forces are causing hospitals to reevaluate their existing practices and strategies to adapt to a new environment of care where value, rather than quantity, will be rewarded. Section 3001(a) of the Patient Protection and Affordable Care Act (PPACA) defines the Hospital Value-Based Purchasing (HVBP) program. Under the program, the Medicare payment system will be linked to quality of care provided in inpatient hospital settings. Hospitals that show evidence of eliminating or reducing the occurrence of adverse events (healthcare errors resulting in patient harm), adopting evidence-based care standards and protocols that result in the best outcomes for the most patients and re-engineering hospital processes that improve patients' experience of care will receive higher payments from CMS (Centers for Medicare & Medicaid) than hospitals that don't (CMS, 2013). Moreover, the traditional fee-for-service payment system where hospitals received reimbursement based on the amount of services provided is being slowly replaced by "global payments" or "bundled payments." These payments are fixed-dollar payments for the care that patients may receive in a given time period, such as a month or year. Under this system, providers assume the financial risk for both the occurrence of medical conditions as well as the management of those conditions. Global or bundled payments are intended to contain costs and reduce the use of unnecessary services, encourage integration and coordination of services and may also include added incentives to improve the quality of care (Burns, 2013). Most global payments will include hospital and physician services, diagnostic tests, prescription drugs, and possibly other services such as home healthcare and hospice care. For example, a large health system that owns or affiliates with physician practices will receive a global payment from Medicare or a large health plan for a group of members or enrollees. The health system is responsible for ensuring that these members receive all needed healthcare services. The payments will typically reflect the health status of the population of members. The health system and its network of formally and loosely affiliated physicians and organizations can be known as an Accountable Care Organization ACO). In addition, section 3025 of the PPACA added section 1886(q) to the Social Security Act and established the Hospital Readmissions Reduction Program, which requires CMS to reduce payments to hospitals with excess readmissions (CMS, 2012). Under the program, hospital will not receive payments for patients that are readmitted to the hospital within 30 days of discharge. Therefore, hospitals have to provide better and safer care during the inpatient stay by reducing the risk of infection; monitoring patient medications; focusing on discharge planning; improving communication with patients and caregivers regarding follow-up care; and improving care transition through better communication and collaboration with other community providers (James, 2013).

In response to these changes and forces, hospital and health systems will have huge incentives to constraint costs so as not to exceed the global payment amount and to integrate their healthcare offerings in order to better manage risks and improve quality. In this environment, convenient care services that are well integrated with traditional health services will play an important role. For example, expensive emergency room visits can be prevented by providing access to owned or affiliated retail clinics, urgent care centers, online care or house call services, and risks can be mitigated. Similarly, overwhelmed primary care physician offices can find relief by referring patients to these settings, therefore providing high quality care without exceeding the global payment. It is also possible that some of these settings (such as urgent care centers) may act as readmission prevention clinics where patients are seen after discharge by a non-physician providers that follows protocols ensuring fast and safe recovery.

Under the umbrella of a large hospital or health system or an accountable care organization, electronic health records would allow seamless connections between the various levels, cost savings would be accumulated, and overall value would soar.

While the legislative forces seem to be in place for hospitals and health systems to take advantage of convenient care models, market forces suggest that retailers will not be watching from the sidelines. On the contrary, there is every reason to suggest that retailers have already launched aggressive strategies to dominate the convenient care scene. The push seems to be facilitated by the wide diffusion of high-deductible health plans where consumers are responsible for the majority of their medical costs, with insurance coverage mainly providing protection against catastrophic injury or illness. Many analysts suggest that in this era of consumer-driven healthcare, retailers have significant advantages over traditional healthcare providers. In a recent article, PwC Health Industries Advisory Service analyst Vaughn Kauffman stated: “There are some very distinct advantages for retailers. Their business model has evolved in understanding the wants and needs of consumers. Traditional healthcare organizations, outside of maybe the physician relationship with patients, are still trying to figure out their relationship with the consumer. In fact, the definition of customers is changing from what use to always be thought of as the employer as the customer to the individual as a consumer of healthcare. There is a distinct advantage that retailers have with brand recognition and trust of the brand. You know what you get when you walk into a certain retailer. It is not that same way in healthcare and a lot of traditional companies in healthcare recognize that. We are seeing roles being formed at the senior level such as chief experience officers. They are hiring outside of the industry, particularly in the hospitality industry. The focus is on the customer that other industries' business models have been anchored on. The convenience factor is an advantage as well. How often do you walk into a retailer on a given week versus walking into a hospital setting? The ability to capture the hearts and minds of consumers is much easier for retailers because of the frequency that people walk in, and I don't want to discount the e-commerce presence that organization have. The interactions are much more frequent. Once you get a captive audience there is an ability to drive that engagement to another level" (Commins, 2014b, p.1). One example of a retailer moving aggressively into the healthcare arena is Walgreens. In addition to its Take Care retail clinics, Walgreens announced in 2013 that it was the first national pharmacy chain to be approved by CMS to participate in Accountable Care organizations (ACOs). In fact, the national drugstore company developed three ACOS: Advocare Walgreens Well Network in New Jersey, Diagnostic Clinic Well Network in Florida and Scott & White Walgreens Well Network in Texas. Jeffrey Kang, MD, senior vice president of health and wellness services and solutions for Walgreens, explained: "It's a natural evolution. Over the last five or 10 years, Walgreens has been increasingly moving into the healthcare space" (Punke, 2013, p.1) He suggests that Walgreens can manage population health as well or better than hospitals and health system due to various programs it already has in place:

- "Primary prevention and screening. This includes vaccinations and health screenings for chronic conditions such as diabetes and hypertension.
- Health and wellness. Walgreens stores' programs such as weight loss and nutrition efforts.
- Medication adherence. Walgreens pharmacists can follow up with patients after a hospital discharge to make sure they are executing on physician orders to take certain medications. The chain also offers bedside medication delivery.
- Minor episodic care. In-store clinics staffed by nurse practitioners can treat simple illnesses such as colds, sore throats or urinary tract infections.
- Chronic condition management. Walgreen's pharmacists and Take Care Clinic NPs can help monitor patient adherence to a physician's treatment plan."(Punke, 2013, p.1).

Another important advantage the Walgreens has is its existing army of pharmacists and nurse practitioners who can work side-by-side with physicians and can play an important role in filling the primary care gap.

Another retail giant that is bracing itself for more in involvement in healthcare delivery is Walmart. In January of 2013, Walmart announced that it plans to provide "full primary care services" to consumers nationwide within five to seven years. The announcement came two years after it made headlines for sending 14-page letters to health providers and companies requesting information to help it establish "the largest provider of primary healthcare services in the nation." However, Walmart soon clarified that it was "not building a national, integrated, low-cost primary healthcare platform." In the recent announcement, Marcus Osborn (vice president of health and wellness payer relations) suggested that Walmart was heading towards providing retail clinics in rural areas and underserved, urban areas because the chain has many stores in those areas. It is safe to say that Walmart is likely to be creating frequent shock waves in the healthcare industry in the next few years.

2. CONCLUSION

Healthcare consumers in the United States should feel optimistic about the prospects of healthcare delivery. Newer, more convenient, cheaper, and better performing care models will continue to emerge and spread. The race between hospitals and health systems under legislative pressures and giant retailers spotting strategic opportunities will accelerate innovations and enable convenient care models to move from the margins to become the mainstream way of providing preventative services, treating minor conditions and managing some chronic conditions.

REFERENCES

Burns, J. (2013). Bundled payment. *Hospitals & Health Networks*, (4), 26. PMID:23700754

Centers for Medicare & Medicaid. (2013). *Hospital Value-Based Purchasing*. Available at http://www.cms.gov/Medicare/Quality-Initiatives-Patient-Assessment-Instruments/hospital-value-based-purchasing/index.html?redirect=/hospital-value-based-purchasing/

Centers for Medicare & Medicaid. (2013). *Readmissions Reduction Program*. Available at http://www.cms.gov/Medicare/Medicare-Fee-for-Service-Payment/AcuteInpatientPPS/Readmissions-Reduction-Program.html

Commins, J. (2014a, January 6). Retail Medicine a Big Shift for 2014. *HealthLeaders Media*.

Commins, J. (2014b, February 25). Retail Medicine Syncs with High-Deductible Health Plans. *HealthLeaders*.

Jacobson, P. D., & Jazowski, S. A. (2011). Physicians, the affordable care act and primary care: Disruptive change or business as usual? *Journal of General Internal Medicine*, *26*(8), 934–937. doi:10.1007/s11606-011-1695-8 PMID:21455812

James, J. (2013). Health Policy Brief: Medicare Hospital Readmissions Reduction Program. *Health Affairs*, (November), 12.

Punke, H. (2013, February 7). Walgreens' Strategy Behind ACO Participation. *Becker Hospital Review*.

Rodak, S. (2012, December 3). How Can Retail Health Help Hospitals Meet Health Reform Goals? *Becker Hospital Review*.

KEY TERMS AND DEFINITIONS

Access to Care: The ability of patients to receive healthcare services, depending in the availability of healthcare facilities and providers and the patient's insurance status/ability to pay.

Cost of Care: The amount in dollars spent on healthcare services within a certain healthcare system.

Online Services: Healthcare services provided electronically in real time (synchronous) or through "store & forward" (asynchronous) delivery via images, video and audio.

Quality of Care: The extent to which healthcare services provided to individuals and patient populations improve desired health outcomes.

Retail Clinics: Small clinics located in general merchandise or drug stores and offering a limited scope of diagnostic and treatment services for common medical conditions.

Urgent Care: Healthcare provided on a walk-in, no-appointment basis for acute illnesses or injuries that are not life-threatening.

Worksite Clinics: Small clinics located on employers' campuses and dedicated to serving employees by providing primary care services, health promotion and wellness as well as care for occupational injuries.

Related References

To continue our tradition of advancing medicine, healthcare, and life sciences research, we have compiled a list of recommended IGI Global readings. These references will provide additional information and guidance to further enrich your knowledge and assist you with your own research and future publications

.Abu-Faraj, Z. O. (2012). Bioengineering/biomedical engineering education. In Z. Abu-Faraj (Ed.), *Handbook of research on biomedical engineering education and advanced bioengineering learning: Interdisciplinary concepts* (pp. 1–59). Hershey, PA: Medical Information Science Reference. doi:10.4018/978-1-4666-0122-2.ch001

Achehboune, A., & Driouchi, A. (2014). Potential skilled labor migration, internationalization of education with focus on medical education: The case of Arab countries. In A. Driouchi (Ed.), *Labor and health economics in the Mediterranean region: Migration and mobility of medical doctors* (pp. 83–122). Hershey, PA: Medical Information Science Reference.

Adomi, E. E., Egbaivwie, E., & Ogugua, J. C. (2013). Use of the internet by medical practitioners in private hospitals in Warri, Delta State, Nigeria. In A. Cartelli (Ed.), *Fostering 21st century digital literacy and technical competency* (pp. 213–221). Hershey, PA: Information Science Reference.

Afolabi, M. O., Babalola, O. O., & Ola-Olorun, O. J. (2012). Counselling in pharmacy prac tice: Exploring the use of online counselling interactions to improve medicine use among people living with HIV/AIDS (PLWHA). In B. Popoola, & O. Adebowale (Eds.), *Online guidance and counseling: Toward effectively applying technology* (pp. 91–103). Hershey, PA: Information Science Referenc. doi:10.4018/978-1-61350-204-4.ch007

Ahmad, Y. J., Raghavan, V. V., & Martz, W. B., Jr. (2011). Adoption of electronic health records. In *Clinical technologies: Concepts, methodologies, tools and applications* (pp. 132-146). Hershey, PA: Medical Information Science Reference. doi:10.4018/978-1-60960-561-2.ch109

Al-Dossary, S., Al-Dulaijan, N., Al-Mansour, S., Al-Zahrani, S., Al-Fridan, M., & Househ, M. (2013). Organ donation and transplantation: Processes, registries, consent, and restrictions in Saudi Arabia. In M. Cruz-Cunha, I. Miranda, & P. Gonçalves (Eds.), *Handbook of research on ICTs for human-centered healthcare and social care services* (pp. 511–528). Hershey, PA: Medical Information Science Reference doi:10.4018/978-1-4666-3986-7.ch027

Al-Khudairy, S. (2014). Caring for our aging population: Using CPOE and telehomecare systems as a response to health policy concerns. In C. El Morr (Ed.), *Research perspectives on the role of informatics in health policy and management* (pp. 153–166). Hershey, PA: Medical Information Science Reference.

Albert, A., Serrano, A. J., Soria, E., & Jiménez, N. V. (2010). Clinical decision support system to prevent toxicity in patients treated with Digoxin. In A. Shukla, & R. Tiwari (Eds.), *Intelligent medical technologies and biomedical engineering: Tools and applications* (pp. 1–21). Hershey, PA: Medical Information Science Reference. doi:10.4018/978-1-61520-977-4.ch001

Alexandrou, D. A., & Pardalis, K. V. (2014). SEMantic PATHways: Modeling, executing, and monitoring intra-organizational healthcare business processes towards personalized treatment. In Software design and development: Concepts, methodologies, tools, and applications (pp. 1036-1062). Hershey, PA: Information Science Reference. doi:10.4018/978-1-4666-4301-7.ch050

Alhaqbani, B., & Fidge, C. (2013). A medical data trustworthiness assessment model. In User-driven healthcare: Concepts, methodologies, tools, and applications (pp. 1425-1445). Hershey, PA: Medical Information Science Reference. doi:10.4018/978-1-4666-2770-3.ch071

Ali, S., Abbadeni, N., & Batouche, M. (2012). *Multidisciplinary computational intelligence techniques: Applications in business, engineering, and medicine* (pp. 1–365). Hershey, PA: IGI Global. doi:10.4018/978-1-4666-1830-5

Alonso, J. M., Castiello, C., Lucarelli, M., & Mencar, C. (2013). Modeling interpretable fuzzy rule-based classifiers for medical decision support. In *Data mining: Concepts, methodologies, tools, and applications* (pp. 1064–1081). Hershey, PA: Information Science Reference.

Alonso-Barba, J. I., Nielsen, J. D., de la Ossa, L., & Puerta, J. M. (2012). Learning probabilistic graphical models: A review of techniques and applications in medicine. In R. Magdalena-Benedito, E. Soria-Olivas, J. Martínez, J. Gómez-Sanchis, & A. Serrano-López (Eds.), *Medical applications of intelligent data analysis: Research advancements* (pp. 223–236). Hershey, PA: Information Science Reference. doi:10.4018/978-1-4666-1803-9.ch015

Anderson, J. G. (2010). Improving patient safety with information technology. In K. Khoumbati, Y. Dwivedi, A. Srivastava, & B. Lal (Eds.), *Handbook of research on advances in health informatics and electronic healthcare applications: Global adoption and impact of information communication technologies* (pp. 144–152). Hershey, PA: Medical Information Science Reference.

Anderson, J. G. (2011). Regional patient safety initiatives. In *Clinical technologies: Concepts, methodologies, tools and applications* (pp. 1491-1503). Hershey, PA: Medical Information Science Reference. doi:10.4018/978-1-60960-561-2.ch506

Andonegui, J., Serrano, L., & Eguzkiza, A. (2010). E-health applications in ophthalmic diseases: Ongoing developments. In M. Cruz-Cunha, A. Tavares, & R. Simoes (Eds.), *Handbook of research on developments in e-health and telemedicine: Technological and social perspectives* (pp. 1088–1115). Hershey, PA: Medical Information Science Reference.

Andrés, A. R. (2014). Understanding the migration of medical doctors in the context of Europe. In A. Driouchi (Ed.), *Labor and health economics in the Mediterranean region: Migration and mobility of medical doctors* (pp. 139–157). Hershey, PA: Medical Information Science Reference.

Ann, O. C., & Theng, L. B. (2014). A facial expression mediated natural user interface communication model for children with motor impairments. In G. Kouroupetroglou (Ed.), *Assistive technologies and computer access for motor disabilities* (pp. 254–284). Hershey, PA: Medical Information Science Reference.

Anselma, L., Bottrighi, A., Molino, G., Montani, S., Terenziani, P., & Torchio, M. (2011). Supporting knowledge-based decision making in the medical context: The GLARE approach. [IJKBO]. *International Journal of Knowledge-Based Organizations*, *1*(1), 42–60. doi:10.4018/ijkbo.2011010103

Apostolakis, I., Valsamos, P., & Varlamis, I. (2011). Quality assurance in evidence-based medicine. In A. Moumtzoglou, & A. Kastania (Eds.), *E-health systems quality and reliability: Models and standards* (pp. 86–99). Hershey, PA: Medical Information Science Reference.

Archibald, D., MacDonald, C. J., Hogue, R., & Mercer, J. (2013). Accessing knowledge from the bedside: Introducing the tablet computer to clinical teaching. In C. Rückemann (Ed.), *Integrated information and computing systems for natural, spatial, and social sciences* (pp. 96–109). Hershey, PA: Information Science Reference.

Aspradaki, A. A. (2013). Deliberative democracy and nanotechnologies in health. [IJT]. *International Journal of Technoethics*, *4*(2), 1–14. doi:10.4018/jte.2013070101

Assis-Hassid, S., Reychav, I., Pliskin, J. S., & Heart, T. H. (2013). The effects of electronic medical record (EMR) use in primary care on the physician-patient relationship. In M. Cruz-Cunha, I. Miranda, & P. Gonçalves (Eds.), *Handbook of research on ICTs for human-centered healthcare and social care services* (pp. 130–150). Hershey, PA: Medical Information Science Reference. doi:10.4018/978-1-4666-3986-7.ch007

Atanasov, A. (2011). Quality and reliability aspects in evidence based e-medicine. In A. Moumtzoglou, & A. Kastania (Eds.), *E-health systems quality and reliability: Models and standards* (pp. 100–117). Hershey, PA: Medical Information Science Reference. doi:10.4018/978-1-60960-561-2.ch112

Attalla, D. S. (2011). Health hazards of mobile information communication technologies. In A. Abdel-Wahab, & A. El-Masry (Eds.), *Mobile information communication technologies adoption in developing countries: Effects and implications* (pp. 237–251). Hershey, PA: Information Science Reference.

Au, S., & Gupta, A. (2011). Gastrointestinal motility online educational endeavor. In A. Moumtzoglou, & A. Kastania (Eds.), *E-health systems quality and reliability: Models and standards* (pp. 163–182). Hershey, PA: Medical Information Science Reference.

Azar, A. T. (2013). Overview of biomedical engineering. In Bioinformatics: Concepts, methodologies, tools, and applications (pp. 1-28). Hershey, PA: Medical Information Science Reference. doi:10.4018/978-1-4666-3604-0.ch001

Azar, A. T., & Eljamel, M. S. (2014). Medical robotics. In Robotics: Concepts, methodologies, tools, and applications (pp. 1116-1147). Hershey, PA: Information Science Reference. doi:10.4018/978-1-4666-4607-0.ch054

Bagheri, F. B. (2013). eSelf or computerized self network: A tool for individual empowerment & implementation of optimal healthcare. [IJUDH]. *International Journal of User-Driven Healthcare*, *3*(2), 20–32. doi:10.4018/ijudh.2013040103

Baharadwaj, N., Wadhwa, S., Goel, P., Sethi, I., Arora, C. S., & Goel, A. et al. (2014). De-noising, clustering, classification, and representation of microarray data for disease diagnostics. In R. Srivastava, S. Singh, & K. Shukla (Eds.), *Research developments in computer vision and image processing: Methodologies and applications* (pp. 149–174). Hershey, PA: Information Science Reference.

Baijou, A. (2014). A descriptive overview of the emigration of medical doctors from MENA to EU. In A. Driouchi (Ed.), *Labor and health economics in the Mediterranean region: Migration and mobility of medical doctors* (pp. 192–218). Hershey, PA: Medical Information Science Reference.

Bauer, K. (2010). Healthcare ethics in the information age. In J. Rodrigues (Ed.), *Health information systems: Concepts, methodologies, tools, and applications* (pp. 1761–1776). Hershey, PA: Medical Information Science Reference.

Bauer, K. A. (2013). Caught in the web: The internet and the demise of medical privacy. In User-driven healthcare: Concepts, methodologies, tools, and applications (pp. 1252-1272). Hershey, PA: Medical Information Science Reference. doi:10.4018/978-1-4666-2770-3.ch063

Bayona, S., Espadero, J. M., Fernández, J. M., Pastor, L., & Rodríguez, Á. (2011). Implementing virtual reality in the healthcare sector. In N. Rao (Ed.), *Virtual technologies for business and industrial applications: Innovative and synergistic approaches* (pp. 138–163). Hershey, PA: Business Science Reference.

Begg, M., Dewhurst, D., & Ross, M. (2010). Game informed virtual patients: Catalysts for online learning communities and professional development of medical teachers. In J. Lindberg, & A. Olofsson (Eds.), *Online learning communities and teacher professional development: Methods for improved education delivery* (pp. 190–208). Hershey, PA: Information Science Reference. doi:10.4018/978-1-61520-869-2.ch020

Bennett, E. E., Blanchard, R. D., & Fernandez, G. L. (2012). Knowledge sharing in academic medical centers: Examining the nexus of higher education and workforce development. In V. Wang (Ed.), *Encyclopedia of e-leadership, counseling and training* (pp. 212–232). Hershey, PA: Information Science Reference.

Bera, T. K., & Nagaraju, J. (2014). Electrical impedance tomography (EIT): A harmless medical imaging modality. In R. Srivastava, S. Singh, & K. Shukla (Eds.), *Research developments in computer vision and image processing: Methodologies and applications* (pp. 235–273). Hershey, PA: Information Science Reference.

Berler, A., & Apostolakis, I. (2014). Normalizing cross-border healthcare in europe via new e-prescription paradigms. In C. El Morr (Ed.), *Research perspectives on the role of informatics in health policy and management* (pp. 168–208). Hershey, PA: Medical Information Science Reference.

Beswetherick, J. (2012). Health care information systems and the risk of privacy issues for the disabled. In Cyber crime: Concepts, methodologies, tools and applications (pp. 870-890). Hershey, PA: Information Science Reference. doi:10.4018/978-1-61350-323-2.ch411

Bhattacharya, P., Asanga, A. P., & Biswas, R. (2011). Stomodeum to proctodeum: Email narratives on clinical problem solving in gastroenterology. In R. Biswas, & C. Martin (Eds.), *User-driven healthcare and narrative medicine: Utilizing collaborative social networks and technologies* (pp. 34–53). Hershey, PA: Medical Information Science Reference.

Biswas, R., & Martin, C. M. (2011). *User-driven healthcare and narrative medicine: Utilizing collaborative social networks and technologies*. Hershey, PA: IGI Global.

Biswas, R., Martin, C. M., Sturmberg, J., Mukherji, K., Lee, E. W., & Umakanth, S. (2011). Social cognitive ontology and user driven healthcare. In *Concepts, methodologies, tools and applications* (pp. 1996-2012). Hershey, PA: Medical Information Science Reference. doi:10.4018/978-1-60960-561-2.ch710

Biswas, R., Sturmberg, J., Martin, C. M., Ganesh, A. U., Umakanth, S., & Lee, E. W. (2011). Persistent clinical encounters in user driven e-health care. In *Clinical technologies: Concepts, methodologies, tools and applications* (pp. 1030-1046). Hershey, PA: Medical Information Science Reference. doi:10.4018/978-1-60960-561-2.ch403

Black, N. P., Fromme, H. B., Maniscalco, J., Ferrell, C., Myers, J., & Augustine, E. … Blankenburg, R. (2013). Innovation in patient care and medical resident education: Using blended instruction to transform nighttime patient care from a service model into an educational model. In A. Ritzhaupt, & S. Kumar (Eds.) Cases on educational technology implementation for facilitating learning (pp. 161-176). Hershey, PA: Information Science Reference. doi:10.4018/978-1-4666-3676-7.ch010

Blatt, A. J. (2013). Geospatial applications in disease surveillance: Solutions for the future. [IJAGR]. *International Journal of Applied Geospatial Research*, *4*(2), 1–8. doi:10.4018/jagr.2013040101

Boaduo, N. A., & Boaduo, N. K. (2012). ICTs for enhanced use of indigenous medicinal plants by the Ashante speaking people of Ghana. In R. Lekoko, & L. Semali (Eds.), *Cases on developing countries and ICT integration: Rural community development* (pp. 16–24). Hershey, PA: Information Science Reference.

Boboc, C., & Titan, E. (2014). Inputs from the new economics of migration of medical doctors in eastern and central Europe. In A. Driouchi (Ed.), *Labor and health economics in the Mediterranean region: Migration and mobility of medical doctors* (pp. 241–266). Hershey, PA: Medical Information Science Reference.

Boboc, C., & Ţiţan, E. (2014). Migration of medical doctors, health, medical education, and employment in eastern and central Europe. In A. Driouchi (Ed.), *Labor and health economics in the Mediterranean region: Migration and mobility of medical doctors* (pp. 158–191). Hershey, PA: Medical Information Science Reference.

Bolsin, S., & Colson, M. (2010). IT benefits in healthcare performance and safety. In J. Rodrigues (Ed.), *Health information systems: Concepts, methodologies, tools, and applications* (pp. 71–88). Hershey, PA: Medical Information Science Reference.

Bongers, B., & Smith, S. (2014). Interactivating rehabilitation through active multimodal feedback and guidance. In *Assistive technologies: Concepts, methodologies, tools, and applications* (pp. 1650–1674). Hershey, PA: Information Science Reference.

Borges, A. P., & Laranjeira, E. (2013). Why and how did health economics appear? Who were the main authors? What is the role of ITCs in its development? In M. Cruz-Cunha, I. Miranda, & P. Gonçalves (Eds.), *Handbook of research on ICTs and management systems for improving efficiency in healthcare and social care* (pp. 971–987). Hershey, PA: Medical Information Science Reference. doi:10.4018/978-1-4666-3990-4.ch051

Bourgeois, S., & Yaylacicegi, U. (2012). Electronic health records: Improving patient safety and quality of care in Texas acute care hospitals. In J. Tan (Ed.), *Advancing technologies and intelligence in healthcare and clinical environments breakthroughs* (pp. 18–32). Hershey, PA: Medical Information Science Reference. doi:10.4018/978-1-4666-1755-1.ch002

Brandt, R., & Rice, R. (2012). Dermatological telemedicine diagnoses and andragogical training using web 2.0 mobile medicine video conferencing. In V. Dennen, & J. Myers (Eds.), *Virtual professional development and informal learning via social networks* (pp. 276–293). Hershey, PA: Information Science Reference. doi:10.4018/978-1-4666-1815-2.ch016

Brzezinski, J., Kosiedowski, M., Mazurek, C., Slowinski, K., Slowinski, R., Stroinski, M., & Weglarz, J. (2013). Towards telemedical centers: Digitization of inter-professional communication in healthcare. In M. Cruz-Cunha, I. Miranda, & P. Gonçalves (Eds.), *Handbook of research on ICTs and management systems for improving efficiency in healthcare and social care* (pp. 805–829). Hershey, PA: Medical Information Science Reference. doi:10.4018/978-1-4666-3990-4.ch042

Carlén, U., & Lindström, B. (2012). Informed design of educational activities in online learning communities. In A. Olofsson, & J. Lindberg (Eds.), *Informed design of educational technologies in higher education: Enhanced learning and teaching* (pp. 118–134). Hershey, PA: Information Science Reference.

Carrigan, E., Ugaz, A., Moberly, H. K., Page, J., Alpi, K. M., & Vreeland, C. (2013). Veterinary medicine: All collections great and small. In S. Holder (Ed.), *Library collection development for professional programs: Trends and best practices* (pp. 248–268). Hershey, PA: Information Science Reference.

Caruana, C. J. (2012). The ongoing crisis in medical device education for healthcare professionals: Breaking the vicious circle through online learning. [IJRQEH]. *International Journal of Reliable and Quality E-Healthcare*, *1*(2), 29–40. doi:10.4018/ijrqeh.2012040103

Catapano, G., & Verkerke, G. J. (2012). Artificial organs. In Z. Abu-Faraj (Ed.), *Handbook of research on biomedical engineering education and advanced bioengineering learning: Interdisciplinary concepts* (pp. 60–95). Hershey, PA: Medical Information Science Reference. doi:10.4018/978-1-4666-0122-2.ch002

Chandra, S., Shah, N. K., & Sriganesh, V. (2011). The cochrane students journal club and creating a secondary learning resource for gathering and appraising evidence: An example of rational use of medicines to prevent malaria relapse. [IJUDH]. *International Journal of User-Driven Healthcare*, *1*(4), 31–41. doi:10.4018/ijudh.2011100103

Chang, A. Y., Littman-Quinn, R., Ketshogileng, D., Chandra, A., Rijken, T., & Ghose, S. et al. (2012). Smartphone-based mobile learning with physician trainees in Botswana. [IJMBL]. *International Journal of Mobile and Blended Learning*, *4*(2), 1–14. doi:10.4018/jmbl.2012040101

Charissis, G., Melas, C., Moustakis, V., & Zampetakis, L. (2010). Organizational implementation of healthcare information systems. In M. Cruz-Cunha, A. Tavares, & R. Simoes (Eds.), *Handbook of research on developments in e-health and telemedicine: Technological and social perspectives* (pp. 419–450). Hershey, PA: Medical Information Science Reference.

Chaudhuri, A., Young, J., Martin, C. M., Sturmberg, J. P., & Biswas, R. (2011). Hematology: The river within. In R. Biswas, & C. Martin (Eds.), *User-driven healthcare and narrative medicine: Utilizing collaborative social networks and technologies* (pp. 16–33). Hershey, PA: Medical Information Science Reference.

Chen, J. Y., Xu, H., Shi, P., Culbertson, A., & Meslin, E. M. (2013). Ethics and privacy considerations for systems biology applications in predictive and personalized medicine. In Bioinformatics: Concepts, methodologies, tools, and applications (pp. 1378-1404). Hershey, PA: Medical Information Science Reference. doi:10.4018/978-1-4666-3604-0.ch071

Cherian, E. J., & Ryan, T. W. (2014). Incongruent needs: Why differences in the iron-triangle of priorities make health information technology adoption and use difficult. In C. El Morr (Ed.), *Research perspectives on the role of informatics in health policy and management* (pp. 209–221). Hershey, PA: Medical Information Science Reference.

Chetioui, Y. (2014). Perception by Moroccan physicians of factors affecting their migration decisions. In A. Driouchi (Ed.), *Labor and health economics in the mediterranean region: Migration and mobility of medical doctors* (pp. 337–375). Hershey, PA: Medical Information Science Reference.

Chorbev, I., & Joksimoski, B. (2011). An integrated system for e-medicine (e-health, telemedicine and medical expert systems). In *Clinical technologies: Concepts, methodologies, tools and applications* (pp. 486-507). Hershey, PA: Medical Information Science Reference. doi:10.4018/978-1-60960-561-2.ch218

Ciufudean, C., Ciufudean, O., & Filote, C. (2013). New models for ICT-based medical diagnosis. In M. Cruz-Cunha, I. Miranda, & P. Gonçalves (Eds.), *Handbook of research on ICTs and management systems for improving efficiency in healthcare and social care* (pp. 892–911). Hershey, PA: Medical Information Science Reference. doi:10.4018/978-1-4666-3990-4.ch046

Clark, J. M. (2014). Implementation of electronic records in a medical practice setting. In J. Krueger (Ed.), *Cases on electronic records and resource management implementation in diverse environments* (pp. 211–225). Hershey, PA: Information Science Reference.

Clark, T. (2011). Health and health care grid services and delivery integrating eHealth and telemedicine. In E. Kldiashvili (Ed.), *Grid technologies for e-health: Applications for telemedicine services and delivery* (pp. 36–64). Hershey, PA: Medical Information Science Reference.

Claster, W., Ghotbi, N., & Shanmuganathan, S. (2010). Data-mining techniques for an analysis of non-conventional methodologies: Deciphering of alternative medicine. In W. Pease, M. Cooper, & R. Gururajan (Eds.), *Biomedical knowledge management: Infrastructures and processes for e-health systems* (pp. 82–91). Hershey, PA: Medical Information Science Reference. doi:10.4018/978-1-60566-266-4.ch006

Condaris, C. (2012). Scales to scalpels: Doctors who practice the healing arts of music and medicine. [IJUDH]. *International Journal of User-Driven Healthcare*, *2*(3), 84–84. doi:10.4018/ijudh.2012070109

Corrigan, D., Hederman, L., Khan, H., Taweel, A., Kostopoulou, O., & Delaney, B. (2013). An ontology-driven approach to clinical evidence modelling implementing clinical prediction rules. In A. Moumtzoglou, & A. Kastania (Eds.), *E-health technologies and improving patient safety: Exploring organizational factors* (pp. 257–284). Hershey, PA: Medical Information Science Reference.

Crisóstomo-Acevedo, M. J., & Aurelio Medina-Garrido, J. (2010). Difficulties in accepting telemedicine. In J. Rodrigues (Ed.), *Health information systems: Concepts, methodologies, tools, and applications* (pp. 1628–1639). Hershey, PA: Medical Information Science Reference.

Danforth, D. R. (2010). Development of an interactive virtual 3-D model of the human testis using the second life platform. [IJVPLE]. *International Journal of Virtual and Personal Learning Environments*, *1*(2), 45–58. doi:10.4018/jvple.2010040104

Daniel, V. M. (2011). Genomics and genetic engineering: Playing god? In S. Hongladarom (Ed.), *Genomics and bioethics: Interdisciplinary perspectives, technologies and advancements* (pp. 111–129). Hershey, PA: Medical Information Science Reference.

Daskalaki, A. (2010). *Informatics in oral medicine: Advanced techniques in clinical and diagnostic technologies*. Hershey, PA: IGI Global. doi:10.4018/978-1-60566-733-1

Davis, S. A. (2013). Global telemedicine and eHealth: Advances for future healthcare – Using a systems approach to integrate healthcare functions. In V. Gulla, A. Mori, F. Gabbrielli, & P. Lanzafame (Eds.), *Telehealth networks for hospital services: New methodologies* (pp. 15–32). Hershey, PA: Medical Information Science Reference. doi:10.4018/978-1-4666-2979-0.ch002

de Leeuw, E. (2012). The politics of medical curriculum accreditation: Thoughts, not facts? [IJUDH]. *International Journal of User-Driven Healthcare*, *2*(1), 53–69. doi:10.4018/ijudh.2012010108

De Luca, S., & Memo, E. (2010). Better knowledge for better health services: Discovering guideline compliance. In J. Rodrigues (Ed.), *Health information systems: Concepts, methodologies, tools, and applications* (pp. 233–255). Hershey, PA: Medical Information Science Reference.

DeSimio, T., & Chrisagis, X. (2012). Medical e-reference: A benchmark for e-reference publishing in other disciplines. In S. Polanka (Ed.), *E-reference context and discoverability in libraries: Issues and concepts* (pp. 116–125). Hershey, PA: Information Science Reference.

Dhakal, B., & Ross, S. D. (2011). Medical student perspectives: Journey through different worlds. In R. Biswas, & C. Martin (Eds.), *User-driven healthcare and narrative medicine: Utilizing collaborative social networks and technologies* (pp. 125–133). Hershey, PA: Medical Information Science Reference.

Dong, Y., Lu, H., Gajic, O., & Pickering, B. (2012). Intensive care unit operational modeling and analysis. In A. Kolker, & P. Story (Eds.), *Management engineering for effective healthcare delivery: Principles and applications* (pp. 132–147). Hershey, PA: Medical Information Science Reference.

Doyle, D. (2011). E-medical education: An overview. In A. Shukla, & R. Tiwari (Eds.), *Biomedical engineering and information systems: Technologies, tools and applications* (pp. 219–238). Hershey, PA: Medical Information Science Reference.

Driouchi, A. (2014). Introduction to labor and health economics: Mobility of medical doctors in the Mediterranean region. In A. Driouchi (Ed.), *Labor and health economics in the Mediterranean region: Migration and mobility of medical doctors* (pp. 1–22). Hershey, PA: Medical Information Science Reference.

Driouchi, A. (2014). Medical knowledge, north-south cooperation, and mobility of medical doctors. In A. Driouchi (Ed.), *Labor and health economics in the Mediterranean region: Migration and mobility of medical doctors* (pp. 376–395). Hershey, PA: Medical Information Science Reference.

Duan, X., Wang, X., & Huang, Q. (2014). Medical manipulators for surgical applications. In *Robotics: Concepts, methodologies, tools, and applications* (pp. 608-618). Hershey, PA: Information Science Reference. doi:10.4018/978-1-4666-4607-0.ch030

Dyro, J. F. (2012). Clinical engineering. In Z. Abu-Faraj (Ed.), *Handbook of research on biomedical engineering education and advanced bioengineering learning: Interdisciplinary concepts* (pp. 521–576). Hershey, PA: Medical Information Science Reference. doi:10.4018/978-1-4666-0122-2.ch012

El Morr, C., & Subercaze, J. (2010). Knowledge management in healthcare. In M. Cruz-Cunha, A. Tavares, & R. Simoes (Eds.), *Handbook of research on developments in e-health and telemedicine: Technological and social perspectives* (pp. 490–510). Hershey, PA: Medical Information Science Reference.

Eleni, A., & Maglogiannis, I. (2010). Adoption of wearable systems in modern patient telemonitoring systems. In M. Cruz-Cunha, A. Tavares, & R. Simoes (Eds.), *Handbook of research on developments in e-health and telemedicine: Technological and social perspectives* (pp. 1004–1023). Hershey, PA: Medical Information Science Reference.

Epstein, J. H., Goldberg, A., Krol, M., & Levine, A. (2013). Virtual tools in medical education. In Y. Kats (Ed.), *Learning management systems and instructional design: Best practices in online education* (pp. 364–380). Hershey, PA: Information Science Reference. doi:10.4018/978-1-4666-3930-0.ch019

Eskeland, S., & Oleshchuk, V. (2010). Information security and privacy in medical application scenario. In K. Khoumbati, Y. Dwivedi, A. Srivastava, & B. Lal (Eds.), *Handbook of research on advances in health informatics and electronic healthcare applications: Global adoption and impact of information communication technologies* (pp. 274–287). Hershey, PA: Medical Information Science Reference.

Esposito, A. (2013). The impact of social media on scholarly practices in higher education: Online engagement and ICTs appropriation in senior, young, and doctoral researchers. In B. Pătruţ, M. Pătruţ, & C. Cmeciu (Eds.), *Social media and the new academic environment: Pedagogical challenges* (pp. 342–367). Hershey, PA: Information Science Reference. doi:10.4018/978-1-4666-2851-9.ch017

Facelli, J. C., Hurdle, J. F., & Mitchell, J. A. (2012). Medical informatics and bioinformatics. In Z. Abu-Faraj (Ed.), *Handbook of research on biomedical engineering education and advanced bioengineering learning: Interdisciplinary concepts* (pp. 577–604). Hershey, PA: Medical Information Science Reference. doi:10.4018/978-1-4666-0122-2.ch013

Fairchild, K. D., & Moorman, J. R. (2012). Heart rate characteristics monitoring in the NICU: A new tool for clinical care and research. In W. Chen, S. Oetomo, & L. Feijs (Eds.), *Neonatal monitoring technologies: Design for integrated solutions* (pp. 175–200). Hershey, PA: Medical Information Science Reference. doi:10.4018/978-1-4666-0975-4.ch008

Fakhar, A. (2014). Beyond brain drain: A case study of the benefits of cooperation on medical immigration. In A. Driouchi (Ed.), *Labor and health economics in the Mediterranean region: Migration and mobility of medical doctors* (pp. 294–313). Hershey, PA: Medical Information Science Reference. doi:10.4018/978-1-4666-4979-8.ch044

Farrell, M. (2011). Use of handheld computers in nursing education. In *Clinical technologies: Concepts, methodologies, tools and applications* (pp. 1504-1517). Hershey, PA: Medical Information Science Reference. doi:10.4018/978-1-60960-561-2.ch507

Ferrer-Roca, O. (2011). Standards in telemedicine. In A. Moumtzoglou, & A. Kastania (Eds.), *E-health systems quality and reliability: Models and standards* (pp. 220–243). Hershey, PA: Medical Information Science Reference.

Fiaidhi, J., Mohammed, S., & Wei, Y. (2010). Implications of web 2.0 technology on healthcare: A biomedical semantic blog case study. In S. Kabene (Ed.), *Healthcare and the effect of technology: Developments, challenges and advancements* (pp. 269–289). Hershey, PA: Medical Information Science Reference. doi:10.4018/978-1-61520-733-6.ch016

Fialho, A. S., Cismondi, F., Vieira, S. M., Reti, S. R., Sousa, J. M., & Finkelstein, S. N. (2013). Challenges and opportunities of soft computing tools in health care delivery. In M. Cruz-Cunha, I. Miranda, & P. Gonçalves (Eds.), *Handbook of research on ICTs and management systems for improving efficiency in healthcare and social care* (pp. 321–340). Hershey, PA: Medical Information Science Reference. doi:10.4018/978-1-4666-3990-4.ch016

Freitas, A., Brazdil, P., & Costa-Pereira, A. (2012). Cost-sensitive learning in medicine. In Machine learning: Concepts, methodologies, tools and applications (pp. 1625-1641). Hershey, PA: Information Science Reference. doi:10.4018/978-1-60960-818-7.ch607

Freitas, A., & Costa-Pereira, A. (2010). Learning cost-sensitive decision trees to support medical diagnosis. In T. Nguyen (Ed.), *Complex data warehousing and knowledge discovery for advanced retrieval development: Innovative methods and applications* (pp. 287–307). Hershey, PA: Information Science Reference.

Freitas, L., Pereira, R. T., Pereira, H. G., Martini, R., Mozzaquatro, B. A., Kasper, J., & Librelotto, G. (2013). Ontological representation and an architecture for homecare pervasive systems. In R. Martinho, R. Rijo, M. Cruz-Cunha, & J. Varajão (Eds.), *Information systems and technologies for enhancing health and social care* (pp. 215–234). Hershey, PA: Medical Information Science Reference. doi:10.4018/978-1-4666-3667-5.ch015

Frigo, C. A., & Pavan, E. E. (2014). Prosthetic and orthotic devices. In *Assistive technologies: Concepts, methodologies, tools, and applications* (pp. 549–613). Hershey, PA: Information Science Reference.

Frunza, O., & Inkpen, D. (2012). Natural language processing and machine learning techniques help achieve a better medical practice. In R. Magdalena-Benedito, E. Soria-Olivas, J. Martínez, J. Gómez-Sanchis, & A. Serrano-López (Eds.), *Medical applications of intelligent data analysis: Research advancements* (pp. 237–254). Hershey, PA: Information Science Reference. doi:10.4018/978-1-4666-1803-9.ch016

Fung-Kee-Fung, M., Morash, R., & Goubanova, E. (2011). Evaluating CoPs in cancer surgery. In O. Hernáez, & E. Bueno Campos (Eds.), *Handbook of research on communities of practice for organizational management and networking: Methodologies for competitive advantage* (pp. 456–466). Hershey, PA: Information Science Reference. doi:10.4018/978-1-60566-802-4.ch025

Gabbrielli, F. (2013). Telemedicine R&D influencing incoming strategies and organization models. In V. Gulla, A. Mori, F. Gabbrielli, & P. Lanzafame (Eds.), *Telehealth networks for hospital services: New methodologies* (pp. 250–264). Hershey, PA: Medical Information Science Reference. doi:10.4018/978-1-4666-2979-0.ch017

Ganz, A., Schafer, J., Yu, X., Lord, G., Burstein, J., & Ciottone, G. R. (2013). Real-time scalable resource tracking framework (DIORAMA) for mass casualty incidents. [IJEHMC]. *International Journal of E-Health and Medical Communications*, *4*(2), 34–49. doi:10.4018/jehmc.2013040103

Gao, X. W., Loomes, M., & Comley, R. (2012). Bridging the abridged: The diffusion of telemedicine in Europe and China. In J. Rodrigues, I. de la Torre Díez, & B. Sainz de Abajo (Eds.), *Telemedicine and e-health services, policies, and applications: Advancements and developments* (pp. 451–495). Hershey, PA: Medical Information Science Reference. doi:10.4018/978-1-4666-0888-7.ch017

Gavgani, V. Z. (2011). Ubiquitous information therapy service through social networking libraries: An operational web 2.0 service model. In R. Biswas, & C. Martin (Eds.), *User-driven healthcare and narrative medicine: Utilizing collaborative social networks and technologies* (pp. 446–461). Hershey, PA: Medical Information Science Reference.

Germaine-McDaniel, N. S. (2013). The emerging hispanic use of online health information in the United States: Cultural convergence or dissociation? In User-driven healthcare: Concepts, methodologies, tools, and applications (pp. 1607-1621). Hershey, PA: Medical Information Science Reference. doi:10.4018/978-1-4666-2770-3.ch079

Ghalib, N. (2014). The design and implementation of paperless medical system (PMS) for offshore operating company: A structured approach. In Software design and development: Concepts, methodologies, tools, and applications (pp. 1064-1072). Hershey, PA: Information Science Reference. doi:10.4018/978-1-4666-4301-7.ch051

Gill, S., & Paranjape, R. (2010). A review of recent contribution in agent-based health care modeling. In J. Rodrigues (Ed.), *Health information systems: Concepts, methodologies, tools, and applications* (pp. 356–373). Hershey, PA: Medical Information Science Reference.

Gilligan, J., & Smith, P. (2014). A formal representation system for modelling assistive technology systems. In G. Kouroupetroglou (Ed.), *Disability informatics and web accessibility for motor limitations* (pp. 1–42). Hershey, PA: Medical Information Science Reference.

Goldberg, E. M. (2014). Business continuity and disaster recovery considerations for healthcare technology. In Crisis management: Concepts, methodologies, tools and applications (pp. 1455-1462). Hershey, PA: Information Science Reference. doi:10.4018/978-1-4666-4707-7.ch073

Gonçalves, F., & David, G. (2013). Definition of a retrospective health information policy based on (re)use study. In M. Cruz-Cunha, I. Miranda, & P. Gonçalves (Eds.), *Handbook of research on ICTs and management systems for improving efficiency in healthcare and social care* (pp. 1130–1155). Hershey, PA: Medical Information Science Reference. doi:10.4018/978-1-4666-3990-4.ch059

Gopalakrishnan, R., & Mugler, D. H. (2010). The evolution of hermite transform in biomedical applications. In A. Shukla, & R. Tiwari (Eds.), *Intelligent medical technologies and biomedical engineering: Tools and applications* (pp. 260–278). Hershey, PA: Medical Information Science Reference. doi:10.4018/978-1-61520-977-4.ch013

Goyal, R. K., O'Neill, M., Agostinelli, N., & Wyer, P. (2011). Critical illness and the emergency room. In R. Biswas, & C. Martin (Eds.), *User-driven healthcare and narrative medicine: Utilizing collaborative social networks and technologies* (pp. 63–74). Hershey, PA: Medical Information Science Reference.

Graham, I. W. (2011). The nature of nursing work. In A. Cashin, & R. Cook (Eds.), *Evidence-based practice in nursing informatics: Concepts and applications* (pp. 51–63). Hershey, PA: Medical Information Science Reference.

Greenshields, I., & El-Sayed, G. (2012). Aspects of visualization and the grid in a biomedical context. In Grid and cloud computing: Concepts, methodologies, tools and applications (pp. 1686-1701). Hershey, PA: Information Science Reference. doi:10.4018/978-1-4666-0879-5.ch710

Grimnes, S., & Høgetveit, J. O. (2012). Biomedical sensors. In Z. Abu-Faraj (Ed.), *Handbook of research on biomedical engineering education and advanced bioengineering learning: Interdisciplinary concepts* (pp. 356–436). Hershey, PA: Medical Information Science Reference. doi:10.4018/978-1-4666-0122-2.ch009

Guedouar, R., & Zarrad, B. (2012). Forward projection for use with iterative reconstruction. In A. Malik, T. Choi, & H. Nisar (Eds.), *Depth map and 3D imaging applications: Algorithms and technologies* (pp. 27–55). Hershey, PA: Information Science Reference.

Gullà, V. (2013). Leading the technological innovation in healthcare systems: The telematic medicine approach. In V. Gulla, A. Mori, F. Gabbrielli, & P. Lanzafame (Eds.), *Telehealth networks for hospital services: New methodologies* (pp. 134–153). Hershey, PA: Medical Information Science Reference. doi:10.4018/978-1-4666-2979-0.ch009

Guo, R., Wang, Y., Yan, H., Li, F., Yan, J., & Xu, Z. (2011). Pulse wave analysis of traditional chinese medicine based on hemodynamics principles. In L. Liu, D. Wei, & Y. Li (Eds.), *Interdisciplinary research and applications in bioinformatics, computational biology, and environmental sciences* (pp. 194–203). Hershey, PA: Medical Information Science Reference.

Gupta, A., Goyal, R. K., Joiner, K. A., & Saini, S. (2010). Outsourcing in the healthcare industry: Information technology, intellectual property, and allied aspects. In M. Khosrow-Pour (Ed.), *Global, social, and organizational implications of emerging information resources management: Concepts and applications* (pp. 18–44). Hershey, PA: Information Science Reference. doi:10.4018/978-1-61520-965-1.ch715

Gupta, S., Mukherjee, S., & Roy, S. S. (2013). Modernization of healthcare and medical diagnosis system using multi agent system (MAS): A comparative study. In S. Bhattacharyya, & P. Dutta (Eds.), *Handbook of research on computational intelligence for engineering, science, and business* (pp. 592–622). Hershey, PA: Information Science Reference.

Ha, S. H. (2011). Medical domain knowledge and associative classification rules in diagnosis. [IJKDB]. *International Journal of Knowledge Discovery in Bioinformatics*, *2*(1), 60–73. doi:10.4018/jkdb.2011010104

Haheim, L. L., & Morland, B. (2010). Health technology assessment: Development and future. In J. Rodrigues (Ed.), *Health information systems: Concepts, methodologies, tools, and applications* (pp. 26–41). Hershey, PA: Medical Information Science Reference.

Hai-Jew, S. (2010). An elusive formula: The IT role in behavior change in public health. In T. Yuzer, & G. Kurubacak (Eds.), *Transformative learning and online education: Aesthetics, dimensions and concepts* (pp. 347–373). Hershey, PA: Information Science Reference. doi:10.4018/978-1-61520-985-9.ch022

Haida, M. (2013). Implications of NIRS brain signals. In J. Wu (Ed.), *Biomedical engineering and cognitive neuroscience for healthcare: Interdisciplinary applications* (pp. 120–128). Hershey, PA: Medical Information Science Reference.

Haidegger, T. (2012). Surgical robots: System development, assessment, and clearance. In T. Sobh, & X. Xiong (Eds.), *Prototyping of robotic systems: Applications of design and implementation* (pp. 288–326). Hershey, PA: Information Science Reference. doi:10.4018/978-1-4666-0176-5.ch010

Hajiheydari, N., Khakbaz, S. B., & Farhadi, H. (2013). Proposing a business model in healthcare industry: E-diagnosis. [IJHISI]. *International Journal of Healthcare Information Systems and Informatics*, *8*(2), 41–57. doi:10.4018/jhisi.2013040104

Hanada, E. (2013). Effective use of RFID in medicine and general healthcare. In T. Issa, P. Isaías, & P. Kommers (Eds.), *Information systems and technology for organizations in a networked society* (pp. 335–352). Hershey, PA: Business Science Reference. doi:10.4018/978-1-4666-4062-7.ch018

Hara, H. (2013). Women and health in Japan: The rise and obstacles of gender and sex-specific medicine. In M. Merviö (Ed.), *Healthcare management and economics: Perspectives on public and private administration* (pp. 203–207). Hershey, PA: Medical Information Science Reference. doi:10.4018/978-1-4666-3982-9.ch016

Harnett, B. (2013). Patient centered medicine and technology adaptation. In User-driven healthcare: Concepts, methodologies, tools, and applications (pp. 77-98). Hershey, PA: Medical Information Science Reference. doi:10.4018/978-1-4666-2770-3.ch005

Hatton, J. D., Schmidt, T. M., & Jelen, J. (2013). Adoption of electronic health care records: Physician heuristics and hesitancy. In R. Martinho, R. Rijo, M. Cruz-Cunha, & J. Varajão (Eds.), *Information systems and technologies for enhancing health and social care* (pp. 148–165). Hershey, PA: Medical Information Science Reference. doi:10.4018/978-1-4666-3667-5.ch010

Heaberg, G. (2011). Case study: Research matchmaker, an advanced nursing practice informatics application. In A. Cashin, & R. Cook (Eds.), *Evidence-based practice in nursing informatics: Concepts and applications* (pp. 217–236). Hershey, PA: Medical Information Science Reference.

Hegde, B. (2011). Learning medicine: A personal view. In R. Biswas, & C. Martin (Eds.), *User-driven healthcare and narrative medicine: Utilizing collaborative social networks and technologies* (pp. 184–190). Hershey, PA: Medical Information Science Reference.

Heilman, J. (2012). Creating awareness for using a wiki to promote collaborative health professional education. [IJUDH]. *International Journal of User-Driven Healthcare*, *2*(1), 86–87. doi:10.4018/ijudh.2012010113

Heinzel, A., Fechete, R., Söllner, J., Perco, P., Heinze, G., & Oberbauer, R. et al. (2012). Data graphs for linking clinical phenotype and molecular feature space. [IJSBBT]. *International Journal of Systems Biology and Biomedical Technologies*, *1*(1), 11–25. doi:10.4018/ijsbbt.2012010102

Hernández-Chan, G. S., Rodríguez-González, A., & Colomo-Palacios, R. (2013). Using social networks to obtain medical diagnosis. In M. Cruz-Cunha, I. Miranda, & P. Gonçalves (Eds.), *Handbook of research on ICTs and management systems for improving efficiency in healthcare and social care* (pp. 306–320). Hershey, PA: Medical Information Science Reference. doi:10.4018/978-1-4666-3990-4.ch015

Hine, M. J., Farion, K. J., Michalowski, W., & Wilk, S. (2011). Decision making by emergency room physicians and residents: Implications for the design of clinical decision support systems. In J. Tan (Ed.), *New technologies for advancing healthcare and clinical practices* (pp. 131–148). Hershey, PA: Medical Information Science Reference. doi:10.4018/978-1-60960-780-7.ch008

Hoonakker, P., McGuire, K., & Carayon, P. (2011). Sociotechnical issues of tele-ICU technology. In D. Haftor, & A. Mirijamdotter (Eds.), *Information and communication technologies, society and human beings: Theory and framework (festschrift in honor of Gunilla Bradley)* (pp. 225–240). Hershey, PA: Information Science Reference.

Hopper, K. B., & Johns, C. L. (2012). Educational technology in the medical industry. In Wireless technologies: Concepts, methodologies, tools and applications (pp. 1306-1322). Hershey, PA: Information Science Reference. doi:10.4018/978-1-61350-101-6.ch511

Hsu, P., Tsai, W., & Tsai, C. (2013). Patient safety concerns among emergency medical staff and patients. [IJPHIM]. *International Journal of Privacy and Health Information Management*, *1*(1), 29–52. doi:10.4018/ijphim.2013010103

Huang, K., Geller, J., Halper, M., Elhanan, G., & Perl, Y. (2011). Scalability of piecewise synonym identification in integration of SNOMED into the UMLS. [IJCMAM]. *International Journal of Computational Models and Algorithms in Medicine*, *2*(3), 26–45. doi:10.4018/jcmam.2011070103

Hughes, B. (2012). Managing e-health in the age of web 2.0: The impact on e-health evaluation. In E-marketing: Concepts, methodologies, tools, and applications (pp. 1268-1288). Hershey, PA: Business Science Reference. doi:10.4018/978-1-4666-1598-4.ch074

Hyde, A., Nee, J., Butler, M., Drennan, J., & Howlett, E. (2011). Preferred types of menopause service delivery: A qualitative study of menopausal women's perceptions. [IJHDRI]. *International Journal of Healthcare Delivery Reform Initiatives*, *3*(1), 1–12. doi:10.4018/jhdri.2011010101

Ilie, V., Van Slyke, C., Courtney, J. F., & Styne, P. (2011). Challenges associated with physicians' usage of electronic medical records. In J. Tan (Ed.), *New technologies for advancing healthcare and clinical practices* (pp. 234–251). Hershey, PA: Medical Information Science Reference. doi:10.4018/978-1-60960-780-7.ch014

Inomata, C., & Nitta, S. (2013). Nursing in integrative medicine and nurses' engagement in caring-healing: A discussion based on the practice and study of music therapy and nursing care for patients with neurodegenerative disorders. In J. Wu (Ed.), *Technological advancements in biomedicine for healthcare applications* (pp. 235–239). Hershey, PA: Medical Information Science Reference.

Inthiran, A., Alhashmi, S. M., & Ahmed, P. K. (2012). Medical information retrieval strategies: An exploratory study on the information retrieval behaviors of non-medical professionals. [IJHISI]. *International Journal of Healthcare Information Systems and Informatics*, *7*(1), 31–45. doi:10.4018/jhisi.2012010103

Isern, D., & Moreno, A. (2010). HeCaSe2: A multi-agent system that automates the application of clinical guidelines. In R. Paranjape, & A. Sadanand (Eds.), *Multi-agent systems for healthcare simulation and modeling: Applications for system improvement* (pp. 113–136). Hershey, PA: Medical Information Science Reference.

Ishaq, G. M., Hussain, P. T., Iqbal, M. J., & Mushtaq, M. B. (2013). Risk-benefit analysis of combination vs. unopposed HRT in post-menopausal women. In Bioinformatics: Concepts, methodologies, tools, and applications (pp. 1424-1440). Hershey, PA: Medical Information Science Reference. doi:10.4018/978-1-4666-3604-0.ch073

Iwaki, S. (2013). Multimodal neuroimaging to visualize human visual processing. In J. Wu (Ed.), *Biomedical engineering and cognitive neuroscience for healthcare: Interdisciplinary applications* (pp. 274–282). Hershey, PA: Medical Information Science Reference.

James, R. (2011). Practical pointers in medicine over seven decades: Reflections of an individual physician. In R. Biswas, & C. Martin (Eds.), *User-driven healthcare and narrative medicine: Utilizing collaborative social networks and technologies* (pp. 173–183). Hershey, PA: Medical Information Science Reference.

Janczewski, M. (2010). Healthcare transformation in a net-centric environment. In S. Ghosh (Ed.), *Net centricity and technological interoperability in organizations: Perspectives and strategies* (pp. 99–114). Hershey, PA: Information Science Reference.

Jesus, Â., & Gomes, M. J. (2013). Web 2.0 tools in biomedical education: Limitations and possibilities. In Y. Kats (Ed.), *Learning management systems and instructional design: Best practices in online education* (pp. 208–231). Hershey, PA: Information Science Reference. doi:10.4018/978-1-4666-3930-0.ch011

Ji, Z., Sugi, T., Goto, S., Wang, X., & Nakamura, M. (2013). Multi-channel template extraction for automatic EEG spike detection. In J. Wu (Ed.), *Biomedical engineering and cognitive neuroscience for healthcare: Interdisciplinary applications* (pp. 255–265). Hershey, PA: Medical Information Science Reference.

Jifa, G., Wuqi, S., Zhengxiang, Z., Rui, G., & Yijun, L. (2012). Expert mining and traditional Chinese medicine knowledge. In W. Lee (Ed.), *Systems approaches to knowledge management, transfer, and resource development* (pp. 239–251). Hershey, PA: Information Science Reference. doi:10.4018/978-1-4666-1782-7.ch016

Johnson, D. E. (2012). Electronic medical records (EMR): Issues and implementation perspectives. In A. Kolker, & P. Story (Eds.), *Management engineering for effective healthcare delivery: Principles and applications* (pp. 333–351). Hershey, PA: Medical Information Science Reference.

Johnson, K., & Tashiro, J. (2013). Interprofessional care and health care complexity: Factors shaping human resources effectiveness in health information management. In User-driven healthcare: Concepts, methodologies, tools, and applications (pp. 1273-1302). Hershey, PA: Medical Information Science Reference. doi:10.4018/978-1-4666-2770-3.ch064

Jose, J. (2012). Pharmacovigilance: Basic concepts and applications of pharmacoinformatics. In T. Gasmelseid (Ed.), *Pharmacoinformatics and drug discovery technologies: Theories and applications* (pp. 322–343). Hershey, PA: Medical Information Science Reference. doi:10.4018/978-1-4666-0309-7.ch020

Juzoji, H. (2012). Legal bases for medical supervision via mobile telecommunications in Japan. [IJEHMC]. *International Journal of E-Health and Medical Communications*, *3*(1), 33–45. doi:10.4018/jehmc.2012010103

Juzwishin, D. W. (2010). Enabling technologies and challenges for the future of ubiquitous health the interoperability framework. In S. Mohammed, & J. Fiaidhi (Eds.), *Ubiquitous health and medical informatics: The ubiquity 2.0 trend and beyond* (pp. 596–622). Hershey, PA: Medical Information Science Reference. doi:10.4018/978-1-61520-777-0.ch028

Kabene, S., & Wolfe, M. (2011). Risks and benefits of technology in health care. In *Clinical technologies: Concepts, methodologies, tools and applications* (pp. 13-24). Hershey, PA: Medical Information Science Reference. doi:10.4018/978-1-60960-561-2.ch102

Kabene, S. M. King, Lisa, & Gibson, C. J. (2010). Technology and human resources management in health care. In S. Mohammed, & J. Fiaidhi (Eds.) Ubiquitous health and medical informatics: The ubiquity 2.0 trend and beyond (pp. 574-595). Hershey, PA: Medical Information Science Reference. doi:10.4018/978-1-61520-777-0.ch027

Kabene, S. M., Wolfe, M., & Leduc, R. (2012). Recruitment and retention of healthcare professionals for the changing demographics, culture, and access in Canada. In Human resources management: Concepts, methodologies, tools, and applications (pp. 276-290). Hershey, PA: Business Science Reference. doi:10.4018/978-1-4666-1601-1.ch017

Kadiri, M., & Zouag, N. (2014). The new economics of skilled labor migration: The case of medical doctors in MENA. In A. Driouchi (Ed.), *Labor and health economics in the Mediterranean region: Migration and mobility of medical doctors* (pp. 267–292). Hershey, PA: Medical Information Science Reference.

Kalantri, S. P. (2012). On being a patient. [IJUDH]. *International Journal of User-Driven Healthcare*, *2*(4), 1–4. doi:10.4018/ijudh.2012100101

Kaldoudi, E., Konstantinidis, S., & Bamidis, P. D. (2010). Web 2.0 approaches for active, collaborative learning in medicine and health. In S. Mohammed, & J. Fiaidhi (Eds.), *Ubiquitous health and medical informatics: The ubiquity 2.0 trend and beyond* (pp. 127–149). Hershey, PA: Medical Information Science Reference. doi:10.4018/978-1-61520-777-0.ch007

Kannry, J. L. (2011). Operationalizing the science. In *Clinical technologies: Concepts, methodologies, tools and applications* (pp. 1600-1622). Hershey, PA: Medical Information Science Reference. doi:10.4018/978-1-60960-561-2.ch601

Karayanni, D. (2010). A cluster analysis of physician's values, prescribing behaviour and attitudes towards firms' marketing communications. [IJCRMM]. *International Journal of Customer Relationship Marketing and Management*, *1*(4), 62–79. doi:10.4018/jcrmm.2010100104

Kastania, A., & Moumtzoglou, A. (2012). Quality implications of the medical applications for 4G mobile phones. [IJRQEH]. *International Journal of Reliable and Quality E-Healthcare*, *1*(1), 58–67. doi:10.4018/ijrqeh.2012010106

Kastania, A. N. (2013). Evaluation considerations for e-health systems. In User-driven healthcare: Concepts, methodologies, tools, and applications (pp. 1126-1140). Hershey, PA: Medical Information Science Reference. doi:10.4018/978-1-4666-2770-3.ch057

Kaufman, D. (2010). Simulation in health professional education. In D. Kaufman, & L. Sauvé (Eds.), *Educational gameplay and simulation environments: Case studies and lessons learned* (pp. 51–67). Hershey, PA: Information Science Reference. doi:10.4018/978-1-61520-731-2.ch003

Kazandjian, V. A. (2013). Learning to accept uncertainty as a quality of care dimension. In A. Moumtzoglou, & A. Kastania (Eds.), *E-health technologies and improving patient safety: Exploring organizational factors* (pp. 1–12). Hershey, PA: Medical Information Science Reference.

Kearns, W. D., Fozard, J. L., & Lamm, R. S. (2011). How knowing who, where and when can change health care delivery. In C. Röcker, & M. Ziefle (Eds.), *E-health, assistive technologies and applications for assisted living: Challenges and solutions* (pp. 139–160). Hershey, PA: Medical Information Science Reference. doi:10.4018/978-1-60960-469-1.ch007

Khan, T. (2013). Transformation of a reluctant patient to a proactive health advocate. [IJUDH]. *International Journal of User-Driven Healthcare*, *3*(1), 71–74. doi:10.4018/ijudh.2013010109

Khetarpal, A., & Singh, S. (2012). Disability studies in medical education. [IJUDH]. *International Journal of User-Driven Healthcare*, *2*(2), 44–51. doi:10.4018/ijudh.2012040105

Kim, J. (2011). The development and implementation of patient safety information systems (PSIS). In *Clinical technologies: Concepts, methodologies, tools and applications* (pp. 2054-2072). Hershey, PA: Medical Information Science Reference. doi:10.4018/978-1-60960-561-2.ch804

Kldiashvili, E. (2011). The application of virtual organization technology for eHealth. In E. Kldiashvili (Ed.), *Grid technologies for e-health: Applications for telemedicine services and delivery* (pp. 1–17). Hershey, PA: Medical Information Science Reference.

Kldiashvili, E. (2012). The cloud computing as the tool for implementation of virtual organization technology for eHealth. [JITR]. *Journal of Information Technology Research*, *5*(1), 18–34. doi:10.4018/jitr.2012010102

Kldiashvili, E. (2013). Implementation of telecytology in Georgia. In V. Gulla, A. Mori, F. Gabbrielli, & P. Lanzafame (Eds.), *Telehealth networks for hospital services: New methodologies* (pp. 341–361). Hershey, PA: Medical Information Science Reference. doi:10.4018/978-1-4666-2979-0.ch022

Klemer, D. P. (2010). Advances in biosensors for in vitro diagnostics. In A. Lazakidou (Ed.), *Biocomputation and biomedical informatics: Case studies and applications* (pp. 178–186). Hershey, PA: Medical Information Science Reference.

Kotwani, A. (2013). Transparency and accountability in public procurement of essential medicines in developing countries. In *Supply chain management: Concepts, methodologies, tools, and applications* (pp. 1437–1452). Hershey, PA: Business Science Reference.

Kuehler, M., Schimke, N., & Hale, J. (2012). Privacy considerations for electronic health records. In G. Yee (Ed.), *Privacy protection measures and technologies in business organizations: Aspects and standards* (pp. 210–226). Hershey, PA: Information Science Reference.

Kukar, M., Kononenko, I., & Grošelj, C. (2013). Automated diagnostics of coronary artery disease: Long-term results and recent advancements. In *Data mining: Concepts, methodologies, tools, and applications* (pp. 1043–1063). Hershey, PA: Information Science Reference.

Kumalasari, C. D., Caplow, J. A., & Fearing, N. (2013). Simulation followed by a reflection and feedback session in medical education. In L. Tomei (Ed.), *Learning tools and teaching approaches through ICT advancements* (pp. 68–81). Hershey, PA: Information Science Reference.

Kumar, R., & Srivastava, R. (2014). Detection of cancer from microscopic biopsy images using image processing tools. In R. Srivastava, S. Singh, & K. Shukla (Eds.), *Research developments in computer vision and image processing: Methodologies and applications* (pp. 175–194). Hershey, PA: Information Science Reference.

Kuruvilla, A., & Alexander, S. M. (2010). Predicting ambulance diverson. [IJISSS]. *International Journal of Information Systems in the Service Sector, 2*(1), 1–10. doi:10.4018/jisss.2010093001

Kyriazis, D., Menychtas, A., Tserpes, K., Athanaileas, T., & Varvarigou, T. (2010). High performance computing in biomedicine. In A. Lazakidou (Ed.), *Biocomputation and biomedical informatics: Case studies and applications* (pp. 106–118). Hershey, PA: Medical Information Science Reference.

LaBrunda, M., & LaBrunda, A. (2010). Fuzzy logic in medicine. In M. Khosrow-Pour (Ed.), *Breakthrough discoveries in information technology research: Advancing trends* (pp. 218–224). Hershey, PA: Information Science Reference.

Lagares-Lemos, Á. M., Lagares-Lemos, M., Colomo-Palacios, R., García-Crespo, Á., & Gómez-Berbís, J. M. (2011). DISMON. In *Clinical technologies: Concepts, methodologies, tools and applications* (pp. 995-1007). Hershey, PA: Medical Information Science Reference. doi:10.4018/978-1-60960-561-2.ch324

Lagares-Lemos, Á. M., Lagares-Lemos, M., Colomo-Palacios, R., García-Crespo, Á., & Gómez-Berbís, J. M. (2013). DISMON: Using social web and semantic technologies to monitor diseases in limited environments. In M. Khosrow-Pour (Ed.), *Interdisciplinary advances in information technology research* (pp. 48–59). Hershey, PA: Information Science Reference. doi:10.4018/978-1-4666-3625-5.ch004

Lappas, K. (2014). Functional assessment of persons with motor limitations: Methods and tools. In G. Kouroupetroglou (Ed.), *Disability informatics and web accessibility for motor limitations* (pp. 43–74). Hershey, PA: Medical Information Science Reference.

Lazakidou, A., & Daskalaki, A. (2012). *Quality assurance in healthcare service delivery, nursing and personalized medicine: Technologies and processes*. Hershey, PA: IGI Global.

Leal, S., Suarez, C., Framinan, J. M., Parra, C. L., & Gómez, T. (2010). Virtual reality for supporting surgical planning. In M. Cruz-Cunha, A. Tavares, & R. Simoes (Eds.), *Handbook of research on developments in e-health and telemedicine: Technological and social perspectives* (pp. 614–635). Hershey, PA: Medical Information Science Reference.

Lemma, F., Denko, M. K., Tan, J. K., & Kassegne, S. K. (2011). Envisioning a national e-medicine network architecture in a developing country: A case study. In J. Tan (Ed.), *Developments in healthcare information systems and technologies: Models and methods* (pp. 35–53). Hershey, PA: Medical Information Science Reference.

Li, G., You, M., Xu, L., & Huang, S. (2012). Personalized experience sharing of Cai's TCM gynecology. In A. Lazakidou, & A. Daskalaki (Eds.), *Quality assurance in healthcare service delivery, nursing and personalized medicine: Technologies and processes* (pp. 26–47). Hershey, PA: Medical Information Science Reference.

Lim, V. K. (2012). The process of medical curriculum development in Malaysia. [IJUDH]. *International Journal of User-Driven Healthcare*, *2*(1), 33–39. doi:10.4018/ijudh.2012010105

Lin, H. (2013). Cultivating chan as proactive therapy for social wellness. In M. Cruz-Cunha, I. Miranda, & P. Gonçalves (Eds.), *Handbook of research on ICTs for human-centered healthcare and social care services* (pp. 151–170). Hershey, PA: Medical Information Science Reference. doi:10.4018/978-1-4666-3986-7.ch008

Liu, Q., Poon, C. C., & Zhang, Y. T. (2012). Wearable technologies for neonatal monitoring. In W. Chen, S. Oetomo, & L. Feijs (Eds.), *Neonatal monitoring technologies: Design for integrated solutions* (pp. 12–40). Hershey, PA: Medical Information Science Reference. doi:10.4018/978-1-4666-0975-4.ch002

Llobet, H., Llobet, P., & LaBrunda, M. (2011). Imaging advances of the cardiopulmonary system. In *Clinical technologies: Concepts, methodologies, tools and applications* (pp. 2183-2190). Hershey, PA: Medical Information Science Reference. doi:10.4018/978-1-60960-561-2.ch812

Logeswaran, R. (2010). Neural networks in medicine: improving difficult automated detection of cancer in the bile ducts. In R. Chiong (Ed.), *Nature-inspired informatics for intelligent applications and knowledge discovery: Implications in business, science, and engineering* (pp. 144–165). Hershey, PA: Information Science Reference.

Logeswaran, R. (2011). Neural networks in medicine. In *Clinical technologies: Concepts, methodologies, tools and applications* (pp. 744-765). Hershey, PA: Medical Information Science Reference. doi:10.4018/978-1-60960-561-2.ch308

Long, L. R., Antani, S., Thoma, G. R., & Deserno, T. M. (2011). Content-based image retrieval for advancing medical diagnostics, treatment and education. In J. Tan (Ed.), *New technologies for advancing healthcare and clinical practices* (pp. 1–17). Hershey, PA: Medical Information Science Reference. doi:10.4018/978-1-60960-780-7.ch001

Lueth, T. C., D'Angelo, L. T., & Czabke, A. (2010). TUM-AgeTech: A new framework for pervasive medical devices. In A. Coronato, & G. De Pietro (Eds.), *Pervasive and smart technologies for healthcare: Ubiquitous methodologies and tools* (pp. 295–321). Hershey, PA: Medical Information Science Reference. doi:10.4018/978-1-61520-765-7.ch014

Lui, K. (2013). The health informatics professional. In User-driven healthcare: Concepts, methodologies, tools, and applications(pp. 120-141). Hershey, PA: Medical Information Science Reference. doi:10.4018/978-1-4666-2770-3.ch007

Lui, T., & Goel, L. (2012). A framework for conceptualizing the current role and future trends of information systems in medical training. [IJHISI]. *International Journal of Healthcare Information Systems and Informatics*, *7*(1), 1–12. doi:10.4018/jhisi.2012010101

MacDonald, C. J., McKeen, M., Leith-Gudbranson, D., Montpetit, M., Archibald, D., & Rivet, C. … Hirsh, M. (2013). University of Ottawa department of family medicine faculty development curriculum framework. In K. Patel, & S. Vij (Eds.) Enterprise resource planning models for the education sector: Applications and methodologies (pp. 197-215). Hershey, PA: Information Science Reference. doi:10.4018/978-1-4666-2193-0.ch014

MacGregor, R. C., Hyland, P. N., & Harvie, C. (2010). Associations between driving forces to adopt ICT and benefits derived from that adoption in medical practices in Australia. In M. Cruz-Cunha, A. Tavares, & R. Simoes (Eds.), *Handbook of research on developments in e-health and telemedicine: Technological and social perspectives* (pp. 652–668). Hershey, PA: Medical Information Science Reference.

Mackert, M., Whitten, P., & Holtz, B. (2010). Health infonomics: Intelligent applications of information technology. In J. Rodrigues (Ed.), *Health information systems: Concepts, methodologies, tools, and applications* (pp. 117–132). Hershey, PA: Medical Information Science Reference.

Malik, A. S., & Malik, R. H. (2012). Adolescent medicine curriculum at faculty of medicine, Universiti Teknologi MARA, Malaysia. [IJUDH]. *International Journal of User-Driven Healthcare*, *2*(1), 40–48. doi:10.4018/ijudh.2012010106

Martin, C. M., Biswas, R., Sturmberg, J. P., Topps, D., Ellaway, R., & Smith, K. (2011). Patient journey record systems (PaJR) for preventing ambulatory care sensitive conditions: A developmental framework. In R. Biswas, & C. Martin (Eds.), *User-driven healthcare and narrative medicine: Utilizing collaborative social networks and technologies* (pp. 93–112). Hershey, PA: Medical Information Science Reference.

Masayuki, K., Eiji, K., Tetsuo, T., & Nozomu, M. (2013). Evaluation of olfactory impairment in Parkinson's disease using near-infrared spectroscopy. In J. Wu (Ed.), *Biomedical engineering and cognitive neuroscience for healthcare: Interdisciplinary applications* (pp. 293–302). Hershey, PA: Medical Information Science Reference.

Mazzanti, I., Maolo, A., & Antonicelli, R. (2014). E-health and telemedicine in the elderly: State of the art. In *Assistive technologies: Concepts, methodologies, tools, and applications* (pp. 693–704). Hershey, PA: Information Science Reference.

Medhekar, A., Wong, H. Y., & Hall, J. (2014). Innovation in medical tourism service marketing: A case of India. In A. Goyal (Ed.), *Innovations in services marketing and management: Strategies for emerging economies* (pp. 49–66). Hershey, PA: Business Science Reference.

Medhekar, A., Wong, H. Y., & Hall, J. (2014). Medical tourism: A conceptual framework for an innovation in global healthcare provision. In A. Goyal (Ed.), *Innovations in services marketing and management: Strategies for emerging economies* (pp. 148–169). Hershey, PA: Business Science Reference.

Memmola, M., Palumbo, G., & Rossini, M. (2010). Web & RFID technology: New frontiers in costing and process management for rehabilitation medicine. In J. Symonds (Ed.), *Ubiquitous and pervasive computing: Concepts, methodologies, tools, and applications* (pp. 623–647). Hershey, PA: Information Science Reference.

Menciassi, A., & Laschi, C. (2014). Biorobotics. In Robotics: Concepts, methodologies, tools, and applications (pp. 1613-1643). Hershey, PA: Information Science Reference. doi:10.4018/978-1-4666-4607-0.ch079

Mika, K. (2010). Cybermedicine, telemedicine, and data protection in the United States. In J. Rodrigues (Ed.), *Health information systems: Concepts, methodologies, tools, and applications* (pp. 274–296). Hershey, PA: Medical Information Science Reference.

Mirbagheri, A., Baniasad, M. A., Farahmand, F., Behzadipour, S., & Ahmadian, A. (2013). Medical robotics: State-of-the-art applications and research challenges. [IJHISI]. *International Journal of Healthcare Information Systems and Informatics*, *8*(2), 1–14. doi:10.4018/jhisi.2013040101

Miscione, G. (2013). Telemedicine and development: Situating information technologies in the Amazon. In J. Abdelnour-Nocera (Ed.), *Knowledge and technological development effects on organizational and social structures* (pp. 132–145). Hershey, PA: Information Science Reference.

Mobasheri, A. (2013). Regeneration of articular cartilage: Opportunities, challenges, and perspectives. In A. Daskalaki (Ed.), *Medical advancements in aging and regenerative technologies: Clinical tools and applications* (pp. 137–168). Hershey, PA: Medical Information Science Reference.

Monzon, J. E. (2012). Bioethics. In Z. Abu-Faraj (Ed.), *Handbook of research on biomedical engineering education and advanced bioengineering learning: Interdisciplinary concepts* (pp. 198–237). Hershey, PA: Medical Information Science Reference. doi:10.4018/978-1-4666-0122-2.ch005

Morais da Costa, G. J., Araújo da Silva Nuno, M., & Alves da Silva Nuno, S. (2010). The human centred approach to bionanotechnology in telemedicine: Ethical considerations. In M. Cruz-Cunha, A. Tavares, & R. Simoes (Eds.), *Handbook of research on developments in e-health and telemedicine: Technological and social perspectives* (pp. 311–335). Hershey, PA: Medical Information Science Reference.

Morgade, A. T., Martínez-Romero, M., Vázquez-Naya, J. M., Loureiro, M. P., Albo, Á. G., & Loureiro, J. P. (2011). Development of a knowledge based system for an intensive care environment using ontologies. [JITR]. *Journal of Information Technology Research*, *4*(1), 21–33. doi:10.4018/jitr.2011010102

Morita, A. (2013). The quantitative EEG change in Parkinson's disease. In J. Wu (Ed.), *Biomedical engineering and cognitive neuroscience for healthcare: Interdisciplinary applications* (pp. 225–234). Hershey, PA: Medical Information Science Reference.

Moumtzoglou, A. (2011). E-health as the realm of healthcare quality: A mental image of the future. In A. Moumtzoglou, & A. Kastania (Eds.), *E-health systems quality and reliability: Models and standards* (pp. 291–310). Hershey, PA: Medical Information Science Reference.

Moumtzoglou, A. (2011). E-health as the realm of healthcare quality. In *Clinical technologies: Concepts, methodologies, tools and applications* (pp. 73-92). Hershey, PA: Medical Information Science Reference. doi:10.4018/978-1-60960-561-2.ch105

Moumtzoglou, A. (2011). E-health: A bridge to people-centered health care. In A. Moumtzoglou, & A. Kastania (Eds.), *E-health systems quality and reliability: Models and standards* (pp. 47–63). Hershey, PA: Medical Information Science Reference.

Moumtzoglou, A. (2013). Health 2.0 and medicine 2.0: Safety, ownership and privacy issues. In User-driven healthcare: Concepts, methodologies, tools, and applications (pp. 1508-1522). Hershey, PA: Medical Information Science Reference. doi:10.4018/978-1-4666-2770-3.ch075

Moumtzoglou, A. (2013). Risk perception as a patient safety dimension. In A. Moumtzoglou, & A. Kastania (Eds.), *E-health technologies and improving patient safety: Exploring organizational factors* (pp. 285–299). Hershey, PA: Medical Information Science Reference.

Mourtzikou, A., Stamouli, M., & Athanasiadi, E. (2013). Improvement of clinical laboratory services through quality. [IJRQEH]. *International Journal of Reliable and Quality E-Healthcare*, *2*(2), 38–46. doi:10.4018/ijrqeh.2013040103

Muriithi, M. K., & Mwabu, G. (2014). Demand for health care in Kenya: The effects of information about quality. In P. Schaeffer, & E. Kouassi (Eds.), *Econometric methods for analyzing economic development* (pp. 102–110). Hershey, PA: Business Science Reference.

Murugan, B. O., & Sornam, S. A. (2013). Internet and online medical journal access skills of the medical practitioners of Tamilnadu: A study. In S. Thanuskodi (Ed.), *Challenges of academic library management in developing countries* (pp. 75–82). Hershey, PA: Information Science Reference.

Nadathur, S. G. (2010). Bayesian networks in the health domain. In A. Ali, & Y. Xiang (Eds.), *Dynamic and advanced data mining for progressing technological development: Innovations and systemic approaches* (pp. 342–376). Hershey, PA: Information Science Reference.

Naidoo, V., & Naidoo, Y. (2014). Home telecare, medical implant, and mobile technology: Evolutions in geriatric care. In C. El Morr (Ed.), *Research Perspectives on the role of informatics in health policy and management* (pp. 222–237). Hershey, PA: Medical Information Science Reference.

Najarian, S., & Afshari, E. (2010). Applications of robots in surgery. In A. Shukla, & R. Tiwari (Eds.), *Intelligent medical technologies and biomedical engineering: Tools and applications* (pp. 241–259). Hershey, PA: Medical Information Science Reference. doi:10.4018/978-1-61520-977-4.ch012

Nakajima, I. (2012). Cross-border medical care and telemedicine. [IJEHMC]. *International Journal of E-Health and Medical Communications*, *3*(1), 46–61. doi:10.4018/jehmc.2012010104

Nakayasu, K., & Sato, C. (2012). Liability for telemedicine. [IJEHMC]. *International Journal of E-Health and Medical Communications*, *3*(1), 1–21. doi:10.4018/jehmc.2012010101

Narasimhalu, D. (2010). Redefining medical tourism. In S. Becker, & R. Niebuhr (Eds.), *Cases on technology innovation: Entrepreneurial successes and pitfalls* (pp. 267–285). Hershey, PA: Business Science Reference. doi:10.4018/978-1-61520-609-4.ch014

Naulaers, G., Caicedo, A., & Van Huffel, S. (2012). Use of near-infrared spectroscopy in the neonatal intensive care unit. In W. Chen, S. Oetomo, & L. Feijs (Eds.), *Neonatal monitoring technologies: Design for integrated solutions* (pp. 56–83). Hershey, PA: Medical Information Science Reference. doi:10.4018/978-1-4666-0975-4.ch004

Nokata, M. (2014). Small medical robot. In I. Management Association (Ed.),Robotics: Concepts, methodologies, tools, and applications (pp. 638-646). Hershey, PA: Information Science Reference. doi:10.4018/978-1-4666-4607-0.ch032

Noteboom, C. (2013). Physician interaction with EHR: The importance of stakeholder identification and change management. In S. Sarnikar, D. Bennett, & M. Gaynor (Eds.), *Cases on healthcare information technology for patient care management* (pp. 95–112). Hershey, PA: Medical Information Science Reference.

Noury, N., Bourquard, K., Bergognon, D., & Schroeder, J. (2013). Regulations initiatives in France for the interoperability of communicating medical devices. [IJEHMC]. *International Journal of E-Health and Medical Communications*, *4*(2), 50–64. doi:10.4018/jehmc.2013040104

O'Hanlon, S. (2013). Avoiding adverse consequences of e-health. In A. Moumtzoglou, & A. Kastania (Eds.), *E-health technologies and improving patient safety: Exploring organizational factors* (pp. 13–26). Hershey, PA: Medical Information Science Reference.

O'Leary, D. E. (2012). An activity theory analysis of RFID in hospitals. In Z. Luo (Ed.), *Innovations in logistics and supply chain management technologies for dynamic economies* (pp. 148–166). Hershey, PA: Business Science Reference. doi:10.4018/978-1-4666-0267-0.ch010

O'Neill, L., Talbert, J., & Klepack, W. (2010). Physician characteristics associated with early adoption of electronic medical records in smaller group practices. In J. Rodrigues (Ed.), *Health information systems: Concepts, methodologies, tools, and applications* (pp. 1503–1512). Hershey, PA: Medical Information Science Reference.

Ogawa, T., Ikeda, M., Suzuki, M., & Araki, K. (2014). Medical practical knowledge circulation based on purpose-oriented service modeling. In M. Kosaka, & K. Shirahada (Eds.), *Progressive trends in knowledge and system-based science for service innovation* (pp. 400–424). Hershey, PA: Business Science Reference.

Oliveira, T. C., Oliveira, M. D., & Peña, T. (2013). Towards a post-implementation evaluation framework of outpatient electronic drug prescribing. In M. Cruz-Cunha, I. Miranda, & P. Gonçalves (Eds.), *Handbook of research on ICTs and management systems for improving efficiency in healthcare and social care* (pp. 133–155). Hershey, PA: Medical Information Science Reference. doi:10.4018/978-1-4666-3990-4.ch007

Orizio, G., & Gelatti, U. (2012). Human behaviors in online pharmacies. In Z. Yan (Ed.), *Encyclopedia of cyber behavior* (pp. 661–670). Hershey, PA: Information Science Reference. doi:10.4018/978-1-4666-0315-8.ch056

Otero, A., Félix, P., & Barro, S. (2010). Current state of critical patient monitoring and outstanding challenges. In M. Cruz-Cunha, A. Tavares, & R. Simoes (Eds.), *Handbook of research on developments in e-health and telemedicine: Technological and social perspectives* (pp. 981–1003). Hershey, PA: Medical Information Science Reference.

Ozturk, Y., & Sharma, J. (2013). mVITAL: A standards compliant vital sign monitor. In IT policy and ethics: Concepts, methodologies, tools, and applications (pp. 515-538). Hershey, PA: Information Science Reference. doi:10.4018/978-1-4666-2919-6.ch024

Pal, K., Ghosh, G., & Bhattacharya, M. (2014). Biomedical watermarking: An emerging and secure tool for data security and better tele-diagnosis in modern health care system. In R. Srivastava, S. Singh, & K. Shukla (Eds.), *Research developments in computer vision and image processing: Methodologies and applications* (pp. 208–234). Hershey, PA: Information Science Reference.

Paolucci, F., Ergas, H., Hannan, T., & Aarts, J. (2011). The effectiveness of health informatics. In *Clinical technologies: Concepts, methodologies, tools and applications* (pp. 25-49). Hershey, PA: Medical Information Science Reference. doi:10.4018/978-1-60960-561-2.ch103

Parasher, A., Goldschmidt-Clermont, P. J., & Tien, J. M. (2012). Healthcare delivery as a service system: Barriers to co-production and implications of healthcare reform. In A. Kolker, & P. Story (Eds.), *Management engineering for effective healthcare delivery: Principles and applications* (pp. 191–214). Hershey, PA: Medical Information Science Reference.

Parry, D. (2010). Coding and messaging systems for women's health informatics. In J. Rodrigues (Ed.), *Health information systems: Concepts, methodologies, tools, and applications* (pp. 2192–2205). Hershey, PA: Medical Information Science Reference.

Parry, D. (2012). Computerised decision support for women's health informatics. In Machine learning: Concepts, methodologies, tools and applications (pp. 1404-1416). Hershey, PA: Information Science Reference. doi:10.4018/978-1-60960-818-7.ch513

Payne, G. W. (2011). The role of blended learning in 21st century medical education: Current trends and future directions. In A. Kitchenham (Ed.), *Blended learning across disciplines: Models for implementation* (pp. 132–146). Hershey, PA: Information Science Reference. doi:10.4018/978-1-60960-479-0.ch008

Penchovsky, R. (2013). Engineering gene control circuits with allosteric ribozymes in human cells as a medicine of the future. In Bioinformatics: Concepts, methodologies, tools, and applications (pp. 860-883). Hershey, PA: Medical Information Science Reference. doi:10.4018/978-1-4666-3604-0.ch047

Pestana, O. (2014). Information value and quality for the health sector: A case study of search strategies for optimal information retrieval. In G. Jamil, A. Malheiro, & F. Ribeiro (Eds.), *Rethinking the conceptual base for new practical applications in information value and quality* (pp. 116–133). Hershey, PA: Information Science Reference.

Peterson, C., & Willis, E. (2011). Social construction of chronic disease: Narratives on the experience of chronic illness. In R. Biswas, & C. Martin (Eds.), *User-driven healthcare and narrative medicine: Utilizing collaborative social networks and technologies* (pp. 395–409). Hershey, PA: Medical Information Science Reference.

Petoukhov, S., & He, M. (2010). Biological evolution of dialects of the genetic code. In S. Petoukhov, & M. He (Eds.), *Symmetrical analysis techniques for genetic systems and bioinformatics: Advanced patterns and applications* (pp. 50–64). Hershey, PA: Medical Information Science Reference.

Petty, G. C., & Joyner, D. H. (2012). The efficacy of continuing education technology for public health physicians practicing in remote areas. In V. Wang (Ed.), *Encyclopedia of e-leadership, counseling and training* (pp. 453–467). Hershey, PA: Information Science Reference.

Phua, C., Roy, P. C., Aloulou, H., Biswas, J., Tolstikov, A., & Foo, V. S. … Xu, D. (2014). State-of-the-art assistive technology for people with dementia. In Assistive technologies: Concepts, methodologies, tools, and applications (pp. 1606-1625). Hershey, PA: Information Science Reference. doi:10.4018/978-1-4666-4422-9.ch085

Portela, F., Cabral, A., Abelha, A., Salazar, M., Quintas, C., & Machado, J. … Santos, M. F. (2013). Knowledge acquisition process for intelligent decision support in critical health care. In R. Martinho, R. Rijo, M. Cruz-Cunha, & J. Varajão (Eds.) Information systems and technologies for enhancing health and social care (pp. 55-68). Hershey, PA: Medical Information Science Reference. doi:10.4018/978-1-4666-3667-5.ch004

Postolache, O., Girão, P., & Postolache, G. (2013). Seismocardiogram and ballistocardiogram sensing. In A. Lay-Ekuakille (Ed.), *Advanced instrument engineering: Measurement, calibration, and design* (pp. 223–246). Hershey, PA: Engineering Science Reference. doi:10.4018/978-1-4666-4165-5.ch017

Premkumar, K. (2011). Mobile learning in medicine. In A. Kitchenham (Ed.), *Models for interdisciplinary mobile learning: Delivering information to students* (pp. 137–153). Hershey, PA: Information Science Reference. doi:10.4018/978-1-60960-511-7.ch008

Price, M. (2011). A bio-psycho-social review of usability methods and their applications in healthcare. In *Clinical technologies: Concepts, methodologies, tools and applications* (pp. 1874-1899). Hershey, PA: Medical Information Science Reference. doi:10.4018/978-1-60960-561-2.ch704

Prigione, A. (2012). Stem cell-based personalized medicine: From disease modeling to clinical applications. In Computer engineering: Concepts, methodologies, tools and applications (pp. 1855-1866). Hershey, PA: Engineering Science Reference. doi:10.4018/978-1-61350-456-7.ch803

Quinaz, F., Fazendeiro, P., Castelo-Branco, M., & Araújo, P. (2013). Soft methods for automatic drug infusion in medical care environment. In M. Cruz-Cunha, I. Miranda, & P. Gonçalves (Eds.), *Handbook of research on ICTs and management systems for improving efficiency in healthcare and social care* (pp. 830–854). Hershey, PA: Medical Information Science Reference. doi:10.4018/978-1-4666-3990-4.ch043

Quoniam, L., & Lima de Magalhães, J. (2014). Perception of the information value for public health: A case study for neglected diseases. In G. Jamil, A. Malheiro, & F. Ribeiro (Eds.), *Rethinking the conceptual base for new practical applications in information value and quality* (pp. 211–232). Hershey, PA: Information Science Reference.

Raghupathi, W. (2010). Designing clinical decision support systems in health care: A systemic view. In M. Hunter (Ed.), *Strategic information systems: Concepts, methodologies, tools, and applications* (pp. 652–661). Hershey, PA: Information Science Reference.

Raghupathi, W., & Nerur, S. (2012). The intellectual structure of health and medical informatics. In J. Tan (Ed.), *Advancing technologies and intelligence in healthcare and clinical environments breakthroughs* (pp. 1–16). Hershey, PA: Medical Information Science Reference. doi:10.4018/978-1-4666-1755-1.ch001

Räisänen, T., Oinas-Kukkonen, H., Leiviskä, K., Seppänen, M., & Kallio, M. (2010). Managing mobile healthcare knowledge: Physicians' perceptions on knowledge creation and reuse. In J. Rodrigues (Ed.), *Health information systems: Concepts, methodologies, tools, and applications* (pp. 733–749). Hershey, PA: Medical Information Science Reference.

Raval, M. S. (2011). Data hiding in digitized medical images: From concepts to applications. In A. Daskalaki (Ed.), *Digital forensics for the health sciences: Applications in practice and research* (pp. 29–47). Hershey, PA: Medical Information Science Reference. doi:10.4018/978-1-60960-483-7.ch003

Ravka, N. (2014). Informatics and health services: The potential benefits and challenges of electronic health records and personal electronic health records in patient care, cost control, and health research – An overview. In C. El Morr (Ed.), *Research perspectives on the role of informatics in health policy and management* (pp. 89–114). Hershey, PA: Medical Information Science Reference.

Reyes Álamo, J. M., Yang, H., Babbitt, R., & Wong, J. (2010). Support for medication safety and compliance in smart home environments. In J. Rodrigues (Ed.), *Health information systems: Concepts, methodologies, tools, and applications* (pp. 2091–2110). Hershey, PA: Medical Information Science Reference.

Ribeiro, C., Monteiro, M., Corredoura, S., Candeias, F., & Pereira, J. (2013). Games in higher education: Opportunities, expectations, challenges, and results in medical education. In S. de Freitas, M. Ott, M. Popescu, & I. Stanescu (Eds.), *New pedagogical approaches in game enhanced learning: Curriculum integration* (pp. 228–247). Hershey, PA: Information Science Reference. doi:10.4018/978-1-4666-3950-8.ch012

Rocci, L. (2010). Biomedical technoethics. In R. Luppicini (Ed.), *Technoethics and the evolving knowledge society: Ethical issues in technological design, research, development, and innovation* (pp. 128–145). Hershey, PA: Information Science Reference. doi:10.4018/978-1-60566-952-6.ch007

Rockland, R., Kimmel, H., Carpinelli, J., Hirsch, L. S., & Burr-Alexander, L. (2014). Medical robotics in k-12 education. In Robotics: Concepts, methodologies, tools, and applications (pp. 1096-1115). Hershey, PA: Information Science Reference. doi:10.4018/978-1-4666-4607-0.ch053

Rodrigues, J. J. (2012). *Emerging communication technologies for e-health and medicine*. Hershey, PA: IGI Global. doi:10.4018/978-1-4666-0909-9

Rodrigues, J. J. (2013). *Digital advances in medicine, e-health, and communication technologies*. Hershey, PA: IGI Global. doi:10.4018/978-1-4666-2794-9

Rodrigues, J. J. (2014). *Advancing medical practice through technology: Applications for healthcare delivery, management, and quality*. Hershey, PA: IGI Global.

Rodríguez-González, A., García-Crespo, Á., Colomo-Palacios, R., Gómez-Berbís, J. M., & Jiménez-Domingo, E. (2013). Using ontologies in drug prescription: The SemMed approach. In J. Wang (Ed.), *Intelligence methods and systems advancements for knowledge-based business* (pp. 247–261). Hershey, PA: Information Science Reference.

Rojo, M. G., & Daniel, C. (2011). Digital pathology and virtual microscopy integration in e-health records. In *Clinical technologies: Concepts, methodologies, tools and applications* (pp. 1235-1262). Hershey, PA: Medical Information Science Reference. doi:10.4018/978-1-60960-561-2.ch415

Rompas, A., Tsirmpas, C., Anastasiou, A., Iliopoulou, D., & Koutsouris, D. (2013). Statistical power and sample size in personalized medicine. [IJSBBT]. *International Journal of Systems Biology and Biomedical Technologies*, *2*(2), 72–88. doi:10.4018/ijsbbt.2013040105

Rosiek, A. B., & Leksowski, K. (2011). Quality assurance and evaluation of healthcare reform initiatives: Strategy for improving the quality of health care services in public health care units, management model that allows the providing of high quality health care and efficient brand-building. [IJHDRI]. *International Journal of Healthcare Delivery Reform Initiatives*, *3*(3), 42–53. doi:10.4018/jhdri.2011070104

Ross, S. (2011). A lexicon for user driven healthcare. [IJUDH]. *International Journal of User-Driven Healthcare*, *1*(1), 50–54. doi:10.4018/ijudh.2011010107

Ross, S. D. (2011). Multiple paths in health care. In R. Biswas, & C. Martin (Eds.), *User-driven healthcare and narrative medicine: Utilizing collaborative social networks and technologies* (pp. 113–124). Hershey, PA: Medical Information Science Reference.

Rosu, S. M., & Dragoi, G. (2014). E-health sites development using open source software and OMT methodology as support for family doctors' activities: A Romanian case study. In M. Cruz-Cunha, F. Moreira, & J. Varajão (Eds.), *Handbook of research on enterprise 2.0: Technological, social, and organizational dimensions* (pp. 72–88). Hershey, PA: Business Science Reference.

Ruiz-Fernandez, D., & Soriano-Paya, A. (2011). A distributed approach of a clinical decision support system based on cooperation. In *Clinical technologies: Concepts, methodologies, tools and applications* (pp. 1782-1799). Hershey, PA: Medical Information Science Reference. doi:10.4018/978-1-60960-561-2.ch612

Ryan, P. (2012). Paying for performance: Key design features and the bigger picture. [IJPPHME]. *International Journal of Public and Private Healthcare Management and Economics*, *2*(2), 1–16. doi:10.4018/ijpphme.2012040101

Sainz de Abajo, B., & Ballestero, A. L. (2012). Overview of the most important open source software: Analysis of the benefits of OpenMRS, OpenEMR, and VistA. In J. Rodrigues, I. de la Torre Díez, & B. Sainz de Abajo (Eds.), *Telemedicine and e-health services, policies, and applications: Advancements and developments* (pp. 315–346). Hershey, PA: Medical Information Science Reference. doi:10.4018/978-1-4666-0888-7.ch012

Salcido, G. J., & Delgado, E. C. (2013). Intelligent agent to identify rheumatic diseases. In M. Cruz-Cunha, I. Miranda, & P. Gonçalves (Eds.), *Handbook of research on ICTs and management systems for improving efficiency in healthcare and social care* (pp. 451–473). Hershey, PA: Medical Information Science Reference. doi:10.4018/978-1-4666-3990-4.ch023

Schallenberg, S., Petzold, C., Riewaldt, J., & Kretschmer, K. (2013). Regulatory T cell-based immunotherapy: Prospects of antigen-specific tolerance induction. In A. Daskalaki (Ed.), *Medical advancements in aging and regenerative technologies: Clinical tools and applications* (pp. 112–136). Hershey, PA: Medical Information Science Reference.

Scheepers-Hoeks, A., Klijn, F., van der Linden, C., Grouls, R., Ackerman, E., & Minderman, N. … Korsten, E. (2013). Clinical decision support systems for ‘making it easy to do it right. In Data mining: Concepts, methodologies, tools, and applications (pp. 1461-1471). Hershey, PA: Information Science Reference. doi:10.4018/978-1-4666-2455-9.ch076

Seçkin, G. (2012). Cyber behaviors of self health care management. In Z. Yan (Ed.), *Encyclopedia of cyber behavior* (pp. 722–734). Hershey, PA: Information Science Reference. doi:10.4018/978-1-4666-0315-8.ch061

Serrano, M., Elmisery, A., Foghlú, M. Ó., Donnelly, W., Storni, C., & Fernström, M. (2013). Pervasive computing support in the transition towards personalised health systems. In J. Rodrigues (Ed.), *Digital advances in medicine, e-health, and communication technologies* (pp. 49–64). Hershey, PA: Medical Information Science Reference. doi:10.4018/978-1-4666-2794-9.ch003

Shachak, A., & Reis, S. (2010). The computer-assisted patient consultation: Promises and challenges. In S. Kabene (Ed.), *Healthcare and the effect of technology: Developments, challenges and advancements* (pp. 72–83). Hershey, PA: Medical Information Science Reference. doi:10.4018/978-1-61520-733-6.ch005

Shachak, A., & Reis, S. (2011). The computer-assisted patient consultation. In *Clinical technologies: Concepts, methodologies, tools and applications* (pp. 160-171). Hershey, PA: Medical Information Science Reference. doi:10.4018/978-1-60960-561-2.ch111

Shankar, P. R. (2011). Medical Humanities. In R. Biswas, & C. Martin (Eds.), *User-driven healthcare and narrative medicine: Utilizing collaborative social networks and technologies* (pp. 210–227). Hershey, PA: Medical Information Science Reference.

Shanmuganathan, S. (2010). A stroke information system (SIS): Critical issues and solutions. In W. Pease, M. Cooper, & R. Gururajan (Eds.), *Biomedical knowledge management: Infrastructures and processes for e-health systems* (pp. 177–191). Hershey, PA: Medical Information Science Reference. doi:10.4018/978-1-60566-266-4.ch012

Shegog, R. (2010). Application of behavioral theory in computer game design for health behavior change. In J. Cannon-Bowers, & C. Bowers (Eds.), *Serious game design and development: Technologies for training and learning* (pp. 196–232). Hershey, PA: Information Science Reference. doi:10.4018/978-1-61520-739-8.ch011

Shendge, S., Deka, B., & Kotwani, A. (2012). A cross-sectional evaluation of illness perception about asthma among asthma patients at a referral tertiary care public chest hospital in Delhi, India. [IJUDH]. *International Journal of User-Driven Healthcare*, *2*(3), 32–43. doi:10.4018/ijudh.2012070104

Shimoyama, I., Shimada, H., & Ninchoji, T. (2013). Kanji perception and brain function. In J. Wu (Ed.), *Biomedical engineering and cognitive neuroscience for healthcare: Interdisciplinary applications* (pp. 266–273). Hershey, PA: Medical Information Science Reference.

Shrestha, S. (2013). Clinical decision support system for diabetes prevention: An illustrative case. In S. Sarnikar, D. Bennett, & M. Gaynor (Eds.), *Cases on healthcare information technology for patient care management* (pp. 308–329). Hershey, PA: Medical Information Science Reference.

Shukla, A., Tiwari, R., & Rathore, C. P. (2011). Intelligent biometric system using soft computing tools. In A. Shukla, & R. Tiwari (Eds.), *Biomedical engineering and information systems: Technologies, tools and applications* (pp. 259–276). Hershey, PA: Medical Information Science Reference.

Sibinga, C. T., & Oladejo, M. A. (2013). Bridging the knowledge gap in management and operations of transfusion medicine: Planning, policy and leadership issues. [JCIT]. *Journal of Cases on Information Technology*, *15*(1), 69–82. doi:10.4018/jcit.2013010105

Slavens, B., & Harris, G. F. (2012). Biomechanics. In Z. Abu-Faraj (Ed.), *Handbook of research on biomedical engineering education and advanced bioengineering learning: Interdisciplinary concepts* (pp. 284–338). Hershey, PA: Medical Information Science Reference. doi:10.4018/978-1-4666-0122-2.ch007

Sliedrecht, S., & Kotzé, E. (2013). Patients with a spinal cord injury inform and co-construct services at a spinal cord rehabilitation unit. In User-driven healthcare: Concepts, methodologies, tools, and applications (pp. 1054-1072). Hershey, PA: Medical Information Science Reference. doi:10.4018/978-1-4666-2770-3.ch053

Sood, R., & Ananthakrishnan, N. (2012). Reforming medical curriculum in India in recent years: Conflicts of political, regulator, educationist and professional natures and strategies for their resolution. [IJUDH]. *International Journal of User-Driven Healthcare*, *2*(1), 1–13. doi:10.4018/ijudh.2012010101

Springer, J. A., Beever, J., Morar, N., Sprague, J. E., & Kane, M. D. (2011). Ethics, Privacy, and the future of genetic information in healthcare information assurance and security. In M. Dark (Ed.), *Information assurance and security ethics in complex systems: Interdisciplinary perspectives* (pp. 186–205). Hershey, PA: Information Science Reference.

Srivastava, S. (2011). Medical transcription a pioneer in the healthcare informatics. In A. Shukla, & R. Tiwari (Eds.), *Biomedical engineering and information systems: Technologies, tools and applications* (pp. 239–258). Hershey, PA: Medical Information Science Reference.

Srivastava, S., Sharma, N., & Singh, S. (2014). Image analysis and understanding techniques for breast cancer detection from digital mammograms. In R. Srivastava, S. Singh, & K. Shukla (Eds.), *Research developments in computer vision and image processing: Methodologies and applications* (pp. 123–148). Hershey, PA: Information Science Reference.

Stanescu, L., & Burdescu, D. D. (2010). Medical hybrid learning tools. In F. Wang, J. Fong, & R. Kwan (Eds.), *Handbook of research on hybrid learning models: Advanced tools, technologies, and applications* (pp. 355–370). Hershey, PA: Information Science Reference.

Staudinger, B., Ostermann, H., & Staudinger, R. (2011). IT-based virtual medical centres and structures. In *Clinical technologies: Concepts, methodologies, tools and applications* (pp. 2035-2046). Hershey, PA: Medical Information Science Reference. doi:10.4018/978-1-60960-561-2.ch802

Stefaniak, J. E. (2013). Resuscitating team roles within Wayburn health system. In A. Ritzhaupt, & S. Kumar (Eds.), *Cases on educational technology implementation for facilitating learning* (pp. 130–145). Hershey, PA: Information Science Reference. doi:10.4018/978-1-4666-3676-7.ch008

Stein, R. A. (2012). Direct-to-consumer genetic testing: Interdisciplinary crossroads. [JITR]. *Journal of Information Technology Research*, *5*(1), 35–67. doi:10.4018/jitr.2012010103

Stergachis, A., Keene, D., & Somani, S. (2013). Informatics for medicines management systems in resource-limited settings. In *Supply chain management: Concepts, methodologies, tools, and applications* (pp. 634–645). Hershey, PA: Business Science Reference.

Stevens, D., & Kitchenham, A. (2011). An analysis of mobile learning in education, business, and medicine. In A. Kitchenham (Ed.), *Models for interdisciplinary mobile learning: Delivering information to students* (pp. 1–25). Hershey, PA: Information Science Reference. doi:10.4018/978-1-60960-511-7.ch001

Stolba, N., Nguyen, T. M., & Tjoa, A. M. (2010). Data warehouse facilitating evidence-based medicine. In T. Nguyen (Ed.), *Complex data warehousing and knowledge discovery for advanced retrieval development: Innovative methods and applications* (pp. 174–207). Hershey, PA: Information Science Reference.

Sugaretty, D. (2014). Risk management in a pandemic crisis at a global non profit health care organization. In Crisis management: Concepts, methodologies, tools and applications (pp. 1253-1270). Hershey, PA: Information Science Reference. doi:10.4018/978-1-4666-4707-7.ch063

Sugi, T., Goto, K., Goto, S., Goto, Y., Yamasaki, T., & Tobimatsu, S. (2013). Topography estimation of visual evoked potentials using a combination of mathematical models. In J. Wu (Ed.), *Biomedical engineering and cognitive neuroscience for healthcare: Interdisciplinary applications* (pp. 129–141). Hershey, PA: Medical Information Science Reference.

Sujan, H., Borrero, S., & Cranage, D. (2014). Good treats: Eating out not just for joy but also for well-being. In A. Goyal (Ed.), *Innovations in services marketing and management: Strategies for emerging economies* (pp. 118–135). Hershey, PA: Business Science Reference.

Swennen, M. H. (2011). The gap between what is knowable and what we do in clinical practice. In R. Biswas, & C. Martin (Eds.), *User-driven healthcare and narrative medicine: Utilizing collaborative social networks and technologies* (pp. 335–356). Hershey, PA: Medical Information Science Reference. doi:10.4018/978-1-60960-561-2.ch705

Szewczak, E. J., & Snodgrass, C. R. (2011). Business associates in the national health information network: Implications for medical information privacy. In I. Lee (Ed.), *E-business applications for product development and competitive growth: Emerging technologies* (pp. 186–198). Hershey, PA: Business Science Reference.

Tabrizi, N. T., Torabi, Z., Bastani, P., Mokhtarkhani, M., Madani, N., Parnian, N., & Hajebrahimi, S. (2013). Assessing the perception of pain and distress of female patients undergoing routine urethral catheterization in cesarean delivery. [IJUDH]. *International Journal of User-Driven Healthcare*, *3*(2), 78–84. doi:10.4018/ijudh.2013040109

Tanaka, H., & Furutani, M. (2013). Sleep management promotes healthy lifestyle, mental health, QOL, and a healthy brain. In J. Wu (Ed.), *Biomedical engineering and cognitive neuroscience for healthcare: Interdisciplinary applications* (pp. 211–224). Hershey, PA: Medical Information Science Reference.

Tang, X., Gao, Y., Yang, W., Zhang, M., & Wu, J. (2013). Audiovisual integration of natural auditory and visual stimuli in the real-world situation. In J. Wu (Ed.), *Biomedical engineering and cognitive neuroscience for healthcare: Interdisciplinary applications* (pp. 337–344). Hershey, PA: Medical Information Science Reference.

Tashiro, M., Okamura, N., Watanuki, S., Furumoto, S., Furukawa, K., & Funaki, Y. … Yanai, K. (2011). Quantitative analysis of amyloid ß deposition in patients with Alzheimer's disease using positron emission tomography. In J. Wu (Ed.), Early detection and rehabilitation technologies for dementia: Neuroscience and biomedical applications (pp. 220-230). Hershey, PA: Medical Information Science Reference. doi:10.4018/978-1-60960-559-9.ch029

Taylor, B. W. (2014). Decision-making and decision support in acute care. In C. El Morr (Ed.), *Research perspectives on the role of informatics in health policy and management* (pp. 1–18). Hershey, PA: Medical Information Science Reference.

Thatcher, B. (2012). Intercultural rhetorical dimensions of health literacy and medicine. In *Intercultural rhetoric and professional communication: Technological advances and organizational behavior* (pp. 247–282). Hershey, PA: Information Science Reference.

Tiwari, S., & Srivastava, R. (2014). Research and developments in medical image reconstruction methods and its applications. In R. Srivastava, S. Singh, & K. Shukla (Eds.), *Research developments in computer vision and image processing: Methodologies and applications* (pp. 274–312). Hershey, PA: Information Science Reference.

Toro-Troconis, M., & Partridge, M. R. (2010). Designing game-based learning activities in virtual worlds: Experiences from undergraduate medicine. In Y. Baek (Ed.), *Gaming for classroom-based learning: Digital role playing as a motivator of study* (pp. 270–280). Hershey, PA: Information Science Reference. doi:10.4018/978-1-61520-713-8.ch016

Trojer, T., Katt, B., Breu, R., Schabetsberger, T., & Mair, R. (2012). Managing privacy and effectiveness of patient-administered authorization policies. [IJCMAM]. *International Journal of Computational Models and Algorithms in Medicine*, *3*(2), 43–62. doi:10.4018/jcmam.2012040103

Übeyli, E. D. (2010). Medical informatics: Preventive medicine applications via telemedicine. In M. Cruz-Cunha, A. Tavares, & R. Simoes (Eds.), *Handbook of research on developments in e-health and telemedicine: Technological and social perspectives* (pp. 475–489). Hershey, PA: Medical Information Science Reference.

Übeyli, E. D. (2011). Telemedicine and biotelemetry for e-health systems. In *Clinical technologies: Concepts, methodologies, tools and applications* (pp. 676-692). Hershey, PA: Medical Information Science Reference. doi:10.4018/978-1-60960-561-2.ch304

Vahe, M., Zain-Ul-Abdin, K., & Türel, Y. K. (2012). Social media as a learning tool in medical education: A situation analysis. In V. Dennen, & J. Myers (Eds.), *Virtual professional development and informal learning via social networks* (pp. 168–183). Hershey, PA: Information Science Reference. doi:10.4018/978-1-4666-1815-2.ch010

Vivekananda-Schmidt, P. (2013). Ethics in the design of serious games for healthcare and medicine. In S. Arnab, I. Dunwell, & K. Debattista (Eds.), *Serious games for healthcare: Applications and implications* (pp. 91–106). Hershey, PA: Medical Information Science Reference.

von Lubitz, D. (2010). Healthcare among the people: Teams of leaders concept (ToL) and the world of technology-oriented global healthcare. In S. Kabene (Ed.), *Healthcare and the effect of technology: Developments, challenges and advancements* (pp. 145–177). Hershey, PA: Medical Information Science Reference. doi:10.4018/978-1-61520-733-6.ch010

von Lubitz, D. (2011). The teams of leaders (Tol) concept: The grid, the mesh, and the people in the world of information and knowledge-based global healthcare. In E. Kldiashvili (Ed.), *Grid technologies for e-health: Applications for telemedicine services and delivery* (pp. 65–104). Hershey, PA: Medical Information Science Reference.

Vouyioukas, D., & Maglogiannis, I. (2010). Communication issues in pervasive healthcare systems and applications. In A. Coronato, & G. De Pietro (Eds.), *Pervasive and smart technologies for healthcare: Ubiquitous methodologies and tools* (pp. 197–227). Hershey, PA: Medical Information Science Reference. doi:10.4018/978-1-61520-765-7.ch010

Walczak, S., Brimhall, B. B., & Lefkowitz, J. B. (2010). Nonparametric decision support systems in medical diagnosis: Modeling pulmonary embolism. In M. Hunter (Ed.), *Strategic information systems: Concepts, methodologies, tools, and applications* (pp. 1483–1500). Hershey, PA: Information Science Reference.

Walczak, S., Brimhall, B. B., & Lefkowitz, J. B. (2011). Diagnostic cost reduction using artificial neural networks. In *Clinical technologies: Concepts, methodologies, tools and applications* (pp. 1812-1830). Hershey, PA: Medical Information Science Reference. doi:10.4018/978-1-60960-561-2.ch614

Wang, G., Cong, A., Gao, H., Zhang, J., Weir, V. J., Xu, X., & Bennett, J. (2012). Medical imaging. In Z. Abu-Faraj (Ed.), *Handbook of research on biomedical engineering education and advanced bioengineering learning: Interdisciplinary concepts* (pp. 634–712). Hershey, PA: Medical Information Science Reference. doi:10.4018/978-1-4666-0122-2.ch015

Watanabe, Y., Tanaka, H., & Hirata, K. (2013). Evaluation of cognitive function in migraine patients: A study using event-related potentials. In J. Wu (Ed.), *Biomedical engineering and cognitive neuroscience for healthcare: Interdisciplinary applications* (pp. 303–310). Hershey, PA: Medical Information Science Reference.

Watfa, M. K., Majeed, H., & Salahuddin, T. (2012). Healthcare applications for clinicians. In M. Watfa (Ed.), *E-healthcare systems and wireless communications: Current and future challenges* (pp. 49–69). Hershey, PA: Medical Information Science Reference.

Weigel, F. K., Rainer, R. K., Hazen, B. T., Cegielski, C. G., & Ford, F. N. (2012). Use of diffusion of innovations theory in medical informatics research. [IJHISI]. *International Journal of Healthcare Information Systems and Informatics*, *7*(3), 44–56. doi:10.4018/jhisi.2012070104

Whitaker, R. (2013). Securing health-effective medicine in practice: A critical perspective on user-driven healthcare. In R. Biswas (Ed.), *Clinical solutions and medical progress through user-driven healthcare* (pp. 35–50). Hershey, PA: Medical Information Science Reference.

Wilkowska, W., & Ziefle, M. (2011). User diversity as a challenge for the integration of medical technology into future smart home environments. In M. Ziefle, & C. Röcker (Eds.), *Human-centered design of e-health technologies: Concepts, methods and applications* (pp. 95–126). Hershey, PA: Medical Information Science Reference.

Xuan, X., & Xiaowei, Z. (2012). The dilemma and resolution: The patentability of traditional Chinese medicine. [IJABIM]. *International Journal of Asian Business and Information Management*, *3*(3), 1–8. doi:10.4018/jabim.2012070101

Yamamoto, S. (2010). IT applications for medical services in Japan. In W. Pease, M. Cooper, & R. Gururajan (Eds.), *Biomedical knowledge management: Infrastructures and processes for e-health systems* (pp. 327–336). Hershey, PA: Medical Information Science Reference. doi:10.4018/978-1-60566-266-4.ch024

Yan, B., Lei, Y., Tong, L., & Chen, K. (2013). Functional neuroimaging of acupuncture: A systematic review. In J. Wu (Ed.), *Biomedical engineering and cognitive neuroscience for healthcare: Interdisciplinary applications* (pp. 142–155). Hershey, PA: Medical Information Science Reference.

Yang, J. (2014). Towards healthy public policy: GIS and food systems analysis. In C. El Morr (Ed.), *Research perspectives on the role of informatics in health policy and management* (pp. 135–152). Hershey, PA: Medical Information Science Reference.

Yang, W., Gao, Y., & Wu, J. (2013). Effects of selective and divided attention on audiovisual interaction. In J. Wu (Ed.), *Biomedical engineering and cognitive neuroscience for healthcare: Interdisciplinary applications* (pp. 311–319). Hershey, PA: Medical Information Science Reference.

Yap, K. Y. (2013). The evolving role of pharmacoinformatics in targeting drug-related problems in clinical oncology practice. In User-driven healthcare: Concepts, methodologies, tools, and applications (pp. 1541-1588). Hershey, PA: Medical Information Science Reference. doi:10.4018/978-1-4666-2770-3.ch077

Young, J. W., Thapaliya, P., & Sapkota, S. (2013). Caught in the middle: The divide between conventional and alternative medicine. In R. Biswas (Ed.), *Clinical solutions and medical progress through user-driven healthcare* (pp. 26–34). Hershey, PA: Medical Information Science Reference.

Yu, J., Guo, C., & Kim, M. (2010). Developing a user centered model for ubiquitous healthcare system implementation: An empirical study. In J. Rodrigues (Ed.), *Health information systems: Concepts, methodologies, tools, and applications* (pp. 1243–1259). Hershey, PA: Medical Information Science Reference.

Yu, J., Guo, C., & Kim, M. (2011). Towards a conceptual framework of adopting ubiquitous technology in chronic health care. In J. Tan (Ed.), *Developments in healthcare information systems and technologies: Models and methods* (pp. 214–231). Hershey, PA: Medical Information Science Reference.

Zaheer, S. (2014). Implementation of evidence-based practice and the PARIHS framework. In C. El Morr (Ed.), *Research perspectives on the role of informatics in health policy and management* (pp. 19–36). Hershey, PA: Medical Information Science Reference.

Zhang, H. H., Meyer, R. R., Shi, L., & D'Souza, W. D. (2012). Machine learning applications in radiation therapy. In S. Kulkarni (Ed.), *Machine learning algorithms for problem solving in computational applications: Intelligent techniques* (pp. 59–84). Hershey, PA: Information Science Reference. doi:10.4018/978-1-4666-1833-6.ch005

Zhang, W. (2011). YinYang bipolar quantum bioeconomics for equilibrium-based biosystem simulation and regulation. In *YinYang bipolar relativity: A unifying theory of nature, agents and causality with applications in quantum computing, cognitive informatics and life sciences* (pp. 266–297). Hershey, PA: Information Science Reference. doi:10.4018/978-1-60960-525-4.ch009

Zhang, Z., Gao, B., Liao, G., Mu, L., & Wei, W. (2011). The study of transesophageal oxygen saturation monitoring. In *Clinical technologies: Concepts, methodologies, tools and applications* (pp. 2191-2200). Hershey, PA: Medical Information Science Reference. doi:10.4018/978-1-60960-561-2.ch813

Zhao, B., Zhang, D. S., & Zhao, Y. Z. (2013). Construction competitiveness evaluation system of regional BioPharma industry and case study: Taking Shijiazhuang as an example. In T. Gao (Ed.), *Global applications of pervasive and ubiquitous computing* (pp. 80–88). Hershey, PA: Information Science Reference.

Zheng, K., Padman, R., Johnson, M. P., & Hasan, S. (2010). Guideline representation ontologies for evidence-based medicine practice. In K. Khoumbati, Y. Dwivedi, A. Srivastava, & B. Lal (Eds.), *Handbook of research on advances in health informatics and electronic healthcare applications: Global adoption and impact of information communication technologies* (pp. 234–254). Hershey, PA: Medical Information Science Reference.

Zhou, F., Yan, J., Wang, Y., Li, F., Xia, C., Guo, R., & Yan, H. (2011). Digital auscultation system of traditional Chinese medicine and its signals acquisition: Analysis methods. In L. Liu, D. Wei, & Y. Li (Eds.), *Interdisciplinary research and applications in bioinformatics, computational biology, and environmental sciences* (pp. 183–193). Hershey, PA: Medical Information Science Reference.

Zijlstra, W., Becker, C., & Pfeiffer, K. (2011). Wearable systems for monitoring mobility related activities: From technology to application for healthcare services. In C. Röcker, & M. Ziefle (Eds.), *E-Health, assistive technologies and applications for assisted living: Challenges and solutions* (pp. 244–267). Hershey, PA: Medical Information Science Reference. doi:10.4018/978-1-60960-469-1.ch011

Zimmer, J., Degenkolbe, E., Wildemann, B., & Seemann, P. (2013). BMP signaling in regenerative medicine. In Bioinformatics: Concepts, methodologies, tools, and applications (pp. 1252-1281). Hershey, PA: Medical Information Science Reference. doi:10.4018/978-1-4666-3604-0.ch064

Zouag, N. (2014). Patterns of migration of medical doctors from MENA and ECE to EU economies with descriptive analysis of relatives wages. In A. Driouchi (Ed.), *Labor and health economics in the Mediterranean region: Migration and mobility of medical doctors* (pp. 124–138). Hershey, PA: Medical Information Science Reference.

Zouag, N., & Driouchi, A. (2014). Trends and prospects of the moroccan health system: 2010-2030. In A. Driouchi (Ed.), *Labor and health economics in the Mediterranean region: Migration and mobility of medical doctors* (pp. 314–336). Hershey, PA: Medical Information Science Reference.

Zybeck, K. L. (2013). A question of degrees: Collecting in support of the allied health professions. In S. Holder (Ed.), *Library collection development for professional programs: Trends and best practices* (pp. 145–163). Hershey, PA: Information Science Reference.

Compilation of References

Accenture. (2013). *Retail medical clinics: From foe to friend?* Retrieved from http://www.accenture.com/SiteCollectionDocuments/PDF/Accenture-Retail-Medical-Clinics-From-Foe-to-Friend.pdf

Accreditation Association for Ambulatory Healthcare. (2013). *Accreditation.* Retrieved from http://www.aaahc.org/accreditation/

Adamson, S. C., & Bachman, J. W. (2010). Pilot study of providing online care in a primary care setting. *Mayo Clinic Proceedings*, *85*(8), 704–710. doi:10.4065/mcp.2010.0145 PMID:20516427

Adashi, E. Y., Geiger, H. J., & Fine, M. D. (2010). Health care reform and primary care-The growing importance of the community health center. *The New England Journal of Medicine*, *362*(22), 2047–2050. doi:10.1056/NEJMp1003729 PMID:20427777

Advance Healthcare Network for NPs and PAs. (2012). *What do NPs and PAs think about convenient care?* Retrieved from http://nurse-practitioners-and-physician-assistants.advanceweb.com/Columns/Retail-Health-Report/What-do-NPs-and-PAs-think-about-convenient-care.aspx

Agency for Healthcare Quality and Research. (2008). *Emergency room services - Median and mean expense per person with expense and distribution by source of payment.* Summary Data Table From the Medical Expenditure Panel Survey -Household Component.

Agency for Healthcare Research and Quality. (2011). *The Number of Practicing Primary Care Physicians in the United States.* Retrieved on May 6 2013 from http://www.ahrq.gov/research/findings/factsheets/primary/pcwork1/index.html

Ahmed, A., & Fincham, J. E. (2010). Physician office vs. retail clinic: Patient preferences in care seeking for minor illnesses. *Annals of Family Medicine*, *8*(2), 117–123. doi:10.1370/afm.1052 PMID:20212298

Aiello, M. (2013). *Hospitals, Don't Fear Retail Health Clinics. Join Them.* HealthLeaders Media.

Alexander, A. (2012). MinuteClinic, UT Medicine San Antonio form clinical affiliation. *Drug Store News.* Retrieved from http://www.drugstorenews.com/article/minuteclinic-ut-medicine-san-antonio-form-clinical-affiliation

American Academy of Family Physicians. (2010). *AAFP board revises retail health clinic policy academy opposes ongoing expansions in scope of service*. Retrieved from http://www.aafp.org/news-now/inside-aafp/20100224retail-policy.html

American Academy of Family Physicians. (2012). Ensuring a quality physician-led team for every patient. *Primary Care*, 21.

American Academy of Family Physicians. (2012). *Primary care for the 21st century: Ensuring a quality physician-led team for every patient*. Leawood, KS: Author.

American Academy of Family Physicians. (2013). Retrieved from http://www.aafp.org/home.html

American Academy of Nurse Practitioners. (2011). *Nurse Practitioner Facts*. Retrieved on May 6 2013 from http://www.aanp.org/images/documents/research/2010-2011np%20 facts2012.pdf

American Academy of Pediatrics. (2006). AAP principles concerning retail-based clinics. Retail-Based Clinic Policy Work Group. *Pediatrics*, *118*(6), 2561–2562. doi:10.1542/peds.2006-2681 PMID:17142546

American Academy of Pediatrics. (2013). Retrieved from http://www.aap.org/en-us/Pages/Default.aspx

American Academy of Physician Assistants. (2013). Retrieved on May 6, 2013 from http://www.aapa.org/the_pa_profession/history.aspx

American Board of Urgent Care Medicine (ABUCM). (2013). Available at http://aaucm.org/professionals/boardcertifications/default.aspx

American College of Occupational and Environmental Medicine. (2008). *The Personal Physician's Role in Helping Patients with Medical Conditions Stay at Work or Return to Work*. Elk Grove Village, IL: Author.

American College of Physicians. (2006). *The impending collapse of primary care medicine and its implications for the state of the nation's health care: A report from the American College of Physicians*. Philadelphia: American College of Physicians.

American Medical Association. (2009). *Scope of practice data series: Nurse practitioners*. Chicago: AMA.

American Medical Association. (2013). Retrieved from http://www.ama-assn.org/ama

American Telemedicine Association. (2013). *What is Telemedicine?* Retrieved from http://www.americantelemed.org/learn

American Well. (2012). *Blue Cross and Blue Shield of North Carolina*. Walgreens Take Care Health Systems and American Well Team Up to Provide Telehealth to Workforce.

American Well. (2013). Retrieved from http://www.americanwell.com/howItWorks.html Last accessed 1/3/14

Amirault, B. (2012). *Day in the Life: Running a nurse practitioner house-call practice*. Retrieved from http://www.bartonassociates.com/2012/11/16/nurse-practitioner-day-in-the-life-1/

Anderson, C. (2013). More large employers adding on-site health clinics. *Healthcare Finance News*. Retrieved from: http://www.healthcarefinancenews.com

Angstman, K. B., Bernard, M. E., Rohrer, J. E., Garrison, G. M., & MacLaughlin, K. L. (2012). Repeat retail clinic visits: Impact of insurance coverage and age of patient. *Population Health Management*, *15*(358), 358–361. doi:10.1089/pop.2011.0088 PMID:22788953

Ashwood, J. S., Reid, R. O., Setodji, C. M., Weber, E., Gaynor, M., & Mehtrotra, A. (2011). Trends in retail clinic use among the commercially insured. *The American Journal of Managed Care*, *17*(11), e443–e448. PMID:22200061

Asplin, B. R., & Knopp, R. K. (2001). A room with a view: On-call specialist panels and other health policy challenges in the emergency department. *Annals of Emergency Medicine*, *37*(5), 500–503. doi:10.1067/mem.2001.115174 PMID:11326186

Association of American Medical Colleges Center for Workforce Studies. (2008). *The complexities of physician supply and demand: Projections through 2025*. Washington, DC: Association of American Medical Colleges.

Association of American Medical Colleges Center for Workforce Studies. (2010). *Help wanted: More US doctors*. Washington, DC: Association of American Medical Colleges.

Association of American Medical Colleges. (2002). *The physician workforce: position statement- June 2002*. Washington, DC: Association of American Medical Colleges.

Atlas, S. J., Grant, R., Ferris, T., Chang, Y., & Barry, M. (2009). Patient–physician connectedness and quality of primary care. *Annals of Internal Medicine*, *150*(5), 325–335. doi:10.7326/0003-4819-150-5-200903030-00008 PMID:19258560

Aversa, S. (2013). *Comparing social sentiment on convenient care clinics*. Business-2Community. Retrieved from http://www.business2community.com/social-media/comparing-social-sentiment-on-convenient-care-clinics-0591279#t7OZE2fH8e2wkolg.99

Ayers, A. (2013). *Judges' Debriefing*. University of Alabama at Birmingham, Annual healthcare administration case competition.

Baker, S. E. (1992). The nurse practitioner in malpractice actions: Standards of care and theory of liability. *Health Matrix*, *2*, 325–355. PMID:10124882

Banjo, S. (2012). Wal-Mart lags in clinic race. *Wall Street Journal*. Retrieved from http://online.wsj.com/news/articles/SB100014240527023044586045774906801078448 76

BBC Research. (2012). Retrieved from www.bccresearch.com

Benfield Research. (2011). *Employer & Coalition Market Overview and Trends — Spring 2011*. Retrieved from: http://www.worksitehealth.org/sites/www.worksite-health.org/files/assets/Benfield%202011%20On-site%20Clinic%20Data.pdf

Bennett, K. L., & Phillips, J. P. (2010). Finding, recruiting, and sustaining the future primary care physician workforce: A new theoretical model of specialty choice process. *Academic Medicine*, *85*(10), S81–S88. doi:10.1097/ACM.0b013e3181ed4bae PMID:20881711

Berry, E. (2012). Work-site clinics try to cover employees' medical access gaps. Once limited to major employers that want occupational health services for workers, the clinics are popping up at more employers — and providing more services. *Amednews*. Retrieved from http://www.amednews.com/article/20120618/business/306189965/4/

Bindman, A. B., Grumbach, K., Osmond, D., Komaromy, M., Vranizan, K., & Lurie, N. et al. (1995). Preventable hospitalizations and access to health care. *Journal of the American Medical Association*, *274*(4), 305–311. doi:10.1001/jama.1995.03530040033037 PMID:7609259

Bitterman, R. A. (1992). A critical analysis of the federal COBRA hospital "antidumping law": Ramifications for hospitals, physicians, and effects on access to healthcare. *University of Detroit Mercy Law Review*, *70*, 125–190.

Bodenheimer, T., Berenson, R. A., & Rudolf, P. (2007). The primary care-specialty income gap: Why it matters. *Annals of Internal Medicine*, *146*(4), 301–306. doi:10.7326/0003-4819-146-4-200702200-00011 PMID:17310054

Bodenheimer, T., & Pham, H. H. (2010). Primary care: Current problems and proposed solutions. *Health Affairs (Project Hope)*, *29*(5), 799–805. doi:10.1377/hlthaff.2010.0026 PMID:20439864

Bodenheimer, T., Wagner, E., & Grumbach, K. (2002). Improving primary care for patients with chronic illness. *Journal of the American Medical Association*, *288*(15), 1909–1914. doi:10.1001/jama.288.15.1909 PMID:12377092

Boehringer Ingelheim Pharmaceuticals, Inc. (2010). *Boehringer Ingelheim Pharmacy Satisfaction™: Retail Clinic Outlook*. Retrieved from http://www.pharmacysatisfaction.com/resources/pdf/MI73586TRF_RCO_Appendix.pdf

Bohmer, R. M. J., & Groberg, J. P. (2002, July). *QuickMedx Inc*. (Case 603-049). Harvard Business School.

Bohmer, R. (2007). The rise of in-store clinics: Threat or opportunity? *The New England Journal of Medicine*, *356*(8), 765–768. doi:10.1056/NEJMp068289 PMID:17314334

Borkowski, S. (2012). Solutions for ED Overcrowding: Increasing Urgent Care Centers. *Journal of emergency nursing: JEN: official publication of the Emergency Department Nurses Association*, *38*(2), 116–117. doi:10.1016/j.jen.2011.12.009 PMID:22401611

Boukus, E.R., & Tu, H.T. (2012). *Despite Employer Interest, Workplace Clinic Use Low*. National Institute for Healthcare Reform.

Boulton, G. (2010, January 5). New clinic boosts access: Health center in Lena's market helps low-income residents. *Milwaukee Journal Sentinel*.

Brassard, A., & Smolenski, M. (2011). Removing barriers to advanced practice registered nurse care: Hospital privileges. *AARP Public Policy Institute Insight on the Issues*, *55*, 1–12.

Brown, E. (2011, March 13). Surgeon general discusses health and community. *Los Angeles Times*.

Buerhaus, P. I., Auerbach, D. I., & Staiger, D. O. (2009). The recent surge in nurse employment: Causes and implications. *Health Affairs*, *28*(4), w657–w668. doi:10.1377/hlthaff.28.4.w657 PMID:19525286

Bunn, W. B. III, Pikelny, D., Paralkar, S., Slavin, T., Borden, S. IV, & Allen, H. M. Jr. (2003). The burden of allergies-and the capacity of medications to reduce this nurden-in a heavy manufacturing environment. *Journal of Occupational and Environmental Medicine*, *45*(9), 941–955. doi:10.1097/01.jom.0000090468.73649.50 PMID:14506338

Burns, J. (2013). Bundled payment. *Hospitals & Health Networks*, (4), 26. PMID:23700754

Burns, L. R., David, G., & Helmchen, L. A. (2011). Strategic Response by Providers to Specialty Hospitals, Ambulatory Surgery Centers, and Retail Clinics. *Population Health Management*, *14*(2), 69–77. doi:10.1089/pop.2010.0021 PMID:21091376

Burton, W. N., Morrison, A., & Wertheimer, A. (2003). Pharmaceuticals and worker productivity loss: A critical review of the literature. *Journal of Occupational and Environmental Medicine*, *45*(6), 610–621. doi:10.1097/01.jom.0000069244.06498.01 PMID:12802214

Business Wire. (2013). *Zipnosis Announces Service in New Markets*. Retrieved from http://www.businesswire.com/news/home/20130118005961/en/Zipnosis-Announces-Service-Markets#.UsbhnvRDuSo

Byrne, R. (2009). Worksite Health Clinics Put New Focus On Employee Health. *HealthLeaders-InterStudy's Ohio, Kentucky & Indiana Health Plan Analysis*, *10*(1), 1–5.

C.S. Mott's Children Hospital. (2007). Retail Clinics: An Emerging Source of Healthcare for Children. C.S. *Mott Children's Hospital National Poll on Children's Health.*, *4*(3), 1–2.

California Healthcare Foundation. (2006). *Overuse of emergency departments among insured Californians*. Oakland, CA: Issue Brief.

Callahan, E. (2007, August 20). Retail clinics can be a valuable source partner. *Medical Staff Briefing*.

Care, O. (2012). *Growing your practice through telehealth*. Retrieved from: http://www.mackstudiopro.com/projects/client/AmericanWell/undocumented/videoLibrary_corpSite_v11_NewSite/pdf/OnlineCare_GrowingYourPracticeWithTelehealth.pdf

Carret, M. L., Fassa, A. C., & Domingues, M. R. (2009). Inappropriate use of emergency services: A systematic review of prevalence and associated factors. *Cadernos de Saude Publica*, *25*(1), 7–28. doi:10.1590/S0102-311X2009000100002 PMID:19180283

Casalino, L. P. (2010). A Martian's prescription for primary care: Overhaul the physician's workday. *Health Affairs*, *29*(5), 785–790. doi:10.1377/hlthaff.2010.0133 PMID:20439862

Cassel, C. K. (2012). Retail clinics and drugstore medicine. *Journal of the American Medical Association*, *307*(20), 2151–2152. doi:10.1001/jama.2012.3966 PMID:22618918

Center for Connected Health Policy. (2013). *What is Telehealth?* Retrieved from http://telehealthpolicy.us/what-telehealth

Center for Disease Control and Prevention. 2012. Retrieved April 17, 2013 from http://www.cdc.gov/obesity/index.html

Centers for Medicare & Medicaid. (2013). *Hospital Value-Based Purchasing*. Available at http://www.cms.gov/Medicare/Quality-Initiatives-Patient-Assessment-Instruments/hospital-value-based-purchasing/index.html?redirect=/hospital-value-based-purchasing/

Centers for Medicare & Medicaid. (2013). *Readmissions Reduction Program*. Available at http://www.cms.gov/Medicare/Medicare-Fee-for-Service-Payment/AcuteInpatientPPS/Readmissions-Reduction-Program.html

Centers for Medicare and Medicaid Services. (2013b). *HHS Final Rule and Treasury Notices on Individual Shared Responsibility Provision Exemptions, Minimum Essential Coverage, and Related Topics*. Retrieved from http://www.cms.gov/Newsroom/MediaReleaseDatabase/Fact-Sheets/2013-Fact-Sheets-Items/2013-06-26.html?DLPage=1&DLSort=0&DLSortDir=descending%20and%20a%20guidance%20

Centers for Medicare and Medicaid. 2013. Retrieved from http://www.cms.gov/Medicare/Quality-Initiatives-Patient-Assessment-Instruments/hospital-value-based-purchasing/index.html?redirect=/Hospital-Value-Based-Purchasing/

Champy, J. (2011). *What's really working in business. What it takes to win, big, now! Jim Champy brings together breakthrough approaches to strategy, marketing, and execution!* FT Press.

Chen, C., Xierali, I., Piwnica-Worms, K., & Phillips, R. (2013). The Redistribution Of Graduate Medical Education Positions In 2005 Failed To Boost Primary Care Or Rural Training. *Health Affairs*, *32*(1), 102–110. doi:10.1377/hlthaff.2012.0032 PMID:23297277

Chenewoth, D. H., & Garrett, J. (2006). Cost-Effectiveness Analysis of a Worksite Clinic: Is It Worth the Cost? *AAOHN Journal*, *54*(2), 84–89. PMID:16509183

Cherkin, D. C., Rosenblatt, R. A., Hart, L. G., Schneeweiss, R., & LoGerfo, J. (1987). The use of medical resources by residency- trained family physicians and general internists. Is there a difference? *Medical Care*, *25*(6), 455–469. doi:10.1097/00005650-198706000-00001 PMID:3695655

Chisholm-Burns, M. A., Kim Lee, J., Spivey, C. A., Slack, M., Herrier, R. N., & Hall-Lipsy, E. et al. (2010). US pharmacists' effect as team members on patient care: Systematic review and meta-analyses. *Medical Care*, *48*(10), 923–933. doi:10.1097/MLR.0b013e3181e57962 PMID:20720510

Christensen, C. (1997). *The innovator's dilemma: When new technologies cause great firms to fail*. Boston: Harvard Business School Press.

Christensen, C. M., Bohmer, R., & Kenagy, J. (2000). Will disruptive innovations cure healthcare? *Harvard Business Review*, *78*(5), 102–112. PMID:11143147

Christensen, C., Grossman, J. H., & Hwang, J. (2008). *The innovator's prescription: A disruptive solution for healthcare*. New York: McGraw-Hills.

Cisco. (2013). *Customer Experience Report for Health Care*. Insight Express.

Colihan, K. (2008, August 12). Parents like retail clinics for kids: Survey shows popularity of health clinics located in stores. *WebMD Health News*.

Commins, J. (2013, July 31). MT Health Clinics Are Cost Effective, Not 'Free'. *HealthLeaders Media*.

Commins, J. (2014a, January 6). Retail Medicine a Big Shift for 2014. *HealthLeaders Media*.

Commins, J. (2014b, February 25). Retail Medicine Syncs with High-Deductible Health Plans. *HealthLeaders*.

Consolidated Omnibus Budget Reconciliation Act, Pub. L. No. 99-272; 1986. 100 Stat. 82, codified as amended, 42 US Code, sec. 1395d(d).

Convenient Care Association. (2013). Retrieved from http://www.ccaclinics.org/index.php?option=com_content&view=article&id=4&Itemid=116

Cooper, R. A. (2001). Health care workforce for the twenty-first century: The impact of nonphysician clinicians. *Annual Review of Medicine*, *52*(1), 51–61. doi:10.1146/annurev.med.52.1.51 PMID:11160767

Cooper, R. A. (2004). Weighing the evidence for expanding physician supply. *Annals of Internal Medicine*, *141*(9), 705–714. doi:10.7326/0003-4819-141-9-200411020-00012 PMID:15520427

Costello, D. (2008). A checkup for retail medicine. *Health Affairs*, *27*(5), 1299–1303. doi:10.1377/hlthaff.27.5.1299 PMID:18780914

Council on Graduate Medical Education. (2007). *New paradigms for physician training for improving access to health care*. Eighteenth Report. Rockville, MD: COGME. Retrieved on March 24, 2010 from: http://www.cogme.gov/18thReport/default.htm

Courneya, P. T., Palattao, K. J., & Gallagher, J. M. (2013). HealthPartners' online clinic for simple conditions delivers savings of $88 per episode and high patient approval. *Health Affairs*, *32*(2), 385–392. doi:10.1377/hlthaff.2012.1157 PMID:23381532

Craven, G., & Ober, S. (2009). Massachusetts nurse practitioners step up as one solution to the primary care access problem. A political success story. *Policy, Politics & Nursing Practice*, *10*(2), 94–100. doi:10.1177/1527154409344627 PMID:19783534

Cunningham, P. (2011). *Nonurgent Use of Hospital Emergency Departments*. Statement Before the U.S. Senate. Health, Education, Labor and Pensions Committee Subcommittee on Primary Health and Aging Hearing on — Diverting Non-urgent Emergency Room Use: Can It Provide Better Care and Lower Costs?

D. R. *Walk-inMedical Clinics*. (2013). Retrieved from http://www.drwalkin.com/

Daugherty, A. (2012). Worksite clinics: Which model is right for you? *Advisory Board*. Retrieved from http://www.advisory.com/Research/Marketing-and-Planning-Leadership-Council/Service-Line-Transformation/2012/04/Worksite-clinics-Which-model-is-right-for-you

Deloitte Center for Health Solutions. (2008). *Growth of retail clinics: 2008 survey of healthcare consumers*. Author.

Deloitte Center for Health Solutions. (2008). *Retail clinics: Facts, trends and implications*. Author.

Deloitte Center for Health Solutions. (2009). *Retail clinics: Update and implications*. Author.

Deloitte Center for Health Solutions. (2012). *Survey of US Health Consumers*. Retrieved from http://www.deloitte.com/assets/dcom-unitedstates/local%20assets/documents/health%20reform%20issues%20briefs/us_chs_issuebrief_2012consumersurvey_061212.pdf

Dierick-van Daele, A. T., Metsemakers, J. F., Derckx, E. W., Spreeuwenberg, C., & Vrijhoef, H. J. (2009). Nurse practitioners substituting for general practitioners: Randomized controlled trial. *Journal of Advanced Nursing*, *65*(2), 391–401. doi:10.1111/j.1365-2648.2008.04888.x PMID:19191937

Dolan, P. L. (2009, March 30). Seasonal slump shutters 89 MinuteClinic Locations. *American Medical News*. Retrieved from http://www.ama-assn.org/amednews/2009/03/30/bisa0330.htm

Donaldson, R. (2009). The Lassa ward: One man's fight against one of the world's deadliest diseases. New York: St. Martin's Press.

Donaldson, M. S., Yordy, K. D., Lohr, K. N., & Vanselow, N. A. (1996). *Primary care: America's health in a new era*. Washington, DC: National Academy Press.

Dunn, L. (2011). From Treating the Sick to Managing Community Health: Hospitals' New Role in Managing Population Health. *Becker's Hospital Review*. Retrieved from http://www.beckershospitalreview.com/hospital-management-administration/from-treating-the-sick-to-managing-community-health-hospitals-new-role-in-managing-population-health.html

Dunn, L. (2010). Quotes on Healthcare in the Midst of Reform. *Top (Madrid)*, *10*.

Eder, R. (2005). A crowded market emerges to fill growth prescription. *Drug Store News*. Retrieved from http://business.highbeam.com/413375/article-1G1-135665176/crowded-market-emerges-fill-growth-prescription

Eibner, C. E., Hussey, P. S., Ridgeley, M. S., & McGlynn, E. A. (2009). *Controlling healthcare spending in Massachusetts, an analysis of options*. Rand Health.

Fairview Clinics. (2014). Retrieved from https://fairview.zipnosis.com/

Families U. S. A. (2011). *Understanding the New Health Reform Law: Fact Sheet*. Retrieved from http://www.familiesusa.org/assets/pdfs/health-reform/coverage-for-young-adults.pdf

Family Van. (2014). Retrieved from http://www.familyvan.org/about/

Feder, J. L. (2011). Charting A Life-and-Health Cycle And Expanded Primary Care Options For Patients In Wisconsin. *Health Affairs*, *30*(3), 387–389. doi:10.1377/hlthaff.2011.0062 PMID:21383347

Fenn, S. (2008). Integrating retail clinics into the hospital system. *Frontiers of Health Services Management*, *24*(3), 33–36. PMID:18435359

Fenn, S. (2008). Integrating Retail clinics into the Hospital System. *Frontiers of Health Services Management*, *24*(3), 33–36. PMID:18435359

Ferrer, R. L., Hambidge, S. J., & Maly, R. C. (2005). The essential role of generalists in health care systems. *Annals of Internal Medicine*, *142*(8), 691–699. doi:10.7326/0003-4819-142-8-200504190-00037 PMID:15838088

Fiscella, K., Meldrum, S., Franks, P., Shields, C. G., Duberstein, P., McDaniel, S. H., & Epstein, R. M. (2004). Patient Trust. *Medical Care*, *42*(11), 1049–1055. doi:10.1097/00005650-200411000-00003 PMID:15586831

Fluckinger, D. (2013). Health Systems involvement in online care Telemedicine clinics: Could they cannibalize primary care practices? *Search Health IT*. Retrieved from http://searchhealthit.techtarget.com/feature/Telemedicine-clinics-Could-they-cannibalize-primary-care-practices

Fluckinger, D. (2013a). Telemedicine clinics: Could they cannibalize primary care practices? *Search Health IT*. Retrieved from http://searchhealthit.techtarget.com/feature/Telemedicine-clinics-Could-they-cannibalize-primary-care-practices

Fluckinger, D. (2013b). Telemedicine reimbursement transcending party politics in some states. *Search Health IT*. Retrieved from http://searchhealthit.techtarget.com/healthitexchange/healthitpulse/telemedicine-reimbursement-transcending-party-politics-in-some-states/

Ford, J. (2011). Online healthcare: A new wave in convenience. *Advance for NPs & PAs*, *2*(4), 17. PMID:21661286

Fottler, M., & Malvey, D. (2010). *The retail revolution in healthcare*. Santa Barbara, CA: Praeger.

Friedberg, M. W., Hussey, P. S., & Schneider, E. C. (2010). Primary care: A critical review of the evidence on quality and costs of health care. *Health Affairs (Project Hope)*, *29*(5), 766–772. doi:10.1377/hlthaff.2010.0025 PMID:20439859

Fronstin, P. (2011). Findings from the 2011 EBRI/MGA Consumer Engagement in Health Care Survey. *EBRI Issue Brief*, *365*, 1–26. PMID:22312794

Fuld & Company. (2009). *The growth of on-site health clinics on-site clinics are expected to serve over 10% of the under 65s by 2015*. White Paper Press.

Gallegos, A. (2007). Retail medicine: The cure for healthcare disparities? *Journal of Healthcare Management*, *52*(4), 227–234. PMID:17695958

Garbutt, J. M., Mandrell, K. M., Allen, M., Sterkel, R., Esptein, J., & Kreusser, K. et al. (2013). Parents' experiences with pediatric care at retail clinics. *Journal of the American Medical Association Pediatrics.*, *167*(9), 845–850. PMID:23877236

Gardner, A. (2013). *Popularity of 'walk-in" retail health clinics growing: Poll trend driven by convenience, low cost and shortage of primary care doctors, Harris Interactive/HealthDay survey finds*. HealthDay. Retrieved from http://consumer.healthday.com/general-health-information-16/doctor-news-206/popularity-of-walk-in-retail-health-clinics-growing-poll-672127.html

Garson, A. Jr, Green, D. M., Rodriguez, L., Beech, R., & Nye, C. (2012). A new corps of trained grand-aides has the potential to increase the reach of primary care workforce and save money. *Health Affairs*, *31*(5), 1016–1021. doi:10.1377/hlthaff.2011.0859 PMID:22566441

Gartner Industry Research. (2008). *Case Study: A Texas Telemedicine Program Offers Lessons for Governments and Care Delivery Organizations Worldwide*. Retrieved from http://telehealth.utmb.edu/news/Gartner%20case_study_a_texas_telemedic_157582.pdf

Gay, J. G., Paris, V., Devaux, M., & de Looper, M. (2011). *Mortality amenable to healthcare in 31 OECD countries: estimates and methodological issues*. OECD Health Working Papers, No. 55, OECD Publishing.

GBI Research. (2012). *Retail Clinics – 2012 Yearbook*. Author.

Gee, P. (2007a). Compete with retail clinics and the rise of moi-medicine, or risk drowning in the wave of change. *Healthcare strategic management, 25*(2), 4-5, 16.

Gee, P. (2007b). Retail Clinics' Influence on Healthcare. *HealthLeaders Media Corner Office,* 29.

Gee, P. (2004). *Are You Ready for 'Big Box' Healthcare?* HealthLeaders Extra.

Gerencher, K. (2010, February 14). Yes, the uninsured can get care. *Wall Street Journal.*

Giberson, S., Yoder, S., & Lee, M. P. (2011). *Improving patient and health system outcomes through advanced pharmacy practice. A Report to the U.S. Surgeon General.Office of the Chief Pharmacist*. Public Health Service.

Goetzel, R. Z., Anderson, D. R., Whitmer, R. W., Ozminkowski, R. J., Dunn, R. L., & Wasserman, J. (1998). The Relationship Between Modifiable Health Risks and Healthcare Expenditures. *Journal of Occupational and Environmental Medicine*, *40*(10), 843–854. doi:10.1097/00043764-199810000-00003 PMID:9800168

Gold, J. (2012). Hospitals Gamble On Urgent Care Clinics To Keep Patients Healthy. *Kaiser Health News*. Retrieved from http://www.kaiserhealthnews.org/Stories/2012/November/08/urgent-care-clinics.aspx

Goldberg, G. A., & Newhouse, J. P. (1987). Effects of cost sharing on physiological health, health practices, and worry. *Health Services Research*, *22*, 279–306. PMID:3119520

Goldsmith, J.C. (1980). The Healthcare Market: Can hospitals survive? *Harvard Business Review*, *58*, 100–112. PMID:10247957

Goldsmith, J.C. (1980, September/October). The healthcare market: Can hospitals survive? *Harvard Business Review*, 100–112. PMID:10247957

Gonzales, R., Malone, D. C., Maselli, J. H., & Sande, M. A. (2001). Excessive antibiotic use for acute respiratory infections in the U.S. *Clinical Infectious Diseases*, *33*(6), 757–762. doi:10.1086/322627 PMID:11512079

Goolsby, M. J. (2011). 2009-2010 AANP national nurse practitioner sample survey: An overview. *Journal of the American Academy of Nurse Practitioners*, *23*(5), 266–268. doi:10.1111/j.1745-7599.2011.00611.x PMID:21518075

Gorman, K., Miller, R., & Kaspin, L. (2012). *Employer Services: Return on Investment*. Kansas City, MO: Cerner Corporation.

Government Accountability Office. (2009). *Hospital emergency departments: Crowding continues to occur, and some patients wait longer than recommended time frames*. Report to the Chairman, Committee on Finance, U.S. Senate. GAO-09-347.

Grayzel, E. F., Finegan, A., & Ponchak, R. (1997). The value of in-house physical therapy. *Journal of Occupational and Environmental Medicine*, *39*(4), 344–346. doi:10.1097/00043764-199704000-00014 PMID:9113606

Greenfield, S., Nelson, E. C., Zubkoff, M., Manning, W., Rogers, W., & Kravitz, R. L. et al. (1992). Variations in resource utilization among medical specialties and systems of care: Results from the Medical Outcomes Study. *Journal of the American Medical Association*, *267*(12), 1624–1630. doi:10.1001/jama.1992.03480120062034 PMID:1542172

Green, L. V., Savin, S., & Lu, Y. (2013). Primary care physician shortages could be eliminated through the use of teams, nonphysicians and electronic communication. *Health Affairs*, *32*(1), 11–19. doi:10.1377/hlthaff.2012.1086 PMID:23297266

Grossman, E. (2013). *Retail clinics: what the data shows*. Paper presented at Retail Clinician Education Congress. New York, NY.

Grundy, P., Hagan, K. R., Hansen, J. C., & Grumbach, K. (2010). The multi-stakeholder movement from primary care renewal and reform. *Health Affairs*, *29*(5), 791–798. doi:10.1377/hlthaff.2010.0084 PMID:20439863

Gulla, R. (2009, June 26). *MMS physician workforce study finds continued shortages in primary care*. Massachusetts Medical Society News Releases. Retrieved on February 22, 2010 from http://www.massmed.org/AM/Template.cfm?Section=MMS_News_Releases&CONTENTID=31507&TEMPLATE=/CM/ContentDisplay.cfm

Gullo, K. (2005). Many agree on potential benefits of onsite clinics in major retail stores that can provide basic medical services, yet large numbers are also skeptical. *The Wall Street Journal, 14*(21).

Halzack, S. (2012, October 21). Large employers look to on-site health clinics to reduce costs and absenteeism. *The Washington Post*. Retrieved from http://www.washingtonpost.com/business/capitalbusiness/large-employers-look-to-on-site-health-clinics-to-reduce-costs-and-absenteeism/2012/10/19/305f57ac-1924-11e2-aa6f-3b636fecb829_story.html

Hansen-Turton, T., & Ridgway, C. (2013). The future of accessible, affordable, quality healthcare. In J. Riff, S. F. Ryan, & T. Hansen-Turton (Eds.), *Convenient Care Clinics*. New York: Springer Publishing Company.

Hansen-Turton, T., Ridgway, C., Ryan, S. F., & Nash, D. B. (2009). Convenient care clinics: The future of accessible healthcare- The formation years 2006-2008. *Population Health Management*, *12*(5), 231–240. doi:10.1089/pop.2009.0041 PMID:19848565

Hansen-Turton, T., Ritter, A., Begun, H., Berkowitz, S. L., Rothman, N., & Valdez, B. (2006). Insurers' contracting policies on nurse practitioners are primary care providers: The current landscape and what needs to change. *Policy, Politics & Nursing Practice*, *7*(3), 216–226. doi:10.1177/1527154406294339 PMID:17071708

Hansen-Turton, T., Ritter, A., & Torgan, R. (2008). Insurers' contracting policies on nurse practitioners are primary care providers: Two year later. *Policy, Politics & Nursing Practice*, *9*(4), 241–248. doi:10.1177/1527154408319450 PMID:18562764

Hansen-Turton, T., Ryan, S., Miller, K., Counts, M., & Nash, D. (2007). Convenient care clinics: The future of accessible healthcare. *Disease Management*, *10*(2), 61–73. doi:10.1089/dis.2006.636 PMID:17444791

Hansen-Turton, T., Ware, J., & McClellan, F. (2010). Nurse practitioners in primary care. *Temple Law Review*, *82*, 1235–1263.

Harris Interactive. (2007) Most Adults Satisfied with Care at Retail-Based Health Clinics. *Health-Care Poll, 6*(6).

Hauer, K. E., Durning, S. J., Keman, W. N., Fagan, M. J., Mintz, M., & O'Sullivan, P. S. et al. (2008). Factors associated with medical students' career choices regarding internal medicine. *Journal of the American Medical Association*, *300*(10), 1154–1164. doi:10.1001/jama.300.10.1154 PMID:18780844

Hawkins, L. (2011). WhiteGlove seeks to raise $32.5 million in 'Dutch auction' IPO. *Austin American Statesman.* Retrieved from http://www.statesman.com/news/business/whiteglove-seeks-to-raise-325-million-in-dutch-auc/nRZg9/

Hawn, C. (2009). Take two aspirin and tweet me in the morning: How Twitter, Facebook and other social media are reshaping healthcare? *Health Affairs*, *28*(2), 361–368. doi:10.1377/hlthaff.28.2.361 PMID:19275991

Health Research Institute, Price Waterhouse Coopers. (2013). Top Industry. *Issues (National Council of State Boards of Nursing (U.S.))*, 2014.

Health Resources and Services Administration. (n.d.). *Health Center Program Terms and Definitions.* Retrieved April 12, 2013, from http://www.hrsa.gov/grants/apply/assistance/buckets/definitions.pdf

Healthcare.gov. (2013). *What if someone doesn't have health coverage in2014?* Retrieved from https://www.healthcare.gov/what-if-someonedoesnt-have-health-coverage-in-2014/

HealthPartners. (2014). Retrieved from https://www.healthpartners.com/public/care/family-of-care/parknicollet/

Heinzelmann, P.J., Williams, C.M., Lugn, N.E., & Kvedar, J.C. (2005). Clinical Outcomes Associated with Telemedicine/Telehealth. *Telemedicine and eHealth, 11*(3), 329-47.

Hello Health. (2013). Retrieved from http://hellohealth.com/about-myca/

Herritt, B. J. (2012). The House Call: Past, Present and Future. *UTMJ*, *89*(3), 175–177.

Hing, E., & Bhuiya, F. (2012). *Wait time for treatment in hospital emergency departments: 2009 NCHS data brief, no 102*. Hyattsville, MD: National Center for Health Statistics.

Hitti, M. (2007). Waiting room tops patient complaints: Patients generally satisfied with doctor-patient relationship, but both sides have gripes. *WebMD Health News*. Retrieved from http://www.webmd.com/health-insurance/20070108/waiting-room-tops-patient-complaints

Hochheiser, L. I., Woodward, K., & Charney, E. (1971). Effect of the neighborhood health center on the use of pediatric emergency departments in Rochester, New York. *The New England Journal of Medicine*, *285*(3), 148–152. doi:10.1056/NEJM197107152850305 PMID:5087704

Hochstadt, B. (2010). *The Value of On-site Health Centers*. Paper presented at Society for Human Resource Management. New York, NY..

Hofer, A. N., Abraham, J. M., & Moscovice, I. (2011). Expansion of coverage under the Patient Protection and Affordable Care Act and primary care utilization. *The Milbank Quarterly*, *89*(1), 69–89. doi:10.1111/j.1468-0009.2011.00620.x PMID:21418313

Hooker, R. S., Cawley, J. F., & Leinweber, W. (2010). Career flexibility of physician assistants and the potential for more primary care. *Health Affairs*, *29*(5), 880–886. doi:10.1377/hlthaff.2009.0884 PMID:20439875

Hopkins, S. C., Lenz, E. R., Pontes, N. M., Lin, S. X., & Mundinger, M. O. (2005). Context of care or provider training: The impact on preventive screening practices. *Preventive Medicine*, *40*(6), 718–724. doi:10.1016/j.ypmed.2004.09.013 PMID:15850870

Horrocks, S., Anderson, E., & Salisbury, C. (2002). Systematic review of whether nurse practitioners working in primary care can provide equivalent care to doctors. *BMJ (Clinical Research Ed.)*, *324*(7341), 819–823. doi:10.1136/bmj.324.7341.819 PMID:11934775

Horwitz-Bennett, B. (2013, February 4). Burgeoning retail clinics require unique designs. *Healthcare Design*. Retrieved from http://www.healthcaredesignmagazine.com/article/burgeoning-retail-clinics-require-unique-designs?page=3

HouseCall Course. (2013). Retrieved from http://advancedclinicalconsultants.org/the-housecall-course/

Hsia, R. Y., Asch, S. A., Weiss, R. E., Zingmond, D., Liang, L. J., Han, W., & Sun, B. C. (2011). Hospital determinants of emergency department left without being seen rates. *Annals of Emergency Medicine*, *58*(1), 24–32, 32.e3. doi:10.1016/j.annemergmed.2011.01.009 PMID:21334761

Huang, E. S., & Finegold, K. (2013). Seven millions Americans live in areas where demand for primary care may exceed supply by more than 10 percent. *Health Affairs*, *32*(3), 614–621. doi:10.1377/hlthaff.2012.0913 PMID:23426931

Huang, J., & Christensen, C. M. (2008). Disruptive innovation in healthcare delivery: A framework for business-model innovation. *Health Affairs*, *27*(5), 1329–1335. doi:10.1377/hlthaff.27.5.1329 PMID:18780919

Huff, C. (2012). *Going Mobile: On-Site Clinics Hit the Road for Employee Health Screenings*. Retrieved from http://www.workforce.com/article/20120406/NEWS02/120409962/going-mobile-on-site-clinics-hit-the-road-for-employee-health-screenings

Hunter, L. P., Weber, C. E., Morreale, A. P., & Wall, J. H. (2009). Patient satisfaction with retail health clinic care. *Journal of the American Academy of Nurse Practitioners*, *21*(10), 565–570. doi:10.1111/j.1745-7599.2009.00447.x PMID:19796291

Hurley, R. E., Freund, D. A., & Taylor, D. E. (1989). Emergency room use and primary care case management: Evidence from four Medicaid demonstration programs. *American Journal of Public Health*, *79*(7), 843–846. doi:10.2105/AJPH.79.7.843 PMID:2660603

Iglehart, J. K. (2010). Health reform, primary care, and graduate medical education. *The New England Journal of Medicine*, *363*(6), 584–590. doi:10.1056/NEJMhpr1006115 PMID:20660398

Institute of Medicine. (2003). *A shared destiny: community effects of uninsurance*. Washington, DC: National Academies Press.

Institute of Medicine. (2006). *The future of emergency care in the United States health system*. Washington, DC: National Academies Press.

Iora Health. (2014). Retrieved from http://www.iorahealth.com/

Itriage . (2014). Retrieved from http://about.itriagehealth.com/for-consumer/what-is-itriage/

Jacobson, P. D., & Jazowski, S. A. (2011). Physicians, the affordable care act and primary care: Disruptive change or business as usual? *Journal of General Internal Medicine*, *26*(8), 934–937. doi:10.1007/s11606-011-1695-8 PMID:21455812

Jacoby, R., Crawford, A. G., Chaudhari, P., & Goldfarb, N. I. (2011). Quality of care for 2 common pediatric conditions treated by convenient care providers. *American Journal of Medical Quality*, *26*(1), 53–58. doi:10.1177/1062860610375106 PMID:20861514

James, J. (2013). Health Policy Brief: Medicare Hospital Readmissions Reduction Program. *Health Affairs*, (November), 12.

Jaspen, B. (2007, June 25). AMA takes on retail clinics: Doctors groups say patients in danger. *Chicago Tribune*.

Jerant, A., Bertakis, K. D., Fenton, J. J., & Franks, P. (2012). Extended office hours and healthcare expenditures: A national study. *Annals of Family Medicine*, *10*(5), 388–395. doi:10.1370/afm.1382 PMID:22966101

Joint Commission. (2013). *Comprehensive Accreditation Manual for Ambulatory Care*. CAMAC.

Kaiser Family Foundation. (2012). *The uninsured and the difference health insurance makes*. Retrieved from http://kff.org/health-reform/fact-sheet/the-uninsured-and-the-difference-health-insurance/

Kaiser Family Foundation. (2013). *Key facts about the uninsured population*. Retrieved from http://kff.org/uninsured/fact-sheet/key-facts-about-the-uninsured-population/

Kaiser Family Foundation. (2013). Retrieved from http://kff.org/uninsured/

Kaiser Family Foundation. (2013a). *Status of State Action on the Medicaid Expansion Decision*. Retrieved from http://kff.org/health-reform/slide/current-status-of-the-medicaid-expansion-decision/

Kaiser Family Foundation. (2013b). *State decisions for creating health insurance exchanges*. Retrieved from http://kff.org/health-reform/slide/state-decisions-for-creating-health-insurance-exchanges/

Kaissi A. & Charland, T. (2013b). Hospital-owned retail clinics in the United States: Operations, patients and marketing. *Primary Healthcare, 3*(1).

Kaissi, A. (2010a). Hospital- affiliated and hospital-owned retail clinics: Strategic considerations and operational challenges. *Journal of Healthcare Management*, *55*(5), 324–337. PMID:21077582

Kaissi, A. (2010b). The future of retail clinics in a volatile healthcare environment. *The Health Care Manager*, *29*(3), 223–229. doi:10.1097/HCM.0b013e3181e93149 PMID:20686393

Kaissi, A., & Charland, T. (2013). The evolution of retail clinics in the United States, 2006-2012. *The Health Care Manager*, *32*(4), 336–342. doi:10.1097/HCM.0b013e3182a9d73f PMID:24168869

Kaissi, A., & Charland, T. (2013a). How Satisfied are Hospital Systems with their Ownership of Retail Clinics? *Journal of Healthcare Management*, *58*(2), 143–153. PMID:23650698

Kaissi, A., & Charland, T. (2013b). Hospital-Owned Retail Clinics in the United States: Operations, Patients and Marketing. *Primary Healthcare*, *3*(1), 1–5.

Kaissi, A., & Charland, T. (2013c). How satisfied are hospital systems with their ownership of retail clinics? *Journal of Healthcare Management*, *58*(2), 143–153. PMID:23650698

Kalorama Information. (2012*). Retail clinics 2012: Growth of stores, consumer opinion surveys, winning competitors, supplier sales of products to clinics, clinic sales forecasts and trends*. Author.

Kamerow, D. (2007). Retail health clinics-threat or promise? *British Medical Journal*, *335*(21).

Kao, H., Conant, R., Soriano, T., & McCormick, W. (2009). The Past, Present, and Future of House Calls. *Clinics in Geriatric Medicine*, *25*(1), 19–34. doi:10.1016/j.cger.2008.10.005 PMID:19217490

Keehan, S. P., Cuckler, G. A., Sisko, A. M., Madison, A. J., Smith, S. D., & Lizonitz, J. M. et al. (2012). National health expenditure projections: Modest annual growth until coverage expands and economic growth accelerates. *Health Affairs*, *31*(7), 1600–1612. doi:10.1377/hlthaff.2012.0404 PMID:22692089

Kellermann, A. L., Saultz, J., Mehrotra, A., Jones, S. S., & Dalal, S. (2013). Primary care technicians: A solution to the primary care workforce gap. *Health Affairs (Project Hope)*, *32*(11), 1893–1898. doi:10.1377/hlthaff.2013.0481 PMID:24191077

Kirch, D. G., Henderson, M. K., & Dill, M. J. (2012). Physician workforce projections in an era of reform. *Annual Review of Medicine*, *63*(1), 435–445. doi:10.1146/annurev-med-050310-134634 PMID:21888514

Kirkpatrick, B. (2012). *The Healthcare Executive's Guide to Urgent Care Centers and Freestanding EDs*. HealthLeaders Media.

Kissinger, M. (2008). Retail health clinics drive innovation into primary care practices. *The Journal of Medical Practice Management*, *23*(5), 314–319. PMID:18472612

Ku, L., Jones, K., Shin, P., Bruen, B., & Hayes, K. (2011). The states' next challenge-securing primary care for expanded Medicaid populations. *The New England Journal of Medicine*, *364*(6), 493–495. doi:10.1056/NEJMp1011623 PMID:21268720

Landers, S. H., Gunn, P. W., Flocke, S. A., Graham, A. V., Kikano, G. E., Moore, S. M., & Stange, K. C. (2005). Trends in house calls to Medicare beneficiaries. *Journal of the American Medical Association*, *294*(19), 2435–2436. PMID:16287953

Landro, L. (2006). The new force in walk-in clinics: Hospitals and doctors seek slice of burgeoning business; getting referrals at ShopRite. *Wall Street Journal*, 1-4.

Laurant, M., Reeves, D., Hermens, R., Braspenning, J., Grol, R., & Sibbald, B. (2005). Substitution of doctors by nurses in primary care. *Cochrane Database of Systematic Reviews*, (2): CD001271. PMID:15846614

Lavoie-Vaughan, N. (2013). *House Calls as a Practice Venture. Nurse Practitioner and Physician Assistant Advanced Web.* Retrieved from http://nurse-practitioners-and-physician-assistants.advanceweb.com/article/house-calls-as-a-practice-venture-2.aspx

Laws, M., Scott, M.K. (2008). The Emergence Of Retail-Based Clinics In The United States: Early Observations. *Health Affairs*, *27* (95), 1293-1298.

Laws, M., & Scott, M. K. (2008). The emergence of retail-based clinics in the United States: Early observations. *Health Affairs*, *27*(5), 1293–1298. doi:10.1377/hlthaff.27.5.1293 PMID:18780913

Lee, W. (2010, May 19). Online medicine in a hurry. *Minnesota Star Tribune*.

Leese, B., Allgar, V., Heywood, P., Walker, R., Darr, A., Din, I., & West, R. O. B. E. R. T. M. (2006). A new role for nurses as primary care cancer lead clinicians in Primary Care Trusts in England. *Journal of Nursing Management*, *14*(6), 462–471. doi:10.1111/j.1365-2934.2006.00644.x PMID:16919124

Leff, B., & Burton, J. R. (2001). The future history of home care and physician house calls in the United States. *The Journals of Gerontology. Series A, Biological Sciences and Medical Sciences*, *56*(10), M603–M608. doi:10.1093/gerona/56.10.M603 PMID:11584032

Leigh, J. P., Tancredi, D., Jerant, A., Romano, P. S., & Kravitz, R. L. (2012). Lifetime earnings for physicians across specialties. *Medical Care*, *50*(12), 1093–1101. doi:10.1097/MLR.0b013e318268ac0c PMID:22922430

Lenz, E. R., Mundinger, M. O., Hopkins, S. C., Lin, S. X., & Smolowitz, J. L. (2002). Diabetes care processes and outcomes in patients treated by nurse practitioners or physicians. *The Diabetes Educator*, *28*(4), 590–598. doi:10.1177/014572170202800413 PMID:12224199

Lenz, E. R., Mundinger, M., Kane, R., Hopkins, S., & Lin, S. (2004). Primary care outcomes in patients treated by nurse practitioners or physicians: Two-year follow-up. *Medical Care Research and Review*, *61*(3), 332–351. doi:10.1177/1077558704266821 PMID:15358970

Leppel, K. (2010). Factors influencing willingness to use convenient care clinics among baby boomers and older persons. *Healthcare Manage Review*, *35*(1), 13-22.

LeRoy, L., & Solkowitz, S. (1980). The costs and effectiveness of nurse practitioners, prepared for the Office of Technology Assessment, U.S. Congress. Washington, DC: U.S. Government Printing Office. Health Technology Case Study no. 16, Pub. no. OTA-HCS-16.

Lin, D. Q. (2008). Convenient care clinics: Opposition, opportunity, and the path to system integration. *Frontiers of Health Services Management*, *24*(3), 3–11. PMID:18435355

Linklaters. (2011). *Encouraging sustainable innovation in health*. White Paper. Retrieved from http://quickcheckhealth.com/encouraging-sustainable-innova/

Lohr, K. N., Brook, R., Kamberg, C., Goldberg, G. A., Leibowitz, A., & Keesey, J. et al. (1986). Use of medical care in the RAND Health Insurance Experiment: diagnosis- and service-specific analyses in a randomized controlled trial. *Medical Care*, *24*, S1–S87. PMID:3093785

Mahon, M., & Fox, B. (2011). *New study: U.S. ranks last among high-income nations on preventable deaths, lagging behind as others improve more rapidly* [Press Release]. The Commonwealth Fund Retrieved from http://www.commonwealthfund.org/News/News-Releases/2011/Sep/US-Ranks-Last-on-Preventable-Deaths.aspx

Malvey, D., & Fottler, M. D. (2006). The retail revolution in healthcare: Who will win and who will lose? *Health Care Management Review, 31*(3), 168–178. doi:10.1097/00004010-200607000-00002 PMID:16877884

Margolius, D., & Bodenheimer, T. (2010). Transforming primary care: From past practice to the practice of the future. *Health Affairs, 29*(5), 779–784. doi:10.1377/hlthaff.2010.0045 PMID:20439861

Margolius, D., & Bodenheimer, T. (2011). Redesigning after-hours care. *Annals of Internal Medicine, 155*(2), 131–132. doi:10.7326/0003-4819-155-2-201107190-00011 PMID:21768588

Market Strategies Inc. (2007). *One in ten retail clinic users replacing their primary care physician with retail clinic for treatment of common ailments*. Retrieved from http://www.marketstrategies.com/news/2014/1/One-in-Ten-Retail-Clinic-Users-Replacing-Their-Primary-Care-Physician-With-Retail-Clinic-for-Treatment-of-Common-Ailments.aspx

Market Strategies. (2007). *MinuteClinic – The evolving face of consumerism in healthcare*. Author.

Martin, E. (2003, March). QuickMedx preps to take clinic concept national. *Upsizemag.com.*

Marx, J. (2010). *Rosen's emergency medicine: Concepts and clinical practice* (7th ed.). Philadelphia, PA: Mosby/Elsevier.

Massachusetts Department of Public Health. (2008). Retrieved from www.massleague.org/CHCManual/105CMR140.pdf

Massachusetts Medical Society. (2008). *2008 Physician workforce study*. Waltham, MA: Massachusetts Medical Society.

McCarthy, D., & Klein, S. (2010). *QuadMed: Transforming Employer-Sponsored Healthcare Through Workplace Primary Care and Wellness Programs*. Washington, DC: The Commonwealth Fund.

McDaniel, R. D., & Dishman, E. (2012). *Patient-Centered Medical Home. A Foundation for Delivering Better Care, Better Health, and Better Value*. Sage Growth Partners LLC.

McNeeley, S. (2012). Urgent Care Centers: An Overview. *The American Journal of Chinese Medicine, 9*(2), 80–81.

Medicaid.gov. (22013). *Keeping America Healthy-Telemedicine*. Retrieved from http://www.medicaid.gov/Medicaid-CHIP-Program-Information/By-Topics/Delivery-Systems/Telemedicine.html

Medicine, M. (2010). *MinuteClinic ends 2009 with more closures*. Retrieved from http://www.merchantmedicine.com/News.cfm?view=77

Medicine, M. (2014). Retrieved from http://www.merchantmedicine.com

Medicine, M. (2011). *ConvUrgent Care Report, 4*(4), 1–4.

Medicine, M. (2011). *ConvUrgentCare Report, 4*(6), 1–6.

Medicine, M. (2011a). *The ConvUrgent Care Report*, *4*(1), 1–6.

Medicine, M. (2013a). *ConVurgentCare Report*, *6*(3), 1–5.

Medicine, M. (2013b). *ConVurgentCare Report.*, *6*(12), 1–6.

Mehrotra, A. (2013). The convenience revolution for treatment of low-acuity conditions. *Journal of the American Medical Association*, *310*(1), 35–36. doi:10.1001/jama.2013.6825 PMID:23821082

Mehrotra, A., & Lave, J. R. (2012). Visits to retail clinics grew fourfold from 2007 to 2009, although their share of overall outpatient visits remains low. *Health Affairs*, *31*(9), 2123–2129. doi:10.1377/hlthaff.2011.1128 PMID:22895454

Mehrotra, A., Liu, H., Adams, J. L., Wang, M. C., Lave, J. R., & Thygeson, M. et al. (2009). Comparing costs & quality of care at retail clinics with that of other medical settings for 3 common illnesses. *Annals of Internal Medicine*, *151*(5), 321–328. doi:10.7326/0003-4819-151-5-200909010-00006 PMID:19721020

Mehrotra, A., Paone, S., Martich, G. D., Albert, S. M., & Shevchik, G. J. (2013). A comparison of care at e-visits and physician office visits for sinusitis and urinary tract infection. *JAMA Internal Medicine*, *173*(1), 72–74. doi:10.1001/2013.jamainternmed.305 PMID:23403816

Mehrotra, A., Paone, S., Martich, G. D., Albert, S. M., & Shevchik, G. J. (2013a). Characteristics of patients who seek care via eVisits instead of office visits. *Telemedicine Journal and e-Health*, *19*(7), 515–519. doi:10.1089/tmj.2012.0221 PMID:23682589

Mehrotra, A., Wang, M. C., Lave, J. R., Adams, J. L., & McGlynn, E. A. (2008). Retail clinics, primary care physicians, and emergency departments: A comparison of patients' visits. *Health Affairs*, *27*(5), 1272–1282. doi:10.1377/hlthaff.27.5.1272 PMID:18780911

Mercer. (2012). *National Survey of Employer-Sponsored Health Plans*. Author.

Merchant Medicine. (2014). Retrieved from http://www.merchantmedicine.com

Mettner, J. (2009). The Doctor Is In (Your Inbox). E-visits can be an efficient way to practice, but they have been slow to catch on. *Minnesota Medicine*. Retrieved from http://www.minnesotamedicine.com/PastIssues/PastIssues2009/January2009/PulseInbox-January2009.aspx

Mettner, J. (2011, April). Virtual Visits Two Twin Cities-based online diagnostic services are bringing relief to patients—and providers. *Minnesota Medicine*. Retrieved from http://www.minnesotamedicine.com/Default.aspx?tabid=3736

Miceli, P. J., & Van Remortel, D. (2003). *Fostering patient loyalty in urgent care settings*. AACN Viewpoint, November/December.

Miller, J. (2007). Right size engineering: MinuteClinic CEO Michael Howe puts retail service suite in context. *Managed HealthCare Executive*. Retrieved from http://managedhealthcareexecutive.modernmedicine.com

Miller, J. M., & Nash, D. B. (2013). Quality metrics and initiatives in the clinic setting. In Convenient Care Clinics. New York: Springer Publishing Company.

MinuteClinic. 2013. Retrieved from http://www.minuteclinic.com/

Mulcahy, A. W., Lowsky, D., Chari, R., Hussey, P. S., Vaiana, M. E., & Kellermann, A. L. (2012). *Flattening the trajectory of health-care spending: Facilitate high-value innovation* (RB-9690/5). Santa Monica, CA: Rand Corporation. Retrieved from http://www.rand.org/pubs/research_briefs/RB9690z5

Mundinger, M. O., Kane, R. L., Lenz, E. R., Totten, A. M., Tsai, W. Y., & Cleary, P. D. et al. (2000). Primary care outcomes in patients treated by nurse practitioners or physicians: A randomized trial. *Journal of the American Medical Association*, *283*(1), 59–68. doi:10.1001/jama.283.1.59 PMID:10632281

National Association for Ambulatory Care (NAFAC). (2013). *National Urgent Care Practice Standards Certification.* Retrieved from http://www.urgentcare.org/CertificationStandards/tabid/134/Default.aspx

National Association for Ambulatory Care. (2012). Available at http://www.urgentcare.org/

National Association of Community Health Centers. (2008). Access transformed: Building a primary care workforce for the 21st century. Bethesda, MD: Author.

National Association of Community Health Centers. (2009). Primary care access: An essential building block of health reform. Bethesda, MD: Author.

National Association of Community Health Centers. (20213). *A sketchbook of community health centers.* Retrieved April 19, 2013 from http://www.nachc.com/client//Chartbook2013.pdf

National Conference of State Legislatures. (2012). *Retail health clinics: State legislatures and laws*. Retrieved from http://www.ncsl.org/research/health/retail-health-clinics-state-legislation-and-laws.aspx

National Headache Foundation. (2006). Emergency room vs. urgent care, a headache sufferer's dilemma. Chicago, IL: Author.

National Institute on Health Care Reform. (2011). *Matching Supply to Demand: Addressing the U.S. Primary Care Workforce Shortage.* NIHCR Policy Analysis No. 7. Retrieved on April 24, 2013 from http://www.nihcr.org/PCP_Workforce

National Residency Matching Program. (2008). *Results and Data: 2008 main residency match.* Retrieved on April 27, 2012 from: http://www.nrmp.org/data/resultsanddata2008.pdf

Naylor, M. D., & Kurtzman, E. T. (2010). The role of nurse practitioners in reinventing primary care. *Health Affairs*, *29*(5), 893–899. doi:10.1377/hlthaff.2010.0440 PMID:20439877

Newbold, P., & O'Neil, M. J. (2008). Small changes lead to large effects. *Frontiers of Health Services Management*, *24*(3), 23–27. PMID:18435357

Newmarker, C. (2008). *MinuteClinic co-founder launches e-medicine startup*. Minneapolis: St. Paul Business Journal Afternoon Edition Newsletter.

Niska, R., Bhuiya, F., & Xu, J. (2010). National hospital ambulatory medical care survey: 2007 emergency department summary. National health statistics reports; no 26. Hyattsville, MD: National Center for Health Statistics.

Niska, R., Bhuiya, F., & Xu, J. (2010). *National hospital ambulatory medical care survey: 2007 emergency department summary. National health statistics reports; no 26.* Hyattsville, MD: National Center for Health Statistics.

NowClinic. (2013a). Retrieved from https://www.mynowclinic.com/riteaid/about_us/overview/

NowClinic. (2013b). Retrieved from https://www.mynowclinic.com/patient/faq/

O'Brien, J. L., Martin, D. R., Heyworth, J. A., & Meyer, N. A. (2009). A phenomenological perspective on advanced practice nurse-physician collaboration within an interdisciplinary healthcare team. *Journal of the American Academy of Nurse Practitioners*, *21*(8), 444–453. doi:10.1111/j.1745-7599.2009.00428.x PMID:19689441

O'Malley, A. S., Gerland, A. M., Pham, H. H., & Berenson, R. A. (2005, November). *Rising pressure: hospital emergency departments as barometers of the healthcare system*, (issue brief no. 101). Center for Studying Health System Change. Retrieved from http://www.hschange.com/CONTENT/799/?words=au167

O'Malley, A. S., Samuel, D., Bond, A. M., & Carrier, E. (2012). After-hours care and its coordination with primary care in the U.S. *Journal of General Internal Medicine*, *27*(11), 1406–1415. doi:10.1007/s11606-012-2087-4 PMID:22653379

O'Reilly, K. B. (2007, March 5). Big retail health clinics agree to AAFP operating guidelines-2007: A newly formed quick-care trade group also aims to collaborate with physician organizations. *American Medical News*.

Ohman-Strickland, P. A., Orzano, A. J., Hudson, S. V., Solberg, L. I., DiCiccio-Bloom, B., & O'Malley, D. et al. (2008). Quality of diabetes care in family medicine practices: Influence of nurse-practitioners and physician's assistants. *Annals of Family Medicine*, *6*(1), 14–22. doi:10.1370/afm.758 PMID:18195310

O'Malley, A. S. (2013). After-hours access to primary care practices linked with lower emergency department use and less unmet medical need. *Health Affairs*, *32*(1), 175–183. doi:10.1377/hlthaff.2012.0494 PMID:23242631

On Site Clinics. (2010). Retrieved from http://onsiteclinics.org/faqs/#sthash.kqKw1Jxk.dpuf

Online Care Anywhere. (2013). Retrieved from http://www.onlinecareanywheremn.com/howitworks.php

Organization for Economic Co-operation and Development. (2012). *OECD Health Data*. Retrieved from http://www.oecd.org/health/health-systems/health-at-a-glance.htm

Paddock, C. (2007, June 26). AMA calls for investigation of retail health clinics. *Medical News Today*.

Palmeri, M., Pipas, C., Wadsworth, E., & Zubkoff, M. (2010). Economic Impact of a primary care career: A harsh reality for medical student and the nation. *Academic Medicine*, *85*(11), 1692–1697. doi:10.1097/ACM.0b013e3181f5b754 PMID:20881829

Parchman, M. L., & Culler, S. (1994). Primary care physicians and avoidable hospitalization. *The Journal of Family Practice*, *39*, 123–128. PMID:8057062

Parente, S. T., & Town, R. (2009). *The impact of retail clinics on cost, utilization and welfare*. University of Minnesota, unpublished paper.

Park, M., Cherry, D., & Decker, S. L. (2011). Nurse practitioners, certified nurse midwives, and physician assistants in physician offices. *NCHS Data Brief*, *69*, 1–8. PMID:22142469

Patient Protection and Affordable Care Act. (2010). Retrieved from http://www.healthcare.gov/law/full/index.html

Patwardhan, A., Davis, J., Murphy, P., & Ryan, S. F. (2012). After-hours access of convenient care clinics and cost savings associated with avoidance of higher-cost sites of care. *Journal of Primary Care & Community Health*, *3*(4), 243–245. doi:10.1177/2150131911436251 PMID:23804168

Pearson, L. J. The Pearson Report 2011. Retrieved on May 9 2012 from http://www.pearsonreport.com/

Pearson, L. J. (2012). *The 2012 Pearson Report: A nation overview of nurse practitioner legislation and healthcare issues*. Monroe Township, N.J.: NP Communication, LLC.

Perman, C. (2012) *Healthcare reform's major hurdle: doctor shortages*. Retrieved from http://www.cnbc.com/id/36036747/Health_Care_Reform_s_Major_Hurdle_Doctor_Shortages

Petterson, S. M., Liaw, W. R., Phillips, R. L., Rabin, D., Meyers, D., & Bazemore, A. W. (2012). Projecting US primary care workforce needs: 2010-2025. *Annals of Family Medicine*, *10*(6), 503–509. doi:10.1370/afm.1431 PMID:23149526

Physician Assistant History Society. (2013). Retrieved on May 6, 2013 from http://www.pahx.org/period02.html

Pitts, S. R., Carrier, E. R., Rich, E. C., & Kellermann, A. L. (2010). Where Americans get acute care: Increasingly, it's not at their doctor's office. *Health Affairs*, *29*(9), 1620–1629. doi:10.1377/hlthaff.2009.1026 PMID:20820017

Pollack, C. E., & Armstrong, K. (2009). The geographic accessibility of retail clinics for underserved populations. *Archives of Internal Medicine*, *169*(10), 945–949. doi:10.1001/archinternmed.2009.69 PMID:19468086

Pollack, C. E., Gidengil, C., & Mehrotra, A. (2010). The growth of retail clinics and the medical home: Two trends in concert or in conflict? *Health Affairs*, *29*(5), 998–1003. doi:10.1377/hlthaff.2010.0089 PMID:20439897

Pollert, P., Dobberstein, D., & Wiisanen, R. (2008). Jumping into the healthcare market: Our experience. *Frontiers of Health Services Management*, *24*(3), 13–21. PMID:18435356

Pollitz, K., Cox, C., Lucia, K., & Keith, K. (2014). *Medical debt among people with health insurance*. Kaiser Family Foundation. Retrieved from http://kff.org/private-insurance/report/medical-debt-among-people-with-health-insurance/

Porter, S. (n.d.). Provision in healthcare reform law gives primary care financial boost. *AAFP New Now*. Retrieved from http://www.aafp.org/online/en/home/publications/news/news-now/practice-management/20100903primcarebonus.html

Post, P. (2007). *Mobile Healthcare for Homeless People: Using Vehicles to Extend Care*. National Healthcare for the Homeless Council. Retrieved from http://www.nhchc.org/wp-content/uploads/2012/02/mobilehealth.pdf. Last accessed 1/4/14

Press Ganey. (2010). *ED Pulse Report*. South Bend, IN: Author.

Prince, T. S., Spengler, S., & Collins, T. (2001). Corporate travel medicine: Benefit analysis of on-site services. *Journal of Travel Medicine*, *8*(4), 163–166. doi:10.2310/7060.2001.22213 PMID:11703899

Pugno, P. A., Schmittling, G. T., Fetter, G. T. Jr, & Kahn, N. B. Jr. (2005). Results of the 2005 national resident matching program: Family medicine. *Family Medicine*, *37*, 555–564. PMID:16145633

Punke, H. (2013, February 7). Walgreens' Strategy Behind ACO Participation. *Becker Hospital Review*.

PwC. (2013). *Medical cost trend: Behind the numbers 2014*. Health Research Institute.

RediClinic. (2013). Retrieved from http://www.rediclinic.com/about/faqs/

Reed, M., Graetz, I., Wang, H., Fung, V., Newhouse, J. P., & Hsu, J. (2012). Consumer-directed health plans with health savings accounts: Whose skin is in the game and how do costs affect care seeking? *Medical Care*, *50*(7), 585–590. doi:10.1097/MLR.0b013e3182495cb3 PMID:22322099

Reid, J. (1996). *A Telemedicine Primer: Understanding the Issues*. Billings, MT: Innovative Medical Communications.

Reid, R. O., Ashwood, J. S., Friedberg, M. W., Weber, E. S., Setodji, C. M., & Mehrotra, A. (2013). Retail clinic visits and receipt of primary care. *Journal of General Internal Medicine*, *28*(4), 504–512. doi:10.1007/s11606-012-2243-x PMID:23070656

Richman, D. (2013). *Harris Interactive: Consumer trends in retail medicine.* Paper presented at Retail Clinician Education Congress. New York, NY.

Richman, D. (2013, May 14). *Consumer trends in retail medicine*. Paper presented at the Retail Clinician Education Congress. New York, NY.

Rieselbach, R. E., Crouse, B. J., & Frohna, J. G. (2010). Teaching primary care in community health centers: Addressing the workforce crisis for the underserved. *Annals of Internal Medicine*, *152*(2), 118–122. doi:10.7326/0003-4819-152-2-201001190-00186 PMID:20008743

Robert Wood Johnson Foundation. (2013). *State-level trends in employer-sponsored health insurance. A state-by-state analysis.* Author.

Roblin, D. W., Howard, D. H., Becker, E. R., Kathleen Adams, E., & Roberts, M. H. (2004, June). (22004). Use of midlevel practitioners to achieve labor cost savings in the primary care practice of an MCO. *Health Services Research*, *39*(3), 607–626. doi:10.1111/j.1475-6773.2004.00247.x PMID:15149481

Rodak, S. (2012). How Can Retail Health Help Hospitals Meet Health Reform Goals? *Becker Hospital Review*. Retrieved from http://www.beckershospitalreview.com/strategic-planning/how-can-retail-health-help-hospitals-meet-health-reform-goals.html

Rodak, S. (2012, December 3). How Can Retail Health Help Hospitals Meet Health Reform Goals? *Becker Hospital Review*.

Rohrer, J. E., Angstam, K. B., & Furst, J. W. (2009a). Impact of retail walk-in care on early return visits by adult primary care patients. *Quality Management in Health Care*, *18*(1), 19–24. doi:10.1097/01.QMH.0000344590.61971.97 PMID:19148026

Rohrer, J. E., Angstman, K. B., Adamson, S. C., Bernard, M. E., Bachman, J. W., & Morgan, M. E. (2010). Impact of online primary care visits on standard costs: A pilot study. *Population Health Management*, *13*(2), 59–63. doi:10.1089/pop.2009.0018 PMID:20415617

Rohrer, J. E., Angstram, K. B., & Bartel, G. A. (2009b). Impact of retail medicine on standard costs in primary care: A semiparametric analysis. *Population Health Management*, *12*(6), 333–335. doi:10.1089/pop.2009.0007 PMID:20038259

Rohrer, J. E., Angstram, K. B., Garrison, G. M., Maxson, J. A., & Furst, J. W. (2013). Family medicine patients who use retail clinics have lower continuity of care. *Journal of Primary Care and Community Health*, *4*(2), 150–153. doi:10.1177/2150131912471683 PMID:23799725

Rohrer, J. E., Garrison, G. M., & Angstman, K. B. (2012). Early Return Visits by Pediatric Primary Care Patients With Otitis Media. *Quality Management in Health Care*, *21*(1), 44–47. doi:10.1097/QMH.0b013e3182418157 PMID:22207018

Rohrer, J. E., Yapuncich, K. M., Adamson, S. C., & Angstam, K. B. (2008). Do retail clinics increase early return visits for pediatric clinics? *Journal of the American Board of Family Medicine*, *21*(5), 475–476. doi:10.3122/jabfm.2008.05.080072 PMID:18772304

Rubenstein, S. (2009). CVS shutters 90 retail clinics for the season. *Wall Street Journal.*

Rudavsky, R., & Mehrotra, A. (2010). Sociodemographic characteristics of communities served by retail clinics. *Journal of the American Board of Family Medicine*, *23*(1), 42–48. doi:10.3122/jabfm.2010.01.090033 PMID:20051541

Rudavsky, R., Pollack, C. E., & Mehrotra, A. (2009). The geographic distribution, ownership, prices, and scope of practice at retail clinics. *Annals of Internal Medicine*, *151*(5), 315–320. doi:10.7326/0003-4819-151-5-200909010-00005 PMID:19721019

Running, A., Kipp, C., & Mercer, V. (2006). Prescriptive patterns of nurse practitioners and physicians. *Journal of the American Academy of Nurse Practitioners*, *18*(5), 228–233. doi:10.1111/j.1745-7599.2006.00120.x PMID:16681710

Rust, G., Ye, J., Baltrus, P., Daniels, E., Adesunloye, B., & Fryer, G. E. (2008). Practical barriers to timely primary care access: Impact on adult use of emergency department services. *Archives of Internal Medicine*, *168*(15), 1705–1710. doi:10.1001/archinte.168.15.1705 PMID:18695087

Ryan, K., & Rahman, A. (2012). Examining factors influencing patient satisfaction with nurse practitioners in rural urgent care centers. *Journal of the American Academy of Nurse Practitioners*, *24*(2), 77–81. doi:10.1111/j.1745-7599.2011.00688.x PMID:22324862

Sackett, D. L. (2009). A landmark randomized healthcare trial: The Burlington trial of the nurse practitioner. *Journal of Clinical Epidemiology*, *62*(6), 567–570. doi:10.1016/j.jclinepi.2009.01.001 PMID:19356898

Salganik, M. W. (2004, August 8). Selling quick fix for minor ailments- health: Clinics promising inexpensive, convenient care are to open in local Target stores. *The Baltimore Sun.* Retrieved from http://articles.baltimoresun.com/2004-08-08/news/0408080212_1_target-health-clinics-pizza-hut

Sanders, B. (2013). *Primary care access- 30 million new patients and 11 months to go: Who will provide their primary care? Report from Chairman Bernard Sanders, Subcommittee on Primary Health and Aging*. U.S. Senate Committee on Health, Education, Labor & Pensions.

Sandstrom, C. (2010). *5 Examples Of Disruptive Innovation*. Retrieved from http://disruptiveinnovation.se/

Scanadu. (2014). Retrieved from http://www.scanadu.com/

Schleiter, K.E. (2010). Retail medical clinics: Increasing access to low cost medical care amongst a developing legal environment. *Annals of Health Law*, *19*(3), 527–575. PMID:21456398

Schoen, C., Osborn, R., Doty, M. M., Bishop, M., Peugh, J., & Murukutla, N. (2007). Toward higher-performance health systems: Adults' healthcare experiences in seven countries, 2007. *Health Affairs*, *26*(6), 717–734. doi:10.1377/hlthaff.26.6.w717

Scott, M.K. (2008a, January 4). Retail clinics- Friend of Foe of the hospital- Part I. The opportunity for hospitals to win with a retail clinic model. *HealthLeaders Media*.

Scott, M.K. (2008b, January 18). Retail clinics- Friend of Foe of the hospital- Part II. Tools to assess the potential impact on patient and physician populations, economics, and brand. *HealthLeaders Media*.

Scott, M. K. (2006). *Healthcare in the express lane: The emergence of retail clinics*. California HealthCare Foundation.

Scott, M. K. (2013). Building and marketing a retail clinic. In J. Riff, S. F. Ryan, & T. Hansen-Turton (Eds.), *Convenient Care Clinics*. New York: Springer Publishing Company.

Scruby, D. J., Denham, S., & Larkin, G. (2001). Economic impact of on-site physical therapy. *Journal of Occupational and Environmental Medicine*, *43*(8), 670–671. doi:10.1097/00043764-200108000-00002 PMID:11515248

Seale, C., Anderson, E., & Kinnersley, P. (2006). Treatment advice in primary care: A comparative study of nurse practitioners and general practitioners. *Journal of Advanced Nursing*, *54*(5), 534–541. doi:10.1111/j.1365-2648.2006.03865.x PMID:16722950

Sherman, B. W., & Fabius, R. J. (2012). Quantifying the Value of Worksite Clini Non-occupational Healthcare Services: A Critical Analysis and Review of the Literature. *JOEM*, *54*(4), 394–403. PMID:22418274

Sherman, B.W. (2010). Worksite Clinics and the Patient-Centered Medical Home: Competition or Collaboration? *The American Journal of Managed Care*, *16*(5), 323–325. PMID:20469952

Smith, K. (2013). *Telehealth: Management of Patient Outcomes and Protecting the Continuity of Care*. Paper presented at Retail Clinician Education Congress. New York, NY.

Smith, D. (2007). Disruptive innovation: Can healthcare learn from other industries? A conversation with Clayton Christensen. *Health Affairs*, *26*(3), 288–295. doi:10.1377/hlthaff.26.3.w288

Smith, S. R. (2011). A recipe for medical schools to produce primary care physicians. *The New England Journal of Medicine*, *364*(6), 496–497. doi:10.1056/NEJMp1012495 PMID:21306236

Son, A. (2013). *IBISWorld Industry Report OD5458*. Urgent Care Centers in the US.

Song, Z., Hill, C., Bennet, J., Vavasis, A., & Oriol, N. E. (2013). Mobile Clinic In Massachusetts Associated With Cost Savings From Lowering Blood Pressure And Emergency Department Use. *Health Affairs (Project Hope)*, *32*(1), 36–44. doi:10.1377/hlthaff.2011.1392 PMID:23297269

Spetz, J., Parente, S. T., Town, R. J., & Bazarko, D. (2013). Scope-of-practice laws for nurse practitioners limit cost savings that can be achieved in retail clinics. *Health Affairs*, *32*(11), 1977–1984. doi:10.1377/hlthaff.2013.0544 PMID:24191089

Spitzer, W. O., Sackett, D. L., Sibley, J. C., Roberts, R. S., Gent, M., & Kergin, D. J. et al. (1974). The Burlington randomized trial of the nurse practitioner. *The New England Journal of Medicine*, *290*(5), 251–256. doi:10.1056/NEJM197401312900506 PMID:4808929

Starfield, B. (1994). Is primary care essential? *Lancet*, *344*(8930), 1129–1133. doi:10.1016/S0140-6736(94)90634-3 PMID:7934497

Starfield, B. (2009). The geographic accessibility of retail clinics for underserved populations – Invited Commentary. *Archives of Internal Medicine*, *169*(10), 950–951. doi:10.1001/archinternmed.2009.110

Starfield, B., Shi, L., & Macinko, J. (2005). Contributions of primary care to health systems and health. *The Milbank Quarterly*, *83*(3), 457–502. doi:10.1111/j.1468-0009.2005.00409.x PMID:16202000

Stempniak, M. (2013, October). Retail clinics: Threat or opportunity? *Hospitals & Health Networks*. PMID:24303633

Stern, David. (2005). Status of Urgent Care in the U.S. *Business Briefing: Emergency Medicine Review.*

Takach, M., & Witger, K. (2009). *Analysis of state regulations and policies governing the operation and licensure of retail clinics*. Washington, DC: National Academy for State Health Policy.

Tang, N., Stein, J., Hsia, R. Y., Maselli, J. H., & Gonzales, R. (2010). Trends and characteristics of US emergency department visits, 1997-2007. *Journal of the American Medical Association*, *304*(6), 664–670. doi:10.1001/jama.2010.1112 PMID:20699458

Taylor, H. (2008). *Innovations in care delivery: Retail clinics. Retail clinics: A new trend in healthcare*. Paper presented at a National Consumers League Stakeholders Forum. New York, NY.

Teladoc. (2014). Retrieved from http://www.teladoc.com/

ter Bogt, N. C., Bemelmans, W. J., Beltman, F. W., Broer, J., Smit, A. J., & van der Meer, K. (2009). Preventing weight gain: One-year results of a randomized lifestyle intervention. *American Journal of Preventive Medicine*, *37*(4), 270–277. doi:10.1016/j.amepre.2009.06.011 PMID:19765497

Terry, K. (2009, May 1). Worksite Clinics - The Next Threat? *Physician Practice*, 1-2.

The Advisory Board Company. (2012). *Member asks: How can we set up a retail clinic partnership?* Retrieved from http://www.advisory.com/Daily-Briefing/2012/11/13/Member-asks

The Commonwealth of Massachusetts. (2006). Retrieved on April 24, 2013 from http://www.malegislature.gov/Laws/SessionLaws/Acts/2006/Chapter58

The Henry J. Kaiser Family Foundation. (2010). *Focus on Health Reform- Summary of new health reform law*. Retrieved on April 24, 2013 from http://www.kff.org/healthreform/upload/8061.pdf

The Kaiser Family Foundation. (2012). *Massachusetts Health care reform: Six years later.* Retrieved on April 24 2013 from: http://www.kff.org/healthreform/upload/8311.pdf

The Patient Protection and Affordable Care Act. (n.d.). Retrieved on April 24, 2013 from http://www.healthcare .gov/law/full/index.html

Thomas, L. (2011). *Early Permanente physicians: making do with makeshift facilities*. Retrieved from http://kaiserpermanentehistory.org/tag/sidney-garfield/

Thygeson, M., Van Vorst, K. A., Maciosek, M. V., & Solberg, L. (2008). Use and costs of care in retail clinics versus traditional care sites. *Health Affairs*, *27*(5), 1283–1292. doi:10.1377/hlthaff.27.5.1283 PMID:18780912

Topol, E. (2012). *The Creative Destruction of Medicine: How the Digital Revolution Will Create Better Health Care*. New York: Basic Books.

Tower Watson. (2012). *2012 On Site Health Center Survey Report*. Author.

Trafford, A. (1983, December19). For doctors, too, it is a surplus. *U.S. News & World Report*, 62–64. PMID:10264129

Truven Health Analytics. (2012). *Data-driven marketing strategy brings new clients to innovative retail clinic*. Retrieved from http://truvenhealth.com/assets/HOSP_11467_0712_HeartlandHealth_CS_Web.pdf

Tu, H. T., & Cohen, G. R. (2008). Checking up on retail-based health clinics: Is the boom ending? *Commonwealth Fund, 1199* (48), 1-11.

Tu, H.T., Boukus, E.R., Cohen, G.R. (2010). *Workplace Clinics: A Sign of Growing Employer Interest in Wellness.* Center for Studying Health System Change.

Tu, H. T., & Boukus, E. R. (2013). *Despite rapid growth, retail clinic use remains modest (Research Brief 29)*. Center for Studying Health System Change.

Tu, H. T., Boukus, E. R., & Cohen, G. R. (2010). *Workplace clinics: A sign of growing employer interest in wellness (Research Brief 17)*. Center for Studying Health System Change.

Turner, D. E. (2010). Worksite primary care: An assessment of cost and quality metrics. *Journal of Occupational and Environmental Medicine*, *52*(6), 573–575. doi:10.1097/JOM.0b013e3181e317b6 PMID:20535088

U.S. Congress, Office of Technology Assessment. (1986). Nurse practitioners, physician assistants, and certified nurse-midwives: a policy analysis. Washington, DC: U.S. Government Printing Office. Health Technology Case Study no. 37, Pub. no. OTA-HCS-37.

U.S. Department of Health and Human Services. (2013). *"What is mHealth?"*. Retrieved from http://www.hrsa.gov/healthit/mhealth.html

U.S. Small Business Administration. (2013). *Employers with 50 or more employees*. Retrieved from http://www.sba.gov/content/employers-with-50-or-more-employees

United States Department of Labor. (2012). *Technical Release No. 2012-01: Frequently Asked Questions from Employers Regarding Automatic Enrollment, Employer Shared Responsibility, and Waiting Periods*. Retrieved from http://www.dol.gov/ebsa/newsroom/tr12-01.html

United States Government Accountability Office. (2008). Primary care professionals: Recent supply trends, projections, and valuation of services. Washington, DC: Author.

Urgent Care Association of America. (2011). (2010). Urgent Care Benchmarking Survey Results. *Structure (London, England)*.

Urgent Care Association of America. (2011). *The case for urgent care*. Naperville, IL: Author.

Urgent Care Association of America. (2013). Available at http://www.ucaoa.org/

Urgent Care College of Physicians. (2013). Available at http://www.uccop.org/

US Department of Health and Human Services Council on Graduate Medical Education. (2005). *Physician workforce policy guidelines for 2000-2020*. Rockville, MD: COGME.

Uscher-Pines, L., Harris, K. M., Burns, R., & Mehrotra, A. (2012). The growth of retail clinics in vaccination delivery in the U.S. *American Journal of Preventive Medicine*, *43*(1), 63–66. doi:10.1016/j.amepre.2012.02.024 PMID:22704748

Uscher-Pines, L., Mehrotra, A., & Chari, R. (2013). On call at the mall: A mixed methods study of U.S. medical malls. *BMC Health Services Research*, *13*(1), 471. doi:10.1186/1472-6963-13-471 PMID:24209495

Uscher-Pines, L., Pines, J., Kellermann, A., Gillen, E., & Mehrotra, A. (2013). Emergency department visits for nonurgent conditions: Systematic literature review. *The American Journal of Managed Care*, *19*(1), 47–59. PMID:23379744

Vaughn, B. T., DeVrieze, S. R., Reed, S. D., & Schulman, K. A. (2010). Can we close the income gap between specialists and primary care physicians? *Health Affairs (Project Hope)*, *29*(5), 933–940. doi:10.1377/hlthaff.2009.0675 PMID:20439883

Vesely, R. (2011). The doctor will see you now—at your office. Workplace health clinics making a resurgence. *Modern Healthcare*, (May): 30.

Virtuwell. (2013). Retrieved from https://www.virtuwell.com/

Walgreens. (2013). Retrieved from http://www.walgreens.com/topic/pharmacy/healthcare-clinic/price-menu.jsp#treatment

Wang, M. C., Ryan, G., McGlynn, E. A., & Mehrotra, A. (2010). Why Do Patients Seek Care at Retail Clinics and What Alternatives Did They Consider. *American Journal of Medical Quality*, *25*(2), 128–134. doi:10.1177/1062860609353201 PMID:20142442

Wasson, J. H., Sauvigne, A. E., Mogielnicki, R. P., Frey, W. G., Sox, C. H., & Gaudette, C. et al. (1984). Continuity of outpatient medical care in elderly men: A randomized trial. *Journal of the American Medical Association*, *252*(17), 2413–2417. doi:10.1001/jama.1984.03350170015011 PMID:6481927

Watson Wyatt. (2008). Realizing the Potential of Onsite Health Centers. Author.

Weinick, R. M., Pollack, C. E., Fisher, M. P., Gillen, E. M., & Mehrotra, A. (2010). *Policy implications of the use of retail clinics*. Rand Health Technical Report.

Weinick, R. M., Bristol, S. J., & DesRoches, C. M. (2009). Urgent care centers in the U.S.: Findings from a national survey. *BMC Health Services Research*, *9*(79), 1–9. PMID:19445656

Weinick, R. M., Bristol, S. J., Marder, J. E., & DesRoches, C. M. (2009). The Search for the Urgent Care Center. *The Journal of Urgent Care Medicine*, *3*, 438–440. http://jucm.com/2009-jan/ucupdate2.shtml

Weinick, R. M., Burns, R. M., & Mehrotra, A. (2010). Many Emergency Department Visits Could Be Managed At Urgent Care Centers And retail clinics. *Health Affairs*, *29*(9), 1630–1636. doi:10.1377/hlthaff.2009.0748 PMID:20820018

Weinick, R., & Bentacourt, R. M. (2007). *No appointment needed- The resurgence of urgent care centers in the United States*. California Healthcare Foundation.

West, C. P., Popkave, C., Schultz, H. J., Weinberger, S. E., & Kolars, J. C. (2006). Changes in career decisions of internal medicine residents during training. *Annals of Internal Medicine*, *145*(10), 774–779. doi:10.7326/0003-4819-145-10-200611210-00010 PMID:17116922

WhiteGlove Health Case Studies. (2014). Retrieved from http://www.whiteglove.com/images/stories/documents/case-study-fully-insured.pdf

WhiteGlove Health. (2014). Retrieved from http://www.whiteglove.com/

Wilson, A. R., Zhou, X. T., Shi, W., Rodin, J., Bargman, E. P., Garrett, N. A., & Sandberg, T. J. (2010). Retail clinics versus office setting: Do patients choose appropriate providers? *The American Journal of Managed Care*, *16*(10), 753–759. PMID:20964471

Wilson, I. B., Landon, B. E., Hirschhorn, L. R., McInnes, K., Ding, L., & Marsden, P. V. et al. (2005). Quality of HIV care provided by nurse practitioners, physician assistants, and physicians. *Annals of Internal Medicine*, *143*(10), 729–736. doi:10.7326/0003-4819-143-10-200511150-00010 PMID:16287794

Woodburn, J. D., Smith, K. L., & Nelson, G. D. (2007). Quality of care in the retail healthcare setting using national clinical guidelines for acute pharyngitis. *American Journal of Medical Quality*, *22*(6), 457–462. doi:10.1177/1062860607309626 PMID:18006426

World Bank. (2013). *Life expectancy at birth*. Retrieved from http://data.worldbank.org/indicator/SP.DYN.LE00.IN

World Bank. (2013). Retrieved from http://data.worldbank.org/indicator/SH.XPD.PCAP

World Health Organization. (2013). *E-health*. Retrieved from http://www.who.int/trade/glossary/story021/en/

Yard, E. E., & Comstock, R. D. (2009). An epidemiologic comparison of injuries presenting to a pediatric emergency department and local urgent care facilities. *Journal of Safety Research*, *40*(1), 63–69. doi:10.1016/j.jsr.2008.12.004 PMID:19285588

Yee, C. M. (2010, April 13). HCMC is late entry in retail clinic race. *Minnesota Star Tribune*.

Yee, T., Boukus, E., Cross, D., & Samuel, D. (2013). Primary care workforce shortages: Nurse practitioner scope-of-practice-laws and payment policies. *National Institute for Healthcare Reform Research Brief*, *13*, 1–7.

Yee, T., Lechner, A. E., & Boukus, E. R. (2013). *The Surge in Urgent Care Centers: Emergency Department Alternative or Costly Convenience? (Research Brief 26)*. Center for Studying Health System Change.

Zamosky, L. (2010, June 7). The doctor's in-box. *Los Angeles Times*. Retrieved from http://www.latimes.com/health/la-he-doctor-emails-20100607,0,639147.story#ixzz2pIdYp0mP

Zentner, J., Dellinger, C., Adkins, W., & Greene, J. (1995). Nurse practitioner provided primary care: Managing healthcare costs in the workplace. *AAOHN Journal*, *43*, 52–53. PMID:7695807

About the Author

Amer Kaissi is a Professor of Health Care Administration at Trinity University, in San Antonio, Texas. He joined Trinity University in 2003 after earning a PhD degree in Health Services Administration, Research, and Policy from the University of Minnesota. While doing his doctoral work, he worked at Allina Hospitals in Minneapolis, Minnesota. Prior to that, he earned a Masters of Public Health in Hospital Administration from the American University of Beirut in his native Lebanon. At Trinity, Dr. Kaissi teaches courses in Institutional Health Care Management, Health Care Strategic Planning and Marketing, and Health Care Human Resource Management. He also teaches a comparative course on the American and French health care systems, *in French*. His research interests include retail clinics and other convenient care models, strategic planning, quality of care and patient safety, and application of organizational theories to health care settings. He has published extensively on these topics in various administrative and clinical peer-reviewed journals. Dr. Kaissi works with hospital systems and physician practices on strategic planning and marketing projects.

Appendix

LIST OF KEY INFORMANTS

Through professional relationships of the author, we approached these individuals and set up the interviews. The interviews were done by phone between January and March of 2013, and lasted between 45 to 90 minutes, using structured open-ended questions developed by the author (below).

Lee Resnick, M.D., Chief Operating Officer/Chief Medical Officer WellStreet Urgent Care- Atlanta, Georgia
Tom Pascuzzi, M.D., President MD urgent Care, MD Urgent Care- Albuquerque, New Mexico
Stephen Lazzari, Director, Fast Care Development, Bellin Health- Green Bay, Wisconsin
Webster Golinkin, Chief Executive Officer, RediClinic- Houston, Texas
Kevin Palattao, Vice President of HealthPartners Clinics & Virtuwell, Health Partners/virtuwell- Minneapolis, Minnesota
Lauren Cates, Senior Vice President of Market Development & Operational Planning Presbyterian Health System- Albuquerque, New Mexico
Stephen Jones, Vice President of Carolinas Physician Network, Carolinas Health System- Charlotte, North Carolina
Tammy Mallow, Corporate Director of Urgent Care, The Schumacher Group- Lafayette, Louisiana
Mark Clayton, Senior Vice President of Business Development, St. Davids' HealthCare- Austin, Texas
William Rice, M.D., Senior vice president of clinical innovation/Co-founder, St. Davids' HealthCare / White Glove – Austin, Texas
Ateev Mehrotra, M.D., Lecturer/ Affiliated Adjunct Staff; Professor, Pardee RAND Graduate School, Harvard Medical School- Boston, Massachusetts /Pardee RAND Graduate School, Santa Monica, California

Questions:

1. Tell me a bit about yourself, your background, how did you get involved in (urgent care, retail clinics, worksite clinics, online clinics)?
2. Tell me about your organization, when was it founded, how large is it?

3. What are some the major challenges faced by your clinic(s)?
4. What do you do to insure quality of care?
5. Who are your main customers?
6. What do you do to keep costs down?
7. How much do you charge per visit?
8. What are your expectation/forecasts for growth for your clinic(s)? for the field itself?
9. What do you think the implications of the Affordable Care Act will be on your organization? On the field?
10. What do you think the implications of the primary care physician shortage will be on your organization? On the field?
11. Are there any resources you can share?
12. Any other comments?

Index

T

U

W

www.ingramcontent.com/pod-product-compliance
Lightning Source LLC
LaVergne TN
LVHW060424300926
849162LV00006B/1519
* 9 7 8 1 4 6 6 6 6 3 5 5 8 *